THE AILING CITY

THE AILING CITY

Health, Tuberculosis, and Culture

in Buenos Aires, 1870–1950

DIEGO ARMUS

DUKE UNIVERSITY PRESS

Durham and London

2011

© 2011 DUKE UNIVERSITY PRESS

All rights reserved. Printed in the United

States of America on acid-free paper ∞

Designed by Amy Ruth Buchanan

Typeset in Minion by Tseng Information Systems, Inc.

Library of Congress Cataloging-in-Publication Data

appear on the last printed page of this book.

CONTENTS

.... ❋ ....

FIGURES

ACKNOWLEDGMENTS

.... ✳ ....

Initially, this book set out to provide a "total history" of tuberculosis in Buenos Aires: a history capable of opening a window from which to see how disease and health became part of life in the city through metaphors and discourses as well as through actual, concrete policies and experiences. It started out as a doctoral dissertation under the supervision of Tulio Halperín Donghi at the University of California, Berkeley. As soon as the investigation started, it became evident that those intentions were overly ambitious due to my own limitations and, more importantly, the scarcity or absence of sources and documents.

Many questions I posed, greatly influenced by the new histories of tuberculosis and the exciting interpretative frameworks provided by social history and cultural studies, could only be answered on the basis of generalizations and without a specific human and temporal anchoring in the history of Buenos Aires. And I was looking for something else, certainly different, a narrative where a strong empirical foundation could dialogue with broader questions relevant in any effort to understand the coming of modernity. In other words, I wanted to avoid producing a narrative articulated around stimulating and provocative issues but with few literary texts, some journalistic references, and a couple of quotes taken from medical academic journals. The dissertation ended up expressing these necessary concessions and adjustments: initial attempts at totality were somewhat left aside and I had to accept a narrower, more modest horizon through my interpretation of the fragmentary world that could be reassembled by means of the available sources.

After years in the making, a period in which I focused my work on other projects that also, often times, touched on the history of health and disease, I decided to refine and expand the dissertation and transform it into a book. First published in Spanish as *La ciudad impura: Salud, tuberculosis y cultura en Buenos Aires, 1879–1950* (Buenos Aires: Edhasa, 2007), this English version differs from the Spanish one in the content's organization, the additions for a non-Argentine readership, and certainly the general tone.

For both versions I am in debt to many institutions that graciously supported my work. Awards from the Center for Latin American Studies at Berkeley, the Inter-American Foundation, the Andrew W. Mellon Foundation, the Rockefeller Foundation Bellagio Center, and the Eugene M. Lang Faculty Fellowship at Swarthmore—all of them—allowed me to comfortably write as well as to dig in many libraries and archives in Buenos Aires; Córdoba; Amsterdam; New York; Washington, D.C.; California; and Swarthmore.

Many people facilitated identifying valuable sources of information. I am particularly grateful to Adriana Alvarez, Angela Aisenstein, Marcelo Baiardi, Diego Bussola, Adrian Carbonetti, Graciela Fainstein, Mark Healey, Dana Jonas, Ana Laura Martin, Francine Massielo, Lía Munilla, María Silvia Di Liscia, Mirta Lobato, Dante Peralta, Ofelia Pianetto, Graciela Queirolo, Beatriz Seibel, Eli Tedesco, and Cecilia Toussounian. Others made my stays in Buenos Aires—short but frequent—particularly pleasant: Clara Gertz, Bernardo Armus, Marcela Armus, and Nesti Segal.

For this English version, I am sincerely appreciative to Eric Behrens, Jane Brodie, Paulo Drinot, Melissa Fricke, John Lear, Robin Myers, Pola Oloixarac, and Steve Palmer. The award from the Constance Hungerford Faculty Support Fund at Swarthmore College facilitated the inclusion in the book of some of the imagery I have found while researching for this book. At Duke University Press I benefited from the encouragement and patience of Valerie Millholland as well as the professional support and advice of Miriam Angress, Katherine Courtland, Gisela Fosado, and Mark Mastromarino. My gratitude goes also to my copy editor Larry Kenney who, I am sure, had to work hard on the manuscript.

Three scholars have been decisive in what I would like this book to be. And I am deeply thankful to them. Back in time and in Buenos Aires, Jorge Enrique Hardoy helped me to discover the city as an amazing historical artifact and Leandro Gutiérrez encouraged me to interrogate it in social and cultural terms. At Berkeley and thereafter, Tulio Halperín Donghi has been an advisor, guide, and an astounding source of intellectual provocation and ways of thinking about the past.

My last word goes for Lauri, for all these years together and for those to come—who knows where.

The Ailing City is not only for Teo and Vera but also for Vera and Teo.

A History of Tuberculosis in Modern Buenos Aires

In 1955 Elda G. was ten years old and lived in a Buenos Aires neighborhood with her parents, who were Italian immigrants and practically illiterate. One winter day she felt a sharp pain in her back, near her right lung. A week later she was convinced she had "caught" tuberculosis. Even though she had no fever, blood sputum, or violent cough, Elda was sure she had tuberculosis and was dying. She was stricken with fear. She dwelled on the stories her parents had told her about a relative who had died of tuberculosis ten years before Elda was born. Between the stories and her back pain, Elda created images and sensations that were, for a time, the focus of her inner world. In the end, Elda's fear of death was stronger than her efforts to hide or secretly manage her distressing feelings. When her mother found out about her fears, she prayed (or at least she told Elda she did) that "God would move the disease to my body and that her "suffering [would] end soon. If someone has to die, let it be me." Her mother's reaction worsened Elda's fears; the possibility of her mother getting sick on her account frightened her more than having the disease herself. She began to obsess about whether her mother was losing weight or manifesting other symptoms.

A couple of months later, after a visit to the doctor revealed that nothing was wrong with her, Elda's lung pain ceased. "Now, four decades later, I can't tell whether the story was true, or just the workings of a child's imagination," she says.[1]

During Elda's childhood, tuberculosis was no longer the major cause of death it had once been; the enigmatic aura that had surrounded the disease for seven or eight decades had vanished. Though it was an unshakable part of people's memory regardless of their social status, class, or condition, tuberculosis was no longer a pressing public health issue in modern Buenos Aires. It was becoming a disease of the past, one that, in the worst-case scenario, weakened bodies and complicated lives but didn't kill.

This book explores the uncertainties prevalent before the discovery and widespread use of antibiotics to treat tuberculosis. It sees these uncertainties as a mirror or, even better, a kaleidoscope, for some crucial social and cultural concerns in Buenos Aires between 1870 and 1950, from new industrial work routines to rapid demographic growth and its consequences for housing, urban services, and living conditions; from the meanings and benefits of social citizenship to new concerns about the reproduction of the workforce; from efforts geared toward building a healthy "national race" to the tensions between images of the city and its future and the real city in the making. In so doing, and pivoting over those issues that shaped the emergence of a modern urban world, the book inquires into the emergence and consolidation of an increasingly medicalized society marked by fear of contagion, state intervention in private life, and by various attempts to reform, care for, and control people's morality, sociability, sexuality, and daily habits. The undeniable ubiquity of tuberculosis in this medicalization process fed a sort of subculture with an array of individual and social experiences, metaphors, and associations that was decisive in articulating the political worries and initiatives of the social hygiene movement and, later, the public health system.

An examination of this subculture shows that the social meanings of tuberculosis went far beyond the pathology itself. Throughout the nineteenth century phthisis had been a part of life in Buenos Aires. However, it was not until the last third of that century, with the development of modern bacteriology and the isolation of Koch's bacillus, that phthisis became tuberculosis and gave rise to a subculture that endured until the arrival of antibiotics at the end of the forties and early fifties. Between 1870 and 1950 tuberculosis not only spread and killed people, but was also a recurrent topic in newspaper and magazine articles. Moreover, it was a metaphor used in literary and political narratives, tango lyrics, and sociological essays, a concern for doctors and public health specialists, and a stigmatizing experience for those who contracted the disease—as well as a source of fear, even panic, for those who thought they might.

The Ailing City recreates some of this world. It examines how tuberculosis was used to speak not only about disease and health, but also about a wide range of other concerns. It tackles the relationships between history, health, and disease in a narrative style that has developed over the past two or three decades and has made an impact on contemporary historiography around the world.[2] On the one hand, these efforts aim to renovate the traditional history of medicine. On the other, they see disease as a very promising object of study for the social sciences and the humanities. Indeed, disease is one of the many new subfields of inquiry that reveal the fragmentary character of current historical studies, which are more concerned with addressing specific themes and topics than with offering an overarching account of the past. These narratives understand disease not solely in terms of viruses and bacteria, that is, in terms of biomedicine. As an influential scholar in the field has noted, diseases represent an opportunity to develop and legitimate public policies; to facilitate and justify the creation, development, and use of science, technologies, and institutions; to channel social anxieties; and to structure the relationships between the sick and health care providers. This approach to the history of disease assumes that an illness, sickness, or pathology does not exist until there is a consensus that it does—that is, once a disease has been perceived as such, once it has been named and has provoked specific answers and reactions.[3]

This way of writing about diseases—stressing their discovery, life, and death—is the basis for a revamped history of medicine, history of public health, and sociocultural history of disease. These three ways of writing about disease from a historical perspective entail different focuses, concurrences, and juxtapositions. The revamped history of medicine, or biomedical history, distances itself from a self-celebratory narrative centered on famous physicians and instead connects the tensions between the natural history of a certain pathology and the uncertain development of biomedical knowledge; it aims not only to contextualize the scientific, social, cultural, and political environments in which some doctors, institutions, and treatments triumph over others and win a place in history, but also to discuss what has been forgotten and why.

The history of public health typically focuses on power, politics, public policy, and medical practice. In this approach, public medicine is usually portrayed as a progressive phenomenon, aimed at providing effective treatments for diseases that have affected the modern world. The relationships between health care institutions and social, political, and economic structures are at the core of a narrative mainly concerned with issues of collective health rather than individual bodies. It studies political actions aimed at preserving or restoring public health and usually focuses on periods when the state or international agencies or certain sectors of society or key actors—mainly public health specialists—have undertaken concrete initiatives. In these narratives, medical and epidemiological questions are as important as political, economic, cultural, scientific, and technological concerns. More generally, public health history looks at itself as a useful, mission-oriented enterprise focused on and able to explore the past in order to find the needed empirical evidence that supposedly will narrow, in a nonspecific way, the inevitable uncertainties in decision-making processes about collective health.

The sociocultural history of disease is the result of the work of historians, demographers, sociologists, anthropologists, and cultural critics. These scholars have discovered the complexity and rich possibilities of exploring health and disease as historical problems as well as ways of discussing related and broader issues. This history is only vaguely linked with biomedicine. It focuses on specific metaphors and experiences associated with certain diseases; healing practices, including those not firmly positioned in the realm of biomedicine; and medicalization and professionalization processes. It also discusses acceptance or resistance to disciplinary discourses and medicosocial control strategies; the role of the state and civil society in the making of the health care institutions and infrastructure and their influence on material living conditions and the effects of those conditions on mortality trends; the increasing presence of a culture of hygiene on peoples' daily habits as a way to participate in the modern world; and the emergence of health as a social entitlement.

Beyond their differences, and at the same time underlining their shared agendas, these ways of writing the history of diseases and health understand biomedicine as a field riddled with uncertainties. From these perspectives, biomedical issues are imbued with human subjectivity and consequently have manifold social, cultural, political, and economic implications. The narratives that grow out of these historiographies are sometimes highly empiricist, devoting most of their efforts to measuring, for instance, the extension of potable water networks, the number of beds available at hospitals, or the total number of people vaccinated. At other times they praise or criticize the role played by institutions, doctors, and health care specialists, elaborating interpretations that may ignore, or not, the mediations between health care actions and the requirements of the economic system. Or they reconstruct the discovery of a biomedical novelty, assuming it will be easily socialized among most of the sick suffering a certain disease when in fact for quite some time the majority of them were not even patients whose health and pain were addressed at a biomedical institution. Or they aim to uncover the normalizing and disciplinary dimensions of modern medicine, most frequently in the discursive realm and paying little attention to the real impact these discourses had on peoples' experiences and daily lives. Occasionally the emphasis of the biomedical history, the history of public health, and the social and cultural history of disease are part of an almost undifferentiated historical narrative.

Occasionally the agendas are more defined and the mutual influences less apparent. And in recent years there has been a growth of historical studies interested in developing creative analytical frameworks that assess and contextualize not only the disciplinary aspects of medicine and public health but also its humanitarian dimensions, the role of the state and civil society, the diversity of healing practices, and the perspective of the sick.

Studies of disease and health that focus on the Argentine past reflect some of these historiographical developments and narrative styles.[4] In assessing the history of public health in the country some scholars have insisted on identifying a ruling elite and dependent political and economic power structures either not capable of or not interested in creating and efficiently distributing resources and health services. Those critical of this schematic application of the dependency model took note of both the achievements and limitations inherent in modern public health projects. They attempted to show how, at certain times, the outcome has not been entirely negative and, moreover, that the peripheral condition of Argentina has not always been an obstacle to the state's ability to become an active agent in building and consolidating a basic health infrastructure and even in reducing mortality rates, particularly when it comes to infectious diseases. Other scholars view health and medical issues as a sort of epiphenomenon or as a byproduct of economic relations. They argue that the lives of the poor have always been marked by misfortune, largely because public health care initiatives were aimed merely at increasing productivity and guaranteeing the reproduction of the workforce. Though not always empirically convincing, these explanations abound. According to some studies, the elite fostered only the health and sanitation reforms that afforded them some safety or that reproduced dependent capitalism. Others saw public health policies as the outcome of a negotiation between various political agents and institutions, stressing that the contents of these policies have not been structurally predetermined but historically produced. Still others focused solely on the metaphors of health and illness or on their cultural implications; discussing disease and medicine as modernity's normalizing instruments; and key resources of broader efforts to develop knowledge and disciplinary languages in order to control and regulate individual and social bodies, to label difference, and to legitimize ideological and cultural systems. Like other national historiographies, both past and current, many of these analytical frameworks and theories, when read and applied rigidly, did not pay enough attention to particularities of time and space and ultimately cannot creatively delve into the specific web of meanings and experiences shaped by the state's public policies, biomedical knowledge, daily life, and people's reactions. In any case, this modern historiography of health and disease in Argentina emerged and grew steadily during the last two decades of the twentieth century, mainly focused on Buenos Aires, though also concerned with other cities and regions. These modest yet dynamic developments within Argentine historiography are part of worldwide trends that have consolidated a vibrant field of studies focused on disease, health, and biomedicine.

Tuberculosis as a Matter of Historical Inquiry

Whether framed by the revamped history of medicine, the history of public health, or the sociocultural history of disease—or by a combination of the three—during the second half of the twentieth century tuberculosis became a topic of great interest to scholars concerned with exploring disease and health in contexts of urbanization, industrialization, and modernization. There are now city, regional, or national histories of tuberculosis for places as diverse as, for example, Japan, the United States, Canada, France, South Africa, India, England, Australia, Brazil, Papua Guinea, and Spain.[5] In Argentine historiography and in the historiography of Buenos Aires, interest in tuberculosis is also rising.[6] *The Ailing City* is part of this growing field.

These studies, focused primarily on the eight or nine decades before the discovery of an effective treatment—that is, from 1860 to 1950—are not a result of the fears and anxieties brought on by the emergence, in the late twentieth century, of drug-resistant tuberculosis. Neither are they a result of increasing mortality owing to tuberculosis in industrial societies, postindustrial and developing countries, and in poor countries where tuberculosis was never eradicated in the first place. The renewed interest in tuberculosis does not lie either in the association between tuberculosis and autoimmune deficiency syndrome (AIDS), drug abuse, and poverty, or in the cure and prevention campaigns supported by international organizations, private foundations, and governments.

The new historiography of tuberculosis was, rather, built on studies that preceded it, studies in which disease was discussed as a phenomenon involving human beings—beyond a specific geographic region—but mainly referring to the now-industrialized Northern Hemisphere. That earlier narrative attempted to reconstruct the milestones in the search for an effective cure and the actions of famous scientists.[7] Somewhat in keeping with this agenda—that is, aspiring to a global history of tuberculosis that, in fact, took into account only a small portion of the world—the pioneering work of René and Jean Dubos, published in the early 1950s, was crucial to creating a tension between that rather heroic narrative and an interest in the social conditions in which tuberculosis was rooted.[8] The Duboses' work significantly influenced the studies of tuberculosis during the seventies and eighties, histories that consciously avoided a global view of the disease. They aimed, instead, at anchoring its history in a determined geography—a country, region, or city—and period of time. These studies were an alternative to transhistoric narratives—the bacillus is the same; the disease does not differ, let's say, throughout the nineteenth century and the twentieth—or narratives that ignored specific geographical and historical contexts. Some of these contemporary studies of tuberculosis are part of an increasing historicist approach to public health, mainly attempting to reconstruct antituberculosis campaigns from the past, which were perceived as early examples of effective (or ineffective) forms of preventive medicine. At the same time, some of these studies convincingly assumed the notion that tuberculosis is deeply connected to demographic, social, and cultural issues. In such studies, these issues could be approached from diverse and sometimes critical interpretative frameworks drawn from the works of Thomas McKeown, Mary Douglas, Michel Foucault, Norbert Elias, and Susan Sontag.

In assessing the relative importance of medical and nonmedical factors in the decline of tuberculosis mortality in England during the late nineteenth century and early twentieth, McKeown affirmed that medical interventions were not decisive: the decline of mortality had begun long before the appearance and widespread use of preventive measures and effective cures. The decline of tuberculosis mortality, especially in cities, should be explained as the result not of changes in medicine or public health, but of nutritional and socioeconomical factors. This provocative approach drew many followers. It also led to detailed studies aimed at revising McKeown's thesis. Some defended the relative importance of medical interventions and sanitation policy in enhancing the achievements of bacteriology as well as increasing the efficacy of public health. Others combined the two interpretations, pointing out that the benefits of public health policies or medical care were not actually that widespread and that they had a positive effect only on the wealthy, the middle classes, and skilled workers.[9] The debate continues, and though there are still studies that credit a single decisive factor with the decline of tuberculosis mortality, more and more interpretations see it as the result of a vast range of interconnected variables. For example, improvements in nutrition can be understood only in relation to broader socioeconomic factors, such as income levels, public health measures that guarantee food hygiene, and access to potable water.

Works by Douglas, Foucault, and Elias lay the ground for a new approach

to the history of tuberculosis, including material life conditions and their relationship to the cultural dimensions of contagion and contamination; biopoli-
tics; disciplinary discourses; issues of exclusion, identity, and difference; daily
hygiene and the dissemination of norms and habits; state and civil society
roles in confronting tuberculosis; consensus and coercion in public health
policies; public urgencies; and individual rights.[10]

Sontag explored the cultural representations of tuberculosis in European
literature, where it was depicted as a romantic disease of refined, sophisticated
souls; in such texts, consumption and tuberculosis constitute a sort of spiritual
promotion. Sontag's emphasis on the romantic dimension of tuberculosis was
followed by studies that explored other, mainly twentieth-century representations. Tuberculosis emerged as a disease of the masses, reclaiming metaphors
and associations articulated by the sick themselves, by new literary narratives,
and by those waving the banners of social change or those self-appointed to
speak on behalf of workers. This more nuanced scenario encouraged studies
that intentionally sought to investigate the tensions between the worlds of experience around the disease and those created by literary, medical, and media
discourses.[11]

Today, tuberculosis is defined as an infectious disease caused by the Koch
bacillus. Lungs are not the only organs or tissues that might be affected by the
bacillus, but pulmonary tuberculosis has been and continues to be the most
widespread form of the disease. People with active tuberculosis are the source
of contagion: when coughing and sneezing, they release into the air droplets
full of bacilli. Most of these droplets are harmless because their size prevents
them from penetrating the pulmonary alveoli in the lungs of the person who
inhales them. Droplets fall on many surfaces, though mostly on the ground,
where they do not entail major risk. Once they dry up, the droplets can release
dry, very light particles which contain one to three bacilli that survive in the
air. These particles are small enough to penetrate the alveoli in the lungs of a
healthy individual. The ensuing infectious process may or may not lead to the
disease.

Generally, during the first three months after infection, a primary wound
appears on the lungs. The wound may heal thanks to defense cells capable of
destroying the bacillus, or it may calcify after the formation of a small inflam-
mation—the tubercle—that contains bacilli. If this happens, the bacilli don't
spread, and the usually asymptomatic infection can be detected only by means
of the tuberculin skin test. Unless the person is treated with modern therapies
that destroy the bacilli, the infected individual will have a latent infection that
might become active owing to diminished immunity caused by other diseases,

physical or emotional stress, or poor diet. A decline in immunity allows the bacilli to cross through the walls of the tubercles and spread the infection to the lungs and neighboring tissues. Sometimes the primary wound is not contained in a tubercle. In this case, it spreads to the lungs over a period of six to twelve months and to other parts of the body through the circulatory or the lymphatic system. This process weakens the body considerably and, if untreated, leads to death.

The factors that cause infection and the factors that lead to disease are not the same. For infection to occur there must be prolonged close contact with a person whose sputum contains a great deal of bacilli. Poorly ventilated rooms—where particles carrying bacilli may circulate without being exposed to sunlight, which kills them—increase risk. Tuberculosis infection may become active if several factors, mostly related to the age of the individual and how recently infection occurred, conspire. Regardless of age, tuberculosis develops during the first and second year after exposure. The speed of the process is affected by the strength of the infected person's immune system; children under the age of three, young adults, and pregnant women are the most vulnerable.[12]

Levels of resistance have been and continue to be a topic of discussion. The question revolves around who doesn't get infected, who gets infected but doesn't get sick, who gets infected and does get sick, who gets sick and then heals, and who gets sick and dies. Some have insisted on the importance of socioeconomic and psychosocial factors; others, on nutrition and issues related to the frequency and degree of exposure to bacilli by certain individuals and social groups. These factors are usually combined and consequently it is very difficult to identify a single causal connection for a social disease like tuberculosis. Such limitations are also evident in ideas about the genetic propensity of certain individuals or social groups.[13] These considerations reveal some of the obstacles faced by both current epidemiological analysis and historical studies of tuberculosis.

The Ailing City *in the History of Tuberculosis of Modern Buenos Aires*

From the last third of the nineteenth century to the 1950s, the period studied in this book, pulmonary tuberculosis was one of the largest killers in absolute numbers in Buenos Aires. It was also endowed with a vast number of social and cultural meanings. Despite the dubiousness of historical statistics, the evolution of tuberculosis in Buenos Aires during that period was very similar to that in many European and North American cities of equal size. Between

1878 and 1889 the mortality rate fluctuated from 230 to 300 per 100,000 inhabitants; the rate then drops for some years and, at the beginning of the 1890s through 1907, reaches a plateau of fewer than 200 per 100,000, though always more than 180. Between 1908 and 1912 records show a moderate decline in mortality rates. Starting in 1912 the mortality level rises again and peaks in 1918, with almost 250 deaths per 100,000 inhabitants. From 1919 to 1932 the mortality rate is largely steady. Though there is a modest decline, it never falls to fewer than 170. From 1933 through the mid-1940s the decline is constant and after 1947 the rate plummets.

In 1953, the tuberculosis mortality rate was 29 per 100,000 inhabitants. Compared with general mortality, the decline in the rate for tuberculosis is less pronounced until 1930, and it speeds up during the thirties and forties. During the last third of the nineteenth century tuberculosis mortality was somewhat overshadowed by other infectious and contagious diseases. But by the beginning of the twentieth century, mortality due to infectious and contagious diseases was largely under control. In 1928 tuberculosis was the second cause of death. Two decades later, after a steady decline, it was the fifth cause of death, after cardiovascular diseases, cancer, and cerebral-vascular and respiratory diseases. Throughout, mortality in men was higher than in women. Starting at the end of the 1920s the mortality rates for both men and women declined, but the tendency was more marked in women: in 1928, for every 100 men who died of tuberculosis, 72.9 women did, and by 1947 the figure was only 63.3. During this period the group most affected was men between the ages of twenty and twenty-nine, though their relative number tended to decrease along with the overall decline of tuberculosis mortality and the concomitant displacement of mortality to older people.[14]

Explaining these shifts in tuberculosis mortality is more difficult than reconstructing them. As stated in a study from the mid-1930s, the causes for the decline were "as complex as tuberculosis epidemiology."[15] Several narratives developed primarily in the twenties and thirties aimed at establishing the decisive role of what were then called biological and socio-environmental factors.[16] In hindsight, some of these narratives appear arbitrary, even ludicrous; others seem reasonable; still others seem to attempt a true exploration of the disease and its causality. All of them, in different ways, were borne of a prolonged period marked by undeniable biomedical uncertainty. In this book I aim to delve into these uncertain times—that is, those decades when the disease was part of the life of the city but biomedicine was unable to deliver an efficient therapy—and connect them to a number of problems involving both the history of tuberculosis in Buenos Aires and the history of its modernity. I intend not to explain the gradual decline of tuberculosis mortality over time but to unveil how those long decades marked by broader social and cultural anxieties associated tuberculosis with many problems and issues whose nature was not strictly biomedical. I seek to provide a sort of record of the images, implications, and concrete experiences that were the stuff of a subculture which, over seven or eight decades, gave tuberculosis its meaning and defined its role in Buenos Aires. In other words, I contend that from 1870 to 1950 tuberculosis was a way of speaking not only about biomedical issues but also about other matters, matters not necessarily medical and more directly located in the social and cultural realms.

The Ailing City does not contain an overarching hypothesis. It explores the changes in as well as the relative stability of the tuberculosis subculture in a peripheral and very cosmopolitan city of the Americas. It aims at recreating some dimensions of Buenos Aires life by looking at the practices, discourses, tropes, rituals, and institutions surrounding a disease that, by the end of the nineteenth century, was becoming a major public health concern. This book's narrative is intentionally eclectic. It delves alike into elite and popular cultures and experiences, medical opinions expressed by professionals as well as explanations informally articulated by laypeople. It explores the achievements and shortcomings of welfare and public health initiatives as well as people's new and old habits and the array of norms suggested by experts that had limited influence on people's daily lives. It looks into the experiences of the sick as well as of those who, being sick, at some point in their personal struggle against tuberculosis, became patients dealing with biomedical institutions, doctors, and nurses.

This history of tuberculosis in modern Buenos Aires is not organized chronologically. One chapter does not necessarily introduce the next. Instead, the book offers a sort of inventory of the shifting spectacle of modern life in Buenos Aires from 1870 to 1950. It shows a vision of the city steeped in the cultural residues of this disease. The chapters were written as relatively independent pieces. Some focus on topics present throughout the entire period, while others deal with questions relevant only at a specific moment. The discussion of some issues is very detailed, partly because their connection to the disease is patent. This is the case with the experiences of the sick who received institutionalized and noninstitutionalized forms of therapy; the emergence of a culture of hygiene; eugenics; contagion; and excess. In discussing realms less apparently and directly associated with the history of tuberculosis—for example, urban utopias, racial and gender stereotyping, corsets, soccer, tango lyrics, and the language and design of medication advertisements—my intent is to show how the disease deeply affected and was affected by multiple spheres of life in modern Buenos Aires.

This book shares many concerns and trends easily identified in the current Latin American historiography of diseases and public health. But I believe it stresses other issues, or at least does so with different emphases. Although I address the institutions, agents, and struggles that encouraged and implemented a culture of hygiene to combat tuberculosis, these issues are not at the core of my narrative. In that sense, and only to a certain extent, my book partakes of the growing field of the history of public health.[17] Furthermore, tuberculosis was mainly a domestic public health issue; international concerns and agendas played a role in it, but—as usually happened with so-called tropical diseases in nontemperate cities and regions—they were not decisive in the efforts to control tuberculosis morbidity and mortality. As a result, this book does not share the agenda and concerns of international and global health studies, which, particularly for the first half of the twentieth century in Latin America, are mainly invested in issues of cooperation, negotiation, and disputes between peripheral areas and metropolitan centers that, in the end, facilitated the emergence and consolidation of diverse types of public health systems.[18]

The Ailing City is not a medical history of tuberculosis in Buenos Aires either. Even if the biomedical dimension of the disease serves as a backdrop for many of its discussions—namely, the medical uncertainties about tuberculosis during these decades—I am not concerned with evaluating the effectiveness of any one treatment, exploring how biomedical knowledge and practices produced in the center of the Western world were absorbed or redefined in academic circles of the Argentine capital, or assessing the quality or scientific excellence of those circles and their work.[19]

Finally, the book does not have comparative pretensions. Instead, this history of tuberculosis is deliberately local. It focuses on a wide range of experiences, topics, discourses, and policies that permeated modern Buenos Aires. Some of them are predictable, in no way unique to Buenos Aires history, and consequently also present in exhaustive studies of tuberculosis conducted for cities and countries all over the world. Others are quite specific and confined to the history of Buenos Aires. My intention is to identify both the common features pertaining to a global history of tuberculosis as well as the peculiarities of the tuberculosis subculture in Buenos Aires between 1870 and 1950.

Two other remarks are in order. The first is related to the just-mentioned issue of the local–global dimension in this history of tuberculosis in modern Buenos Aires. In a few cases I do explicitly indicate that a certain process or problem was also a part of the experience of tuberculosis elsewhere.

But by and large I tried to avoid commentaries and digressions that merely stated the same problem elsewhere without much contextualization rather than truly composing them. I also refrained from referring to other scholarly works available on a certain topic for another city or country. Certainly, my interpretations and narrative are informed by a rich and dynamic historiography of tuberculosis. However, I do not see why this kind of study must engage in a dialogue with similar works focused on other places, mainly Western Europe and the United States. In fact, those studies tend to be oblivious to the historiographical production focused on the many peripheries of the modern world; perhaps the exception occurs when the problem is framed as part of the so-called imperial medicines. That dialogue, which I firmly believe is needed, should be part of a global history of tuberculosis that presumably someone will write someday, a history able to deal with similarities as well as differences in the way societies confronted tuberculosis.

My second remark has to do with the frame and topics that organize my discussion of tuberculosis in Buenos Aires: To a large extent my narrative is the result of what primary sources have allowed me to see and to interpret. My empirical investigation is based on oral histories and physicians' case histories; government reports and medical studies; literary texts and newspaper articles; advertisements and tango lyrics; sociological essays published in academic journals and articles published in the workers' press; patients' diaries; doctors' accounts; statistics and congressional discussions; and movies and photographs. The topics around which I organize my analysis are intentionally limited to the information found in those primary sources, whose richness and availability vary greatly. Needless to say, many intriguing topics were part of my initial research agenda but ended up being put aside because there was not enough material to support a sensitive and historically localized discussion.

The organization of *The Ailing City* is different from that of most histories of tuberculosis. The first three chapters focus on the sick. I intentionally avoided the stories of well-known individuals, many of whom were artists, whose consumption or tuberculosis was described, and sometimes perceived and experienced, as a romantic experience. People with tuberculosis in this book are more ordinary individuals from the upper, middle, and lower classes. Capturing their voices and experiences was a highly elusive goal and, to a large extent, a motivation. The emphasis on the tuberculars demanded breaking free of the language and constructs of biomedicine; I sought to see the sick from within as well as from outside the perspectives of institutionalized health care, to go beyond the narratives written by doctors in their quite often detached, unemotional clinical histories. Finding accounts of the tuberculosis experience turned out to be a real challenge. From that fragmented and scarce primary information—namely, an array of narratives whose emphasis and storylines were informed by age, gender, occupation and accessibility to therapeutic options—I tried to reconstruct the experiences of people with tuberculosis as reflected not only in written and oral accounts but also in individual and collective actions. In so doing, I attempted to frame the experience of the sick within the reality of the disease, of their lives, and of society at large.

The first two chapters reconstruct the therapeutic trajectories pursued by a person with tuberculosis, from home care to over-the-counter medicines, visits to herbalists and neighborhood healers, tuberculosis dispensaries, public hospitals, rest cure in a sanatorium, or the doctor's office. These trajectories were neither preestablished nor necessarily similar. For people with tuberculosis the array of treatments was commonly a scenario of complementary alternatives, not rival or competitive ones. This was the case because of the inability of biomedicine to offer an effective cure—and also because of the limited scope of the medicalization process, given the fact that institutionalized medicine had been growing steadily since the end of the nineteenth century but not enough to be able to take care of the majority of people with the disease.

Chapter 3 explores the ways in which tuberculosis inpatients came to grips with medical power and knowledge. Individual and collective actions such as negotiating internment conditions with a sanatorium or hospital director; lobbying Congress; using the media and organizing strikes in order to publicize their needs; abandoning treatments, protesting against some of them, and demanding to try out others they thought were part of their right in spite of the opposition of the medical establishment—all of these reveal patients with not only a dense, complex inner world but also a determination to find a cure. These negotiations, which inevitably included adaptations as well as confrontations, point to a much less passive and submissive patient–physician relationship than is often assumed. Though patients were certainly subordinate to medical doctors' knowledge and practices, that subordination, far from absolute, was limited and often ruptured.

Chapter 4 studies initiatives of the state, medical and professional circles, and civil society that turned tuberculosis into a public issue. It may very well be extremely difficult, even impossible, to measure the extent to which those campaigns were responsible for the declining tuberculosis mortality rate before the mid-1940s, when antibiotics became available, and I do not set out to gauge that impact. Instead, I discuss those initiatives in relation to the expanding value of hygiene. More specifically, I examine a catalogue of detailed indications for daily conduct. Geared toward stopping the spread of tuberculosis, this catalogue aimed at affecting society at large, though how diverse social groups and individuals actually understood and applied those recommendations varied enormously. Interestingly, the value of hygiene had an even greater impact on the discourses of almost all political and ideological groups, from anarchists to social Catholics. This relative consensus seems to suggest that ideological differences did not matter much when it came to hygiene. Consequently, in this chapter and the two that follow it the emphasis is less on the experiences of people with tuberculosis than on the discourses, instruments, and strategies developed by experts and institutions to control tuberculosis mortality and morbidity.

In chapter 5 I look at how social and civic behavior were intended to be regulated through an antituberculosis discourse that emphasized individual responsibility and promoted modern hygienic habits by disseminating information, prescriptive recommendations, and prohibitions. I discuss some of the objects, practices, and institutions around which the campaign against contagion was organized: spitting and dust in the home, schools, and streets; women's corsets; kissing; and eugenic initiatives aimed at governing marriages and pregnancies of people with tuberculosis. There was a backlash against the obsessions and anxieties associated with this campaign and the notion of an omnipresent risk of contagion. Often ironic, these responses coined the term *tuberculophobia*, stressing how devoid of common sense some of the normative efforts, particularly those aimed at the popular sectors of society without taking into account their material life environment, really were.

In chapter 6 I explore the varied, ambiguous, and sometimes arbitrary associations between tuberculosis and sexuality, alcohol, work fatigue, and the housing of the poor. It discusses the dominant ideas about the negative consequences of sexual and alcoholic excesses; overcrowding and promiscuity in the home; long workdays; the poor hygienic labor environment of certain trades; and exploitation in general. Whether the result of personal choice or imposed by others, these excesses saturated perceptions, preconceptions, clichés, and realities which, concurrently, gave meaning to a tuberculosis subculture that lasted until the 1950s.

Chapters 7–9 deal with three topics—immigration, gender, and children's health—that were persistently crisscrossed by tuberculosis as a sociocultural phenomenon. Chapter 7 discusses the role of the disease in the ambitious, but unrealized, project of selecting the supposed best immigrants to forge the ethnically mixed social body of modern Buenos Aires and the Argentine nation. Here I look at the prejudices and stereotypes that connected tuberculosis with certain immigrant groups, indigenous populations, and native-born Argentine women. These negative racial stereotypes contrast with a few positive ones, and together they reveal the arbitrary and unsound nature of the attempts to link natural predispositions to tuberculosis with certain ethnic or national groups.

Chapter 8 examines the associations between women and tuberculosis found in novels, poetry, tango lyrics, movies, and popular theater. These narratives constructed at least three pathological scenarios and characters. The first one links tuberculosis with passions and mental waste. As in the nineteenth-century European novel, the protagonists of these texts are consumptive or neurasthenic. The second considers tuberculosis as the result of overwork. Here, *tísicas*—that is, women suffering from phthisis and tuberculosis, typically seamstresses—are depicted as the victims of an unfair labor system. Finally, in the third, tuberculosis appears as a malady of young women, the *milonguitas*, who dare to stray from the tranquil but limited, self-contained, and submissive world of the home and the neighborhood. Such girls are drawn to the city's nightlife, where they are inevitably punished with death by tuberculosis. Mostly written by men, all of these narratives portray phthisis and tuberculosis as an illness of adventurous, transgressive young women. In such works, men don't get tuberculosis, though in real life they did and usually at a higher rate than women.

In chapter 9 I study the figure of the child supposedly predisposed to tuberculosis and its influence on the development of initiatives designed to strengthen the bodies of those deemed crucial to the future of the nation. The chapter focuses on a number of preventive public health policies for children, such as the protection of newborns from tubercular mothers, physical education at school, and summer camps for allegedly weak, pretubercular children. In chapter 10 I discuss tuberculosis not so much as a dangerous and threatening disease but as an opportunity for discourses on individual and social regeneration. I explore, on the one hand, imagined cities where tuberculosis is under control or even defeated. And, on the other, the hygienic home, an ideal in which order, propriety, and cleanliness are seen as the safeguards of a healthy life, regardless of social and economic conditions.

In the epilogue, I show that the recent reemergence of tuberculosis as a public health issue is not a replica, a second version, of the disease studied in this book. Though there are some similarities, the numerous differences indicate that tuberculosis is not transhistorical and that this disease, like most, has to be understood as a complex historical phenomenon shaped not only by biomedicine. In other words, tuberculosis is much more than a bacillus, and not just because the bacillus of this current cycle of tuberculosis is no longer of the same strain that was successfully controlled by the antibiotics first used on a mass scale in the late 1950s.

This history of tuberculosis in Buenos Aires deals with a time of profound, rapid urban changes that were evident in almost every aspect of the city's life, from demographics to social geography, from politics to culture.[20] Starting in the 1880s and the 1890s, during the Argentine centennial celebration in 1910, throughout the 1920s, and again in the 1940s, witnesses of those changes discussed the making of a cosmopolitan and modern Buenos Aires with commentaries that ranged from enthusiastic and zealous to skeptical.

The city's demographics are eloquent indicators of this process. By the early 1870s Buenos Aires had 200,000 inhabitants; in 1914, that number has risen to more than 1.5 million. It soon had the largest population of any city in Latin America and was second only to New York among cities on the Atlantic seaboard. In 1936 its population reached 2.5 million, and by the early 1950s it was 3 million. For decades transatlantic migration was largely responsible for this rapid demographic growth. Between 1860 and 1930 immigrants from Italy and Spain constituted 80 percent of all immigrants, the rest coming from eastern and western Europe as well as the Middle East. By 1910 three out of every four members of the adult population in Buenos Aires were foreign-born. During the 1930s this began to change: in 1936 a third of the population was foreign, but domestic migration was becoming the real engine of Buenos Aires's demographic growth, and most of the new immigrants were from neighboring South American countries.

By the 1870s Buenos Aires was a quite dense city, its center located by the banks of the river and the port; only a few blocks existed to the north, west, and south. It was, no doubt, a walking city. Quite soon, though, Buenos Aires was on the way to becoming a horse-drawn urban society. The first expansion, during the last third of the nineteenth century, resulted from the incorporation of neighboring towns. By the late 1910s the city had well-defined borders, but its population density was uneven. During those early years of the twentieth century Buenos Aires experienced a major expansion outward. Tramways, first horse-drawn and later electric, as well as the possibility of renting a home or buying, on installments, a piece of land on which eventually to build, facilitated the physical expansion of the city and the making of new neighborhoods populated by immigrants and their Argentine offspring. There were still, however, many unpopulated areas. By the end of the 1930s and during the 1940s the city underwent a second period of expansion, this time associated with domestic migrations and a bus network that increased the value of interstitial and outlying lands that had a weak or nonexistent integration into the urban grid.

Both periods of expansion accommodated workers, craftspeople, employees, and the emerging middle classes. The 1940s and 1950s witnessed urban growth that was no longer contained by the city's legal borders. This led to a large and very popular metropolitan area that surrounded the city itself with more than 2 million inhabitants. At that time, Buenos Aires was just a sliver of what has since become one of the most populated urban areas in Latin America. During the second half of the century the population of the city proper stagnated, and the physical and demographic growth of metropolitan Buenos Aires slowed. However, the fact that by the beginning of the twenty-first century the city itself (as well as what is now called Greater Buenos Aires) houses more than a quarter of the country's population reveals its decisive and perdurable dominant role in national affairs from at least the beginning of the nineteenth century.

By the early 1870s Buenos Aires was already a complex city and the seat of the Buenos Aires Province's government. In 1880 it became the nation's capital and, from then on, local and national politics were quite often indistinguishable. During the period covered in this book Buenos Aires was the only major metropolis in the country; there were just a few midsize and many smaller provincial cities. Along with its port, commercial, and bureaucratic activities, Buenos Aires was developing a manufacturing sector with hundreds of workshops and a few huge industrial factories. Not even during the 1940s and 1950s, at the height of the state's efforts to substitute imports through industrialization, was Buenos Aires transformed into an industrial city. It was, rather, an urban conglomerate with industries initially spread over several neighborhoods and, later, firmly installed on the city outskirts and the metropolitan area.

By the last third of the nineteenth century Buenos Aires had one-story houses with colonial courtyards; large, Frenchified mansions for the rich; more modest Italianate houses; several new massive government buildings; an extraordinary opera house; and a great number of precarious, poorly equipped tenements, shacks, and hovels. In the following decades, despite the absence of an active state policy aimed at constructing houses for the working classes and the poor, the urban landscape was transformed, mainly as a result of individual efforts associated with a widespread process of modest but attainable upward social mobility. By the 1930s Buenos Aires was a sprawling and, for the most part, horizontal city. The downtown, inhabited between the 1880s and the 1940s by the elite, had a relatively high population density, with three- or four-story modern apartment buildings and even a few skyscrapers. It was in the throes of an urban renovation consisting of the construction of public and private buildings and the improvement of the main avenues. Beyond the downtown, both in the neighborhoods and in the emerging metropolitan area, Buenos Aires looked like a sea of one-story houses that, as one moved outward, dissolved into the open spaces of the plains. By the early 1940s most of the city dwellings were of brick; only 10 percent of residential houses were makeshift, most of them near the city limits.

Many other indicators illustrate the speed and magnitude of urban growth during the period discussed: 6,000 street lights in 1910 and 38,000 in 1930; more than 2 dozen radio stations broadcasting during the 1920s; by the end of the 1930s, 200 libraries and 168 movie theaters; 2,000 cars and 40,000 carriages in 1910; and, by the late 1930s, 72 local bus lines transporting more than 1.5 million passengers daily. By 1940 trash collection, drinking water, and sewage systems reached most of the urban grid. Access to these novelties and modern urban services, however, varied from neighborhood to neighborhood, and not everybody enjoyed them to the same degree. But during these seven decades the city underwent a sea change and did so in a way in which integration into the urban social fabric and a limited but real social mobility were possible.

The speed and magnitude of urban growth are evident in other realms of city life. The changes did away with a mid-nineteenth-century distinction between the northern area of the city, which was better serviced and wealthier, and the southern area, often associated with epidemics and lower standards of living. By the 1900s, though, another distinction was taking place: the difference between the *centro*, or downtown, and the *barrios*, outlying neighborhoods. Immigrants and native-born *criollos*, craftspeople and small merchants, teachers and workers, public employees and seamstresses were the members of these very cosmopolitan, yet small and locally oriented, societies. These neighborhoods featured a remarkable social integration, cultural mixing, Argentinization, and an effort to live respectable lives that echoed those of the downtown elite but in a popular fashion. With very few exceptions the neighborhoods were physically alike. Mostly without major social conflicts, in a sort of silent but steady manner, the identities of these neighborhoods were built around their inhabitants' daily experiences, concerns, and practical demands. Among them, the connectivity to the rest of the city; the dominant presence of a factory or a certain trade; spaces for socialization, from public libraries to soccer clubs, from local movie theaters and cafés to neighborhood associations; and the availability or pursuit of basic urban infrastructure, such as sewage, drinking water, trash collection, public schools, and health institutions.

The neighborhood culture revolved around personal relationships, the family, modesty, and the possibilities of public education for upward social mobility. In spite of its inner stratification, neighbors tended to think of their local social world as largely equalitarian; they believed it could be improved through social reform and collective progress as well as individual thrift and industriousness. They confronted and built bridges with the culture of the centro, which they sometimes perceived as progressive and modern and sometimes as a site of decadence and moral decline. Many new channels, including the new journalism, tango lyrics, radio, and movies, facilitated these exchanges and efforts toward integration and differentiation. In the end, the neighborhood both accelerated and softened the modernization of urban life by including the barrio in the city as well as offering a strong sense of identity in a context of increasingly impersonal social relations and fast-paced downtown lifestyles.

But the inhabitants of the neighborhoods, the *vecinos*, were not the only ones living in the barrios. There were also workers, themselves vecinos but also participants in a very dynamic labor movement focused mostly on workplace issues. Until the electoral reform of 1912 only the elite had political rights. Such a context impelled the growth of a workers' movement with strong anarchist leadership that articulated its demands through general strikes and, more broadly, a call to dismantle the existing social and political status quo to make way for a radically new society. This period witnessed many conjunctures of intense social confrontation. But in the 1920s radical protest was progressively decreasing, and state institutions were, to a certain extent, addressing workers' demands, now voiced by socialists, anarcho-syndicalists, and communists. The demands now had a moderate tone, and to a certain extent their desires for widespread, lasting social reform were quite similar—although grounded in the world of work—to those of the vecinos, mainly focused on the neighborhood's needs and more as consumers than producers.

The electoral reform of 1912, which gave political rights to all adult men, was part of a liberal and reformist sociopolitical climate. Before, owing to the rules and constraints of the conservative republic, city politics was mostly the concern of elite politicians and emerging professional groups actively involved in building the city itself and the national state. Only on certain occasions, and not through elections, did the people of Buenos Aires participate in formal politics. But starting in 1917, when electoral reform was enacted in Buenos Aires, the political life of the city became more active and inclusive, with periodic national and municipal elections. Though the president of the nation named the city's mayor, the citizens of Buenos Aires—defined by the new law as male, city residents, and taxpayers—elected representatives to the City Council. This peculiar arrangement was the result of the existence of two spheres of city government, each producing and managing its own discourses, urban policy, and public expenditure priorities. Thus, while the federal government constructed the city's large building for government agencies and most of the hospitals and schools, the municipal government provided basic urban services and supervised others delivered by the private sector. It was also out of this context of political decision-making arrangements that a remarkably equalitarian urban grid was drawn. Initially aimed at containing the city's growth, the urban grid ended up invigorating it, fostering the creation of new neighborhoods and speeding up the settlement of the outskirts. By the 1930s it had laid the basis for a new, vibrant metropolitan area.

The Socialist Party and the Unión Cívica Radical were the most important players in city politics after 1900 as well as in the period after the military coup d'état of 1930, the first in Argentine history. There were also much smaller local political parties, though they never had significant electoral weight. Both major parties tended to see city issues as part of national issues. They usually spoke of local politics in terms of a vague notion of progress for the city, and usually failed to address more specific agendas concerning specific social groups, such as the working or middle classes. Whether they controlled the municipal government or opposed it, the two parties were strongly committed to building efficient machines that were instrumental and decisive in the business of doing national politics in the nation's capital, undoubtedly the most important political district. Neighborhood associations spoke on behalf of the vecinos, articulating an agenda focused on local issues and aimed at influencing and being influenced by the city government and the national political parties.

The rise of tuberculosis as a public and private issue took place in the context of these profound urban changes, and various forces, including the state, new professional groups, organized sectors of the civil society, and political parties, participated with varying degrees of leverage. But, interestingly, the history of tuberculosis does not unfold along the milestones of Argentine political history or those of the social and cultural history of Buenos Aires. In most periodizations of modern Argentine politics, 1930 is a watershed year: it saw the first military coup d'état and the end of the liberal consensus that had organized the turn-of-the-century policy of capitalist, export-oriented economic growth and modernization. In the history of tuberculosis, however, 1930 is not significant in terms of social or health policy, biomedical advances, or changes in mortality.

The history of tuberculosis is not synchronized with the periodization around which Buenos Aires cultural and social history has usually been organized either. This history, generally speaking, divides into two periods: from 1870 to the end of the First World War and from the early 1920s to Juan Domingo Perón's first administration in the second half of the 1940s. Though both periods were marked by a climate of change, the changes during the first one were sudden, intense, and spectacular, whereas during the second they were calmer and less strident.[21] But, as in the case of the political history, the history of tuberculosis I discuss is largely one of continuities. In other words, the two above-mentioned periods that allow organizing some social and cultural phenomena and processes are not particularly useful when attempting to reconstruct the history of this disease. In fact, neither the First World War nor the crisis of 1930 represented a turning point in the history of tuberculosis in Buenos Aires. This book discusses and analyzes a slow process, one in which the pace is determined more by continuity than by change. Recurrences abounded. It is a history of repeated cycles, especially those involving new cures that ultimately frustrated the hopes they awakened. It is a history with an enduring fear of contagion, despite persistent public campaigns aimed at changing conduct and prejudices. It is a history in which most people with tuberculosis do not have access to hospitals, dispensaries, or sanatoriums, all services that, though made more accessible thanks to a steady medicalization of city life, were never sufficient to cope with an increasing demand. It is a history in which desperate tuberculars want to believe in any remedy, whether offered by the medical profession or by alternative, hybrid therapies. Indeed, inertia seems to be one of the most persistent features of this history in which biomedicine tried, futilely, to control and cure the disease.

In the end, this history is aptly represented by the curve of declining tuberculosis mortality: a plateau with a slight downturn that lasted for decades. Not even the arrival of antibiotics significantly affected the curve, mainly because its decline had already been taking place. In the 1950s and 1960s there were people with tuberculosis, but they numbered many fewer than in the first decades of the century, and no doubt few of them died of it. During those years tuberculosis persisted for quite some time in many provinces of the interior of Argentina. But that was no longer the case in Buenos Aires, where, as a biomedical, social, and cultural problem, it was already becoming a matter of the past.

CHAPTER ONE

People with Tuberculosis Looking for Cures

At the beginning of the twentieth century, the reputable physician Clemente Álvarez described what he called the "*via crucis* of the tubercular":

> First, an apparently insignificant cough is treated, at best, with home reme-
> dies or expectorants obtained after consulting with the pharmacist. When
> symptoms worsen, or when one is alarmed by a bloody cough, the sick
> person goes to the doctor. This usually happens several months after the
> onset of the disease. Once the diagnosis is confirmed, the *via crucis* of the
> tubercular begins. On the one hand, treatment requires quitting one's job,
> rest, fresh air, good diet, good hygiene. On the other, the overwhelming de-
> mands of the home force the sick person to keep working in order to sup-
> port his family. Compromises are made; work is temporarily suspended,
> objects of value pawned, and friends and relatives are asked to contribute
> as much as possible. As soon as his condition improves, the person with
> tuberculosis goes back to work to make up the losses. But tuberculosis is
> unforgiving: soon, the person falls sick again, his condition just as bad as
> before or even worse. Relapses vary in number and duration according to
> the intensity of the infection and the patient's lifestyle. Some people know
> that city life affords little chance of recovery, and manage to spend a sea-
> son in the countryside . . . ; however, this does them little good. Short stays,
> lack of medical supervision, and the concerns about leaving the family be-
> hind make this solution largely useless . . . ; next, patients are admitted to
> the hospital, which are generally overcrowded . . . there, they wait—usually
> not very long—for death.[1]

The gloomy scenario described by Álvarez still persisted in the 1920s. Hospital statistics in Buenos Aires show that few tubercular inpatients were cured. At the Hospital Tornú during late 1920s, for instance, 80 percent of hospitalized tuberculars died.[2] Fear was rampant and resilient among those who survived. Perhaps that is why the doctor Antonio Cetrángolo wrote in the mid-1940s that "having, or having had tuberculosis, changes people's lives," an observation he illustrated with the case of one of his former patients who, twenty years after being cured, still wrestled with the idea of how to keep on living in a supposedly disease-infested city like Buenos Aires.[3]

Tuberculosis challenged biomedicine until well into the 1940s. Early diagnosis was difficult, and there were many entirely asymptomatic but ultimately fatal cases. Frequent coughs and sputum, irregular appetite, paleness, and weight loss were some of the possible signs. Only fever was a definite symptom, though it was hard to record at that time and hardly a sure basis for diagnosis. Once diagnosed, tuberculosis could be acute and advance rapidly, leading to death within a matter of weeks; or chronic, slowly weakening the patient over the course of several years; or moderate and controllable but with further recurrences. Of mild cases, particularly those detected early, it was said there was a 50 percent chance of being cured.[4]

Thanks to antibiotics, in the late 1940s and early 1950s the slow decline in the tuberculosis mortality rate since the beginning of the century accelerated, but morbidity remained constant, and people lived longer after contracting the disease. In those years treatment by medical professionals likely displaced that by nonprofessionals. Between the 1870s and the late 1940s the experience of tuberculosis was marked by a lack of effective therapy. Commonly, every tubercular, once home care and self-medication had proven insufficient, devised his or her own course of therapy. These attempts at finding a cure did not follow pre-established steps and were not necessarily practiced by other people with tuberculosis. They could include treatments provided by healers, herbalists, and quacks as well as institutional care at hospitals, sanatoriums, neighborhood antituberculosis dispensaries, and, for those who could afford it, visits to doctors' offices.

Perhaps sick persons with some exposure to formal education were less willing, from the beginning of their recovery efforts, to try alternative treatments. However, once so-called acceptable cures had failed, few could resist trying alternative ones. In any case, over the course of the first half of the twentieth century institutionalized health care became more and more dominant. Biomedical therapies offered a remarkable variety of remedies—some dubious, some innocuous, and some even harmful. Doctors often resorted to changing the medication in order to generate some improvement derived from the psychological action of the change.[5] They might prescribe balms, pills, and invigorating tonics advertised in the newspapers and available at drugstores. In addition, throughout this period doctors recommended the rest cure in the mountains; or an array of preventive or supposedly curative resources, from eating crushed eggshells and inhaling crushed garlic to being injected with sucrose, gold, and calcium salts; or serums and vaccines that were all the rage but only for a single season; or heliotherapy, exposing the body to sunlight; or, starting in the 1920s, specific surgical interventions in the lungs.[6]

Most certainly, from the 1870s to the 1950s death from tuberculosis and health care for people with tuberculosis entered the realm of medicine. In 1880 "terminal consumptives" or the chronically sick could not access an impoverished and precarious, if not downright pathetic, hospital infrastructure. In 1900 the hygienist Samuel Gache reported that rich people with tuberculosis went to great lengths to die at home.[7] However, as the twentieth century proceeded, fewer people died at home, many more died in hospitals, and the figures of the doctor, the nurse, and the social worker became more influential. For the wealthy, home care was followed by seasons in the Swiss Alps, luxury hotels, and private sanatoriums in the city or in the countryside, preferably the Córdoba foothills. Middle- and working-class tuberculars who were able to get some treatment found institutionalized health care restricted to dispensaries and hospitals in Buenos Aires; boardinghouses; or less expensive, sometimes free, Córdoba sanatoriums, usually managed by the state, private individuals, or mutual aid and philanthropic organizations. At least in theory these institutions shared an ambitious agenda aimed not only at curing the sick, but also at radically reforming their lifestyle.

Yet before such institutionalized therapies became real alternatives in the tuberculars' search for a cure, home medicine and self-medication were the two most obvious ways to confront tuberculosis.

Domestic Care: Home Remedies and Over-the-Counter Medication

Remembering his medical practice in poor and middle-class neighborhoods in Buenos Aires during the 1930s and 1940s, José Alejandro López wrote, "If an adult gets sick or has a fever, he's put to bed, given an aspirin and, if in a couple days he doesn't get better, a doctor might be called." His words reveal how medicalization had expanded but also the limits of that expansion.[8] In the intimate environs of the tenement room or the single-family home, the sick, before they consulted a doctor or went to the hospital, were not yet patients. They were, rather, individuals facing more or less confusing symptoms, usually connected at the beginning with ordinary, familiar pains.

The sick person received first aid and attention at home, from cloths soaked in vinegar to potato slices placed on the temples, cups of tea, remedies that could be bought without doctors' prescriptions at the neighborhood drugstore, and leftover medicines people had from previous bouts of similar symptoms. Also at home some very specific antituberculosis prevention measures were taken. María L., whose mother was the youngest of five and the only one not to die of tuberculosis, recalls being forced to "drink cod liver oil mixed with an egg yolk, sugar, and port every day, or to eat finely chopped raw liver that was buttered to make it easier to swallow."[9]

Tuberculars with mild cases who could keep working at least for awhile were, to a great extent, home tuberculars whose care was in the hands of their families and neighbors. By the mid-1930s, the popular biweekly magazine *Ahora* referred to them and elaborated on the home care scenario, indicating that reactions to having a person with tuberculosis in the house went from "understanding and solidarity to marginalization and rejection." Also around that time some doctors—highly critical of the idea that tuberculosis was a very contagious disease—didn't hesitate to encourage "wives to give their husbands the most attentive care at home, without fearing for their own health."[10] Among wealthy families tuberculosis home care consisted of hygiene, relative isolation, a good diet, rest, and the services of trained nurses. Among the less wealthy things were much more complicated. Medical booklets urged people to think about caring for a person with tuberculosis as a collective endeavor: the sick person and his or her relatives had to learn the rituals of rest, of ventilation, and, especially, of personal hygiene, such as properly disposing of a sick person's collected sputum on a daily basis; washing the bed sheets, handkerchiefs, and food utensils separately from those of the rest of the family; and disinfecting the room frequently.[11] However, and despite the discipline of the sick person and the vigilance of the relatives, poor living conditions often worked against such efforts. The physician Eduardo Wilde had warned in a turn-of-the-century hygiene manual about this, pointing out that "in a working-class family where the father has tuberculosis, hygiene is inevitably overshadowed by hardship, poverty, and the risks of contagion."[12]

Other factors contributed to making the household the primary site of health care for tuberculars. In the last third of the nineteenth century and the first years of the twentieth many people, including doctors and the infirm, rejected hospitals as places where one could catch other ills and even die. This attitude also contributed to the widespread preference for home care. In the

1920s, once those prejudices had been overcome, hospitals were overwhelmed by the increasing demands of the chronically ill, most of them with tuberculosis. But because of hospitals' inability to meet these demands, the household once again became a central site of primary health care. In any case, home care for a person with mild tuberculosis was the least onerous option for the family budget, an option supported and encouraged not only by common sense but also by home medicine and home economics manuals, radio broadcasts focused on health issues, and the growing supply of over-the-counter medications.

An article published in 1915 in the magazine *El Hogar* acknowledged the importance of home medicine. It stated that "medical knowledge has become so popularized that is difficult to find a home where it is not applied, whether correctly or incorrectly . . . and the cause for the voracity [for this knowledge] should be found in tuberculosis." The article ended by inviting the reader to become an active agent of his or her own health care and that of his relatives: "The sick person and his family must actively collaborate with the doctor and the hygienic and sanitary ordinances, rather than mechanically carrying out orders and indications; . . . people must be capable of recognizing symptoms and signals that announce health problems . . . and everybody must have the rudiments in order to avoid tuberculosis contagion."[13]

Home medicine manuals were available during the second half of the nineteenth century and well into the twentieth. *Medicina doméstica o sea el arte de conservar la salud, de conocer las enfermedades, sus remedios y aplicación al alcance de todos* (which translates to "domestic medicine, or the art of preserving health, recognizing illnesses, their remedies and application within the reach of everyone") circulated in Buenos Aires during the 1850s. Its lengthy subtitle underlined its role in helping everyone preserve health and recognize and cure diseases. In the 1870s the *Diccionario de medicina popular y ciencias accesorias* by Pedro Chernovitz recommended raw meat, wine, and liquor as a remedy for phthisis and tuberculosis. The *Almanaque medical y guía para la salud* by Dr. Jayne recommended "Jayne's Expectorant, a remedy that could be bought at drugstores and administered at home" following the instructions given in the almanac. In 1918 *El médico en casa: Libro para las madres* by Hugo W. O'Gorman proposed homemade medicines as a complement to doctors' services. In the 1920s the "new and expanded edition" of *Medicina casera* (which translates to "homemade medicine") by Juan Igón was advertised frequently in the socialist newspaper *La Vanguardia*, underlining that the manual contained a list of "all the diseases and the medicinal plants" that cure them and offering instructions on "how to prepare homemade remedies,"

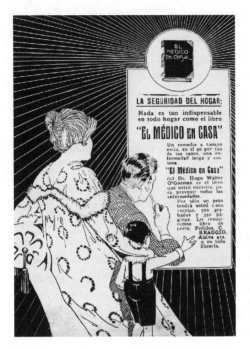

Advertisement announcing a home medicine book entitled *El médico en casa*, written by Hugo Walter O'Gorman. It emphasizes that "a good remedy on time will avert a long disease." (*El Gráfico*, July 3, 1920)

as well as general hygienic principles and tips on "how to create a home drug-store with all the essentials."[14]

In the 1930s Carlos Kozel's book *Salud y curación por yerbas* exalted the use of lemon, flax flour, and bananas to treat tuberculosis.[15] And in the 1940s the *Revista Farmacéutica* informed its readers, most certainly pharmacists, about the advantages of concoctions based on *palo santo* and *culantrillo* as well as other medicinal herbs that were later advertised and sold in pharmacies, a practice that medical journals like *La Semana Médica* compared to the illegal practice of medicine.[16] Starting in the late 1920s radio broadcasts encouraged and supported home medicine. Broadcasting was a resource used by both professional and unlicensed doctors. The Department of Tuberculosis Pathology and Clinic at the University of Buenos Aires Medical School offered a series of conferences on Radio Belgrano in which celebrated specialists presented—in a language they deemed simple and plain—the importance of observing the hygiene code that was supposed to prevent tuberculosis.[17] On the other hand, the radio show called *La hora de la salud* also informed listeners about "diets and formulas to prepare medicines to cure tuberculosis at home" while inviting them to disregard what professional medicine was offering.[18]

Throughout the first half of the twentieth century, advocates of naturalism encouraged home health care. Some anarchists believed in "natural cures" as part of an austere lifestyle in which vegetarianism and ideology merged for the "physical and moral" regeneration of workers.[19] Other voices articulating a message based on commercial, modern, and naturalistic reasons, and certainly with less radical political positions than those of the anarchists, made similar recommendations. For example, the director of the Instituto de Fisioterapia de Buenos Aires criticized "classic pharmacopoeia unable to cure chronic diseases" and advocated that "the best doctor resides within us," while praising home care and recommending treatments based on "electrotherapy, heliotherapy, and phototherapy" that, of course, were offered at his institute as a way of "helping nature in her spontaneous healing process."[20]

Remedies for the Modern Consumer

Increased access to over-the-counter medications was a key factor in reaffirming and renewing the importance of the household in treating tuberculosis. Numerous fortifying medications were supposedly offering cures to vaguely defined maladies like loss of energy, exhaustion, and cachexia, as well as blood diseases, weakness, scrofula, chlorosis, anemia, and tuberculosis. Along with these tonics, laxatives, diuretics, and purgatives there were other over-the-counter remedies to cure venereal diseases, skin problems, headaches, and colds. Taken as a whole, these medicines were probably among the first goods Buenos Aires residents bought as modern consumers, that is, as buyers who could choose between products with similar attributes but different brand names. As the century advanced, the supply of medicines expanded with greater networks of imports, more commercialization, and, to a lesser extent, local production.

In the last three decades of the nineteenth century the pharmaceutical sector depended entirely on foreign suppliers. Local drugstores sent their orders to the mostly French and Italian import agents and then manipulated several ingredients in order to prepare medicines that for awhile were called specifics. As the local market expanded, some of these foreign firms set up concessionaires and local offices. Though this was the dominant business model until the First World War, some drugstores in Buenos Aires began to manufacture preparations using formulas for which they had obtained a license from a foreign company; others followed suit but did so without licenses or with dubious or fake ingredients. The war years made it difficult to import drugs and chemicals, facilitating the local production of serums, vaccines, and specifics. Moreover, the First World War facilitated not only a much greater influx of basic ingredients for preparations made in the United States but also the local development of ways to dissolve, compress, mix, and fractionate them. Once the war was over local pharmaceutical production was temporarily put on hold. In the 1920s imports dominated the market once again; former commercial agents, who used to simply convey the orders of the local drugstores to their headquarters, became exclusive retailers, built large stocks, and began to sell directly to the local pharmacies. In the 1930s a large segment of the exclusive retail concessionaires—by then not only French and Italian, but also American and German—turned into laboratories that produced under license and enjoyed the benefits of increased custom duties on imports that competed with locally produced medications.[21]

Prudencio Dupont's career exemplifies very well the ups and downs of the Argentine pharmaceutical industry. As a representative of a French laboratory, Dupont started selling pharmaceuticals in Buenos Aires. Quite soon he expanded his operations to the provinces as well as to other South American countries. In time, following the changes in the national economy, the Duponts added to their pharmaceutical import business the local production of medicines. By the mid-1940s the family was running the C. Dupont y Cía. laboratory. Ernesto Caillón's career was somewhat similar. In 1888 he began importing patented medicines from France; his company was responsible for bringing to Argentina the *Alquitrán de Guyot*, a product that, well until the twentieth century, was believed to be an effective treatment for tuberculosis. Ernesto's son, Emilio, took over the business in the late 1890s and in 1901 he formed a partnership with León Hamonet. In the 1940s the business was incorporated, though it was still managed by the founder's relatives.[22]

A relatively new advertising industry enhanced the possibilities and massive commercialization of pharmaceutical goods. Newspaper and magazine advertisements from that time reveal not only an expanding market but also a growing sophistication in advertising styles. Gradually, communication strategies came to incorporate novel persuasive tactics, and design became worldlier. However, in spite of the increasing presence of commercial ads in print media read by more and more people during the last three decades of the nineteenth century, the professionalization of advertising was still to come. The first agencies, such as Ravenscroft, Vaccaro, Aymará, Albatros, Exitus, and Cosmos, started their operations at the beginning of the twentieth century.[23] In 1909, when advertising was a relatively consolidated industry, one of these agencies announced its services to the Buenos Aires business world, stressing its ability to "elaborate original ideas in order to multiply sales" as well as to encourage the use of ads in "newspapers, magazines, tramways, trains, and [on] street signs."[24] A decade later, in 1920, an envoy from the U.S. Department of

Commerce described Buenos Aires as a market where advertising agencies had been greatly accepted and were even essential to the city's commercial life. Although he considered the existing ads to be very poor, he indicated that the Buenos Aires market was very receptive to advertising messages.[25] By the 1930s several U.S. agencies, Walter Thompson, Lintas, and McCann Ericsson among them, controlled part of the Buenos Aires advertisement market.

Advertising quickly became a part of daily life in the city, and advertising techniques grew more refined in terms of design and strategy. The new technologies of the graphic industry played a part in this process, as did the development of a new journalism aimed at both reflecting and trying to shape social and cultural changes. In this new context, newspapers and magazines expanded their print runs, which often exceeded one hundred thousand copies. Naturally, this massive supply of print media demanded a reading public—to a great extent, a consequence of the steady growth of public education. This audience's enhanced interests included modern hygienic topics and practices. Newspaper and magazine readers were also protagonists in a hygiene culture that attracted consumers interested in taking care of their health and, later, in their health and beauty. It was in this context that the ubiquitous presence of ads announced the need and advisability of procuring supposedly effective treatments and medicines against tuberculosis.

At first the marketing of these products was limited to simple displays on store shelves and windows, street vendors' shopping carts, street signs, brochures sent in the mail, and announcements in newspapers and magazines. In those early years, advertising was basic: very modest ads without illustrations and employing typography not unlike that used in newspaper articles. Ads appeared in the classified section that listed products and services. They did not attempt to take the reader by surprise or stand out from the rest of the information. On the contrary, the reader had to look for the ad. Early in the twentieth century, ads had become larger and more attractive, efforts were made to improve design, and a new language was beginning to develop. Simple announcements that happened to appear on the same newspaper page began to be passé as commercial advertising quickly found special, more prominent space, to the point that in some weekly magazines a quarter of the pages were given over to commercial publicity.

The new approach to advertising was a distinctive and deliberate effort to dazzle the reader. This could be achieved by placing the ad in an unusual section of the newspaper or magazine, or by making the message bigger and more sophisticated, or by making illustrations more prominent. More and more, ads sought the reader out. Some products were advertised for decades.

In a newspaper ad from 1883 that lacked the style of the modern journalism of the 1920s, the Vino de Peptona Pépsica de Chapoteaut was called a "strengthening antituberculosis tonic for women." The ad, which consisted of no more than fifteen words printed in a single typeface and narrow column, was virtually lost on the page. By 1901 the message had become much more complex, stressing the product's benefits for those "recovering from fevers, diabetes, tuberculosis, dysentery, and tumors." It indicated that "the product was not from Argentina but from laboratories in Paris, Vienna, and Saint Petersburg." More than one hundred words long, the text used five fonts and described the product in great detail. By the end of the 1920s the ad for the Vino de Peptona Pépsica was quite sophisticated. It was bottle-shaped, and the text emphasized the product's strengthening qualities, mentioning that it had been used at the Pasteur Institute in Paris; children as well as adults were listed as being among its potential users.[26]

Advertisements for tonics, pills, syrups, and strengthening emulsions all promised similar benefits, and they were often on the same page in newspapers and magazines; they gave readers similar messages and demanded that they choose. These ads were dramatically different from the department stores' publicity, where women's clothing was often advertised without being associated with a particular brand. In the case of over-the-counter medication, supply-side competition was impossible to ignore. On June 10, 1901, for instance, six supposedly effective antituberculosis medicines struggled to get the reader's attention on the same page of the newspaper *La Prensa*. The most attractive advertisements were for Emulsión Kepler, Fórmula Ferrán, and Somatose. "A perfect solution made from the finest cod liver oil," Emulsión Kepler was presented to the reader as a malt recommended by the "most eminent doctors" to treat "undernourishment, rickets, and lung diseases." Fórmula Ferrán promised to cure tuberculosis within a month, and Somatose, "a tasteless powder made from meat substances and a top-notch rebuilding tonic," was recommended for "people weakened by poor nutrition, people with tuberculosis and children with rickets."[27]

This competitive context led to a refinement in advertising techniques. By the beginning of the century, in an ad that occupied a third of a column, Alquitrán de Guyot was announced as an effective way to "dominate and even cure tuberculosis." The ad used new advertising techniques, including drawings and dialogues between characters with whom readers could easily identify. In 1917 the advertisement reappeared, reaffirming the product's known qualities while warning against imitations. The consumer was instructed to "give enough details and information at the pharmacy when requesting the authentic Alquitrán de Guyot" and to make sure that "on the label Guyot is printed in big letters and in three colors the address Maison L. Frère, 19 rue Jacob, Paris."[28] Emulsión de Scott also warned against "buying a second-rate emulsion to save a couple of cents" and pointed out that "in the end, you can pay dearly for cheap products and, when it comes to health, you can even pay with your life."[29] Since emulsions were relatively common, a deliberate effort was made to stress the quality of this particular brand as well as to appeal to a discerning consumer, a consumer who would not be tempted by counterfeits, fakes, or substitutes.

The forgery of medicines underscored the issues of legitimacy, quality, and origin. For many years, indications of a remedy's foreign origin or its connection with a foreign laboratory were used and abused in advertisements. The assumption was that in the peripheral Buenos Aires the imported condition of a good was a guarantee of quality. And to a great extent that assumption was largely accurate, given the widespread preference for foreign goods among the elite and, to a lesser extent, among the middle and working classes. Along with the laboratory address where the medicine was produced—invariably in European or U.S. cities—recommendations from foreign doctors and scientists, often associated with prestigious institutions, were generally displayed. In fact, the suggestions of these accomplished foreigners were quite vague, such as "used by Dr. Rose in Paris." When, however, advertisements cited Argentine doctors, the testimony on the medicine's effectiveness was much more detailed. Their messages aimed to incite a sense of familiarity in the reader. The advertisements for Píldoras de Catramina Bertelli often ended with a very personalized professional commentary: "I've used these pills and had outstanding results in the treatment of tuberculosis," followed by the doctor's name and the address of his office. Sometimes the doctor's statement was accompanied by consumers' comments, as in the series of ads for Pastillas McCoy, in which the letter of a mother was reproduced: "[My story] bears witness to the beneficial effect of this medicine in improving the health of my tubercular daughter."[30]

Advertisements attempted to legitimize these products by appealing to medicine and science. Quite often this strategy was not only fairly subtle but also very committed to making clear that the product advertised didn't question the validity of medicine but complemented it. In 1920, in an attempt to show that many doctors prescribed these easy-to-get medications, an advertisement for Pastillas Dr. Williams promoted the product's power to cure and avoid "diseases produced by poor blood, weakness, and pulmonary fatigue." The ad invited the reader to "obey the doctor" who recommended these pills but also to keep in mind that they were "over-the-counter medications available in all the good pharmacies."[31] Sometimes the message was exactly the opposite: emphasis was placed on the ineffectiveness of medical treatments. In 1908, again in an ad for Dr. Williams's pills, a young woman reported having felt "a great weakness. I saw many doctors, but it was all in vain. Finally, a friend recommended these pills to me."[32] By the end of the 1920s, in a series of advertisements with changing characters but a single message and tone, a young man affirmed that "after suffering terrible pulmonary tuberculosis, vomiting a great deal of blood, coughing, and fatigue, and after spending six months in the Hospital Tornú and confirming that all the medical treatments were useless, I decided to go for Radiosol Vegetal."[33]

Thanks to a growing awareness of the importance of form, packaging— cans, flasks, bottles—and labels were meticulously reworked with innovative designs. Product format also mattered. Tonics, syrups, powders, and pills abounded. These products were explicitly marketed to people who were reluctant to drink unpleasant tonics. The McCoy pills were advertised as a new way of swallowing cod liver oil. In the mid-1920s Alquitrán de Guyot was promoted as Cápsulas de Guyot de Noruega, indicating that these cod liver pills induced "identical effects" and were the perfect solution for those who couldn't stand "the taste of tar water."[34] On the one hand, then, these medications were geared toward mass commercialization, toward becoming the medicine "that everybody takes." On the other hand, they had to stand out, which explains the deliberate effort to market medications for different tastes. And tastes began to be connected with certain ages and genders. Often medicines that had originally claimed to be designed for everyone later shifted their focus to a particular group—men, women, or children—but barely changed the contents of the ad. Thus, Pastillas McCoy, pills based on cod liver oil, were advertised as "the great solution for poor, weak, skinny children who scream at the mere sight of the loathed bottle of cod liver oil." Sirotan was an "iodine tonic that replaces cod liver oil and that children drink with pleasure." Preparación de Wampole was a medication that provided "relief and sure healing for tuberculosis without foul smells and flavors." And the Vino Nourry was depicted as a tonic with an "agreeable taste for the child's palate."[35]

Some advertisements stressed prevention, recommending liquors to fight colds and coughs that, if not fully cured, seemed to lead inevitably to tuberculosis. Advertisements for Pastillas Montagú preached that "anyone who coughs is exposed to tuberculosis, bothers the people around him, and spreads dangerous germs. . . . Coughing should be against the law."[36] Sometimes advertising emphasized the idea that primary health care was in the hands of the reader. In the 1920s certain advertisements clearly articulated this noninstitutionalized conception of health care and its role in the world of home medicine and over-the-counter medication. One such ad indicated that "a cold paves the way for tuberculosis" and must be "vehemently attacked starting with the first symptoms" by applying the "Untisal method, which is the quickest and most effective medicine because it employs the body's natural and unlimited defenses."[37] Other advertisements postulated that "the person who coughs and doesn't take action conspires deliberately against himself. The pain, sputum, and coughing attacks should convince you that you're incubating a serious disease. Start treatment immediately by taking three spoonfuls of Tomillo Erytoso a day, followed by a cup of tisane and hot milk. With this very simple remedy, you will manage to dominate any ill, no matter how chronic."[38] The notion of a consumer engineering his or her own cure often went hand in hand with the development of a new distribution or commercial technique that professional organizations were quick to criticize. In 1933, for example, the *Revista del Colegio Médico de la Capital* criticized the laboratory La Estrella for mailing forms where people could write down their symptoms and then telling them which "medication made by La Estrella laboratory would cure their particular illness."[39]

Most over-the-counter medicines claiming to cure tuberculosis were just restorative tonics. There were also other types of medicines, like Dr. Kaufmann's sulfuric patch.[40] And during the twenties and thirties electricity-based therapies were quite common, such as Dr. Sanden's electric waistband and Dr. Diaz de Souza's "method based on short electric discharges." An ad announcing "Dr. Souza's method" indicated that "every day more and more tuberculars get cured with this new method."[41]

But most were tonics, elixirs, and rejuvenating wines. Their targets were weakness and fatigue, two complaints that during the 1910s and 1920s were consistently connected with tuberculosis, consumption, neurasthenia, and eventually with coughing, bronchitis, colds, chlorosis, respiratory problems, exhaustion, and flu. By the thirties and forties, advertisements for these tonics placed much less emphasis on tuberculosis, instead making indirect reference to the disease when inviting users to "take care of their respiratory tracts" or indicating the need to pay attention to "coughing and colds that end in terrible diseases." Indeed, some medicines that had been on the market for a long time and were advertised in the 1920s as effective against tuberculosis—such as the Pastillas McCoy, the various concoctions based on cod liver oil, the Tomyllo Eritoso pills, Alquitrán de Guyot, and the Guayacose—were, in the 1930s and 1940s, deemed equally effective against the physical weakness that led to a number of diseases, including tuberculosis. It was said that the impurity and weakness of the blood were the problem and that these tonics were supposed to enrich blood and fortify bodies suffering from the pressures and challenges of modern life. By and large, advertising messages promised the same benefit during both periods: restoring lost vitality. Messages invoked a magic bullet that would control the disease, leveled threats — "if you don't take this, you'll get the disease" — and celebrated the product's energizing effects.

Only occasionally did the dubious promises offered by these medicines lead to debates at meetings of the City Council.[42] Their enduring presence on the market didn't create much trouble, because, among other reasons, so many parties were directly or indirectly involved in the business: laboratories and importers; pharmacists always ready to write prescriptions; practitioners who recommended such tonics and pills to their tubercular patients; and manuals for personal and home hygiene, encouraging consumers to take restorative tonics in order to improve the women's reproductive capacities and men's work abilities. Sectors of the medical profession confronted this peculiar alliance time and again, labeling pharmacists as "intruders in medicine" and generalist physicians treating tuberculars without proper credentials as "university quacks" or "lung specialists in winter and intestine specialists in the summer."[43] As can be expected, the interests of the consumers also mattered. And when it came to dealing with the loss of strength in the case of anemia, tuberculosis, children predisposed to tuberculosis, and weak pregnant women, people had become convinced these tonics could provide some help and were relatively easy to acquire.

In any case, given that all biomedicine had to offer was traditional auscultations and examinations of such symptoms as sputum, cough, fevers, and fatigue, or x-rays that could detect the disease early on but couldn't provide an effective cure, advertisements for syrups, pills, and rebuilding tonics didn't need to do much to attract attention. Though their effectiveness was hard to prove, in many cases the meat and vegetable components in such over-the-counter concoctions, which were sometimes actually quite rich in vitamins, might have helped strengthen weak bodies. Here, perhaps, lies one explanation for why people never stopped buying them. Thanks to advertisements and the advice of neighborhood doctors, quacks, pharmacists, neighbors, and relatives, these harmless remedies successfully became a part of the world of over-the-counter medications without confronting the medical establishment.

The enduring presence, plentiful supply, and quite sophisticated publicity of many over-the-counter remedies were constantly questioned by lung spe-

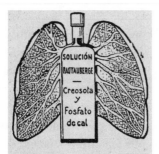

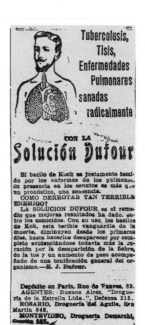

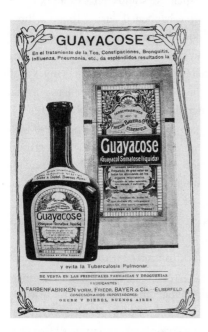

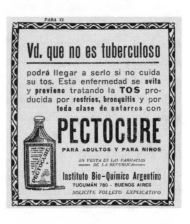

Advertisements announcing over-the-counter medicines for tuberculosis from (clockwise from upper left) *La Nación*, December 7, 1898; *La Nación*, December 12, 1898; *Para Tí*, July 6, 1926; *Para Tí*, July 6, 1926; *Caras y Caretas*, May 21, 1910

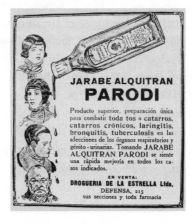

cialists. Though not an open war, two messages directed to tuberculars illustrate this long-lasting dispute. An early twentieth-century advertisement for Píldoras Kynzame promised to restore "the hope of defeating tuberculosis." On the other hand, a recommendation in a brochure from 1927 published by the city government's Asistencia Pública answered the question of "what to do when a person finds out that he or she has tuberculosis" by resoundingly affirming that the only course of action was to "go see a doctor or go to the hospital, get an examination, and promptly follow the doctor's recommendations; don't waste time and money trying out medicines not prescribed by doctors."[44]

Healers, Herbalists, and Quacks

While professional medicine couldn't offer successful, accessible antituberculosis therapies, tuberculars inevitably turned to self-medication and sought treatments practiced outside hospitals, dispensaries, and doctors' offices. From 1870 to 1950—in a fashion similar to what happened during the first three quarters of the nineteenth century, before the bacteriological revolution— herbalists, pharmacists who recommended medicines, empiricists, healers, swindlers, charlatans, midwives, fortunetellers, and quacks were mainstays of health care for vast sectors of society in Buenos Aires. This heterogeneous group, according to its opponents (generally medical doctors) constituted a legion of dangerous, perverse, and illegal pseudoproviders of panaceas who were taking advantage of the sick in their despair and ignorance. This critical view ended up producing a certain stereotype of the healer, a character imagined as a quack who could skillfully combine herbs, magic-wand medicines, and religion in his curing styles: an expert at communicating with the sick, a practitioner of orally transmitted knowledge, and a believer that all sicknesses resulted from the disordered condition of the fluids or humors of the body.

This stereotype of the healer as a quack contrasted with another one that prefigured the image of the university doctor as a solid professional whose judgments were grounded on rational, secular, and biomedical knowledge. Doctors condemned anything that linked medicine with superstition. Whether in a private office or at the hospital, doctors were always committed to a professional practice marked by reasonable material interests and humanitarian responsibilities and obligations.

Undoubtedly, the stereotypes of healers as quacks and of doctors as totally rational and socially sensitive professionals were sometimes close to reality. They were both major players in the entangled world of dubious and generally ineffective antituberculosis therapies offered by popular and professional medicines. Between 1870 and 1950, newspapers and magazines as well as medical journals portrayed plenty of doctors with supposedly impeccable careers. Likewise, they informed readers about healers whose treatments consisted of "purely suggestive therapies" such as "magnetized water," "the laying on of hands," or "the magic ring." Some healers said they could cure anything, while others tended to specialize in a few popular diseases like *daño*, the evil eye, the *pasmo*, and the *jetta*.[45] In 1942 an extended article with numerous photographs was published in *Ahora*. It invited readers to explore this dense world, which the city's commission on illegal medicine was attempting to set right. The highly experienced quacks featured in the article revealed that they were everywhere in the city, that some charged and others didn't, that they were both men and women of all ages, that some had something like a doctor's office or even an institute with preestablished schedules announced in newspapers; others did not advertise and saw their patients at home.[46]

However, very few of those who advertised cures for tuberculosis or whose activities appeared in the print media resembled the quack stereotype largely created by those speaking on behalf of the medical profession. In the 1920s a *manosanta* (hands-on healer, literally "saintly hand") named Hermano Pedro stressed his ability to cure tuberculosis with cold water.[47] But, again, it seems his was a quite unusual case. In fact, most of those who publicly presented themselves as capable of dealing with tuberculosis were the kind of health care practitioners who in other Latin American contexts were labeled as "hybrid healers."[48] Instead of radically alternative practices and visions, hybrid healers combined popular healing traditions and biomedicine. Their actions were part of a health care style that not only offered services outside the boundaries imposed by professional medicine — and, in so doing, obstructed the medicalization of society at large — but also facilitated the extension of some biomedical knowledge and practices to the world of popular and home medicines.

Hybrid healers sought to gain a place in the health services market by displaying many and varied resources, from announcing exceptional former successes to publicizing the infallible effectiveness of a cure; from publishing notes in newspapers to writing short books and brochures that included the testimonials and letters of gratitude sent by those they had cured. These healers circulated remarkably freely at the margins of an urban world increasingly marked by professional medicine and commercialized remedies. In their promotional efforts many stressed the fact that they were foreigners. Emma T., for instance, depicted herself as "having just arrived from Europe, with the latest breakthroughs in modern science," and Celia de R. said she came from

Paraguay cognizant of "the ancient and modern secrets" to defeat tuberculosis. In Emma T.'s case, revered European traditions and science were summoned in an attempt to generate complicity not only in the immigrant population, which was adjusting its lifestyles to the emerging urban modernity, but also in the elite, who were anxiously attempting to reproduce European ways in peripheral Buenos Aires. The target of Celia de R., on the other hand, might have been the Argentine-born population, the local *criollos* who had no recent European family connections. In his advertisements, Carlos Richards emphasized the fact that he was a professor, a title often used by advocates of "naturist cures" who tended to underline the relevance and authority of a supposedly academic diploma. Guillermo Alter promoted himself as a "the only professor who studied at European institutes and cures with the Kuhne Kneip system." Professor E. Alsina claimed to be a member of the Instituto Naturista. Both Alter and Alsina gave to their services an institutionalized hue not shared by most hybrid healers. Many, however, appealed to an almost opposite public presentation. Hermana María, Hermano Pedro, and Don José all stressed that they had specialized knowledge quite different from that of medical doctors.[49] Though religious references appeared in some of the ads placed by hybrid healers, the role of religion seems marginal.

Some healers explicitly promised to cure phthisis and tuberculosis, while others swore to have the solution for blood sputum, fevers, weight loss, and weaknesses.[50] Their promises were at least partly articulated in the language of biomedicine. Joaquín Vazquez, a healer at the beginning of the century who was called a manosanta by *La Semana Médica*, claimed "his magnetic vital fluid" was a unique, polyvalent therapeutic resource capable of curing practically everything. Interestingly, his list of illnesses, which did not include popular diseases like pasmo, apparently replicated the handbook or vademecum of a licensed doctor: "rheumatism, paralysis, depression, asthma, anemia, tuberculosis, bronchitis, hair loss, hip ache, chlorosis, paleness, colics, erisilla, scrofula, phthisis, sterility, bloody sputum, constipation, fever, throat, hemorrhoids, hernia, liver, hysteria, urinary incontinence, insomnia or sleeplessness, headache, madness, menstruation, nervous breakdowns, venereal diseases, weight loss, obesity."[51]

Quite often herbs and, to a lesser extent, balms and concoctions were part of a marketing strategy that combined the services of pharmacists and healers. For a long time the neighborhood drugstore was also a hybrid institution where medicines from very different traditions comfortably shared the shelves. This was largely the case because pharmacists, owing to their own will or clients' demands, ended up diagnosing diseases and prescribing medication even though they were not authorized to do so. Pharmacies were also the places where some healers sold their products, revealing some sort of integration between healer and pharmacist. Naturally, the medical doctors deemed this alliance clear evidence of growing quackery as well as the outgrowth of a commercial activity—trading in medicinal herbs and other over-the-counter-medications—they thought had to be regulated.

Articles in the medical press frequently referred to growing quackery, stating there is always a drugstore willing to sell "quacks' remedies" near the places where they treat their patients.[52] As for the commercial aspect, this was a critical rendition of the gray area where pharmacy, homeopathy, herbal medicine, and many other practices intersected. For instance, an advertisement from 1871 for Dr. Harcourt, a homeopathic doctor, offered "antidotes against tuberculosis" that were "authorized by him and available at the drugstore Botica Imperial." In 1901 a suit against the Bustamante brothers for the "illegal practice of medicine" resulted in a fine. The brothers were charged with advertising in several newspapers on sale "at a private doctor's office . . . highly curative herbs and resins from the Andean mountains" that promised "effective cures authorized by the Departamento Nacional de Higiene." According to the verdict, the Bustamantes couldn't mention the authorization of the Departamento Nacional de Higiene simply because such authorization did not exist. Consequently, they were required to "remove from their advertisement the words 'private doctor's office'" because they were not qualified to "give recommendations" and "receive consultations." In the end, the verdict suggested to the brothers the alternative of associating with a drugstore where they could sell their herbs, a proposal they rejected because it went "against their interests."[53]

Also in 1901 Professor of Hydrotherapy Eliseo Marconi employed a marketing strategy that did not involve pharmacies in selling herbs that cure tuberculosis. In an unusually large advertisement under the caption "Hygienic and Curative Specialties" published in *La Razón* Marconi invited readers to try his "humble little herbs" because their "highly medicinal and nutritive values" cured "venereal diseases, pulmonary tuberculosis—even if hereditary—arthritis, tumors anywhere in the body, cancer, white tumor, nervousness, the diseases of the respiratory tract, and every known sickness and human pain." Marconi informed readers that "any science that comes from nature is more potent than a science that comes from studies," stressing that his cure was natural and did not involve "drugs and operations." His "little herbs" were on sale at his home at Santa Fé 2351, where the sick could also take aromatic baths "for moderate prices." The advertisement ended by declaring

Healer's advertisement announcing his services in a large-circulation newspaper. (*La Razón*, May 1, 1901)

that "[Marconi's] explanations and consolations" were free of charge, that the sick person "would be diagnosed according to his or her facial expressions," and, once examined, informed "whether or not their illness was curable."[54] Other ads promoted "natural medical treatments without medicines of any kind that provide prodigious cures for tuberculosis," like the therapy offered by Doctor Guillermo Brito "at his private office." The self-named Dr. Brito encouraged the sick "not to become desperate" and recommended attacking tuberculosis by "following the Natural Laws."[55]

While these supposed professors and doctors did not resort to the pharmacy and were, in their way, questioning medicine that was unnatural, the herbalist Rogerio Holguín reveals the case of a hybrid healer in which dialogues between popular and certified medicine were more than fluid. Born in Colombia and self-taught, Holguín introduced himself as a practitioner "somewhat familiar with some laconic books of medicine but very fond of the *Diccionario de Medicina Popular* written by Chernoviz." Holguín started preparing "syrups with herbs to treat fevers," learning from the "empiricists that give medical services." In the late nineteenth century and the beginning of the twentieth, Holguín traveled through many South American countries promoting a "vegetal medicine to cure tuberculosis." His life is narrated in his book *Historia del descubrimiento de medicinas vegetales para curar la tuberculosis,* published in 1917. Holguín arrived in Buenos Aires in 1916. At the invitation of his partner, he came to the city to participate in an undertaking organized by another capitalist: the opening of a clinic run by a professional doctor. In his book Holguín says that the tubercular patients treated at that clinic improved, but for reasons he doesn't explain his capitalist partner decided to close the clinic. Months later Holguín treated the son of a "very prestigious gentleman" in the Córdoba foothills who became enthusiastic about Holguín's therapy. Through him Holguin began to be well received in medical circles. He met a doctor who happened to be the director of a hospital for tubercular patients. Soon the two men opened a sanatorium and admitted five women. A month later the sanatorium was closed. By the end of 1916 Holguín returned to Buenos Aires and treated tubercular women at the Hospital Vicente López, until the doctors there decided to dispense with his services. Somewhat annoyed by the way he had been dismissed from the hospital, Holguín stressed his "medical morality" even if he "lacked the academic diploma." In his book he includes letters from patients begging him to continue administering treatment. Marcelina de Oto hoped "to be graced by his kindness." Emilia Almada stated, "I wish, with my whole spirit, to receive your treatment," and Angela Allende and Emilia Bruno asked him to speak to the hospital authorities in order to "get us discharged as soon as possible, because our strength, health and spirit have been restored, thanks first to God and You." The book concludes with a section in which Holguín invites doctors "who are acquainted with science's impotence at fighting tuberculosis" to consider his treatment. "Science," he says, "will be greatly benefited by it."[56] During the twenties and thirties many other healers used medicinal herbs, though they didn't circulate in the hospitals and sanatoriums run by professional doctors as Holguín had. In 1924 "a naturist professor" recommended herbs for "pimples, tuberculosis, and blurry cataracts," and in 1936 a butcher who said he had become a doctor hawked a pomade made from vegetable roots as an effective remedy for tuberculosis.[57]

Some naturopaths stressed the importance of self-cure, lecturing their patients on the benefits of sober lives, a watchful diet, and purging with, predictably, the medicines and treatments they sold.[58] In 1912 a certain Astorga advertised his "vegetarian regime" to "expel the Koch bacillus"; to offer public proof of the effectiveness of his treatment, he asked the dean of the Universidad de Buenos Aires Medical School to inject him with "a dose of microbes." The dean ignored the request, but the issue appeared in the papers, making Astorga a healer who dialogued with the medical academy. Astorga recognized the existence of bacilli and, like other naturalists, he believed that diets based on oranges and other citrus fruits were a way to fight the disease.[59] There was no lack of people who combined natural cures with biomedicine and new technologies. In 1883 Félix Romano was depicted in some newspapers as a charlatan and deemed by others to be a prestigious professional. He invited people with tuberculosis to his "Health House," where they could be treated and cured with "aerotherapy," a fairly common method in Europe that was frowned upon by factions of the local medical establishment.[60] At the turn of the century some people, taking advantage of the fascination aroused by electricity, sold electric waistbands to cure all sorts of organic ills, from neurasthenia, asthma, and tuberculosis to hysteria, pneumonia, and bronchitis.[61] Around that time an advertisement designed to look like a news story reported that Juan Chiloteguy "had found the way to cure tuberculosis with a honey-based injection."[62] In 1928 the newspaper *Crítica* spoke of a German medical school dropout who cured tuberculosis by using sun rays that, when connected with his "extraordinary innate predisposition," turned him into a "source of white, golden, and violet rays." Focusing on "a lung compromised by tuberculosis," the German man managed to "transform the organ and heal the sick."[63] Professor Richards guaranteed, in his brochures, that "no matter how chronic it may be, tuberculosis can be fully cured by means of radio-magnetism, radio-pathology, and natural methods."[64]

Starting in 1882, some official regulations forbade "unauthorized people to announce medical services or specifics to treat certain diseases."[65] These regulations were largely ignored by newspapers and magazines that kept publishing the meticulously designed advertisements for these goods and services, irritating the defenders of academic medicine well into the 1930s.[66] These advertisements evidence the place of hybrid healers in the modern city and also suggest that many of their clients, whether wealthy, middle, or working classes, were literate. They were part of a reading public increasingly exposed to a publishing industry that had been expanding since the end of the nineteenth century. This industry continued to grow in the 1920s, making it easier for healers to publish their own books and brochures, most of the time in very inexpensive editions and on occasion even distributed by mail.[67] Newspapers and magazines became a sort of platform where the biomedical discourses and services coexisted alongside the heterodox discourses and services offered by hybrid healers. Once they started using advertising in the print media, healers' potential share of the market increased significantly and, as a result, many of them became full-time healers. This gave them a greater public presence but also made them more vulnerable to the complaints of the medical profession and the persecution of the police.

Reporting with complicity, indignation, or resignation, the medical press, newspapers and magazines with large print runs, and literature reveal that these hybrid healers were a viable option for rich and poor alike.[68] The failure and impotence of biomedicine led most tuberculars to look for and try other alternatives. But the poor had other motives also. In 1876, when contagion among patients was still common in hospital life, the journal of medicine and surgery *Revista Médico Quirúrgica* affirmed that the poor avoided going to hospitals, which they considered deadly, and ended up "resorting to quacks, charlatans, and healers."[69] Twenty-five years later, once hygiene had improved and the health service network had expanded, embarrassing and stigmatizing therapeutic routines pushed many working people with tuberculosis to consult healers. Unlike very wealthy or just well-to-do tuberculars, who could easily negotiate with their doctors to keep their condition secret, the poor found that in the increasingly sophisticated medical care and control of hospitals and neighborhood dispensaries they were labeled as being sick with tuberculosis. With that stigma came the risk of losing one's job and having one's house or room compulsorily disinfected, which was often experienced as an assault on personal and family respectability. And those who accepted that they had tuberculosis and wanted to receive their health care from hospitals and dispensaries faced the problem of access due to inconvenient and restricted hours for people who worked during the day. Furthermore, most treatments prescribed by doctors—from the customary rest cure at a sanatorium in the foothills to balanced diets and surgery—were quite complicated because of their cost or because access to free, but limited, services required some knowledge or the right contacts in order to take advantage of them.

Healers were an attractive alternative that protected the tubercular from the public exposure implied by professional medicine and its treatments. Indeed, discretion might be one of the reasons many healers prescribed and delivered their medicines by mail.[70] Besides, healers were much less expensive. In the neighborhoods, many part-time healers offered their services for free or indicated that payment, whether in money or goods, was voluntary. In 1909 the popular magazine *PBT* advertised the services of "Mr. CD, who suffered severe tuberculosis and is willing to give away the remedy that cured him."[71] Nevertheless, established, full-time healers acted like modern health care providers, with set schedules and sliding-scale fees. Some, like Hermana María, had disciples who referred their difficult cases to her.[72]

The range of what healers prescribed was vast, from strange, exclusive concoctions to syrups advertised in the papers and even recommended by some medical doctors. At the margins of professional medicine, though drawing on some of its remedies, healers sold hope and possible solutions, two things tuberculars needed the most. Many healers were well acquainted with standard pharmacopeia and often sold their own concoctions and brews or prescribed pills, pomades, and over-the-counter syrups available at the pharmacy. These medications sought to become legitimate in the market, either by invoking science or by the persuasive ability of the healer preaching their beneficial effects. In the last third of the nineteenth century, as well as in the 1940s, the sales skills of healers reinforced the always promising and optimistic messages printed on the labels of specifics, and in so doing, contributed to an inchoate consumer culture of purchasing over-the-counter-medications.[73]

Although there were reports of the negative and even lethal effects that some treatments or remedies had on tuberculars, the herbs, medicines, and simple drinks supplied by healers were by and large pretty innocuous, perhaps even less dangerous than some of the therapies used by biomedicine, like gold salt injections in the 1920s and 1930s and certain surgical techniques.[74] Healers seem to have had a much more empathetic, supportive relationship with the sick than many licensed doctors. Without doubt, there were sensitive doctors capable of dealing with tuberculosis by means of biomedical resources while also providing the sick with affection and respect. And there must also have been unscrupulous, irresponsible, and money-driven healers. Interestingly, doctors were the ones to notice, early on, the way most healers were able to relate to the sick. An article published in *Archivos de Psiquiatría, Criminología y Ciencias Afines* in 1905 recognized that "quacks have more ability to explain how, when, and where an illness was contracted."[75] Almost forty years later, in a tone that hadn't changed significantly, *Ahora* stressed the "consideration, respect, and love" that characterized most healers' practices, and, in 1939, *La Semana Médica* pointed out, "the contagious optimism of the quack," his or her direct talk free of "technical terms and convoluted words." They spoke a language that was similar to "that of the sick, from whom they even accept opinions about the disease."[76] These elements were not always present in the relationship between hospital doctors and their tubercular patients; hence, some explained the persistent presence of healers as the inevitable effect of academic medicine's disregard for emotional factors in the life of tubercular patients. Consulting a healer allowed tuberculars to regain some hope that a cure was possible which, in the end, was what every sick person wanted to hear. In this way, healers' lies and promises were as instrumental as the recurrent and ineffective cures prescribed by doctors.

There were various explanations about when and under what circumstances healers were consulted. Some medical doctors saw a clear itinerary: "[People] start with home medicine, then they go see a quack; only as a last resort do they see a physician."[77] Others assumed that people visited healers after having proven the "impotence of doctors." These people believed the healer clientele included "terminal cases, skeptics and those who didn't believe" in professional medicine, "the ignorant and the silly with an educated spirit who have received the fatal verdict from a doctor," "the incurable guided by the understandable human desire to find a remedy for their pains."[78] Requesting healers' services was often interpreted as a result of a medical practice that "didn't know how to, or just couldn't, provide solutions," a medical practice that was "more expensive" and "unkind," because "doctors are exemplary exponents of proper urban manners at their private offices, but not at the dispensaries and hospitals."[79]

The tubercular may have consulted simultaneously, successively, or alternatively with doctors, pharmacists, and the array of hybrid healers and quacks. This sort of random therapy was also, in part, a result of the fact that the medical profession had yet to define its area of legitimate competence. It was in this context that a sort of gray zone characterized by overlapping and vagueness emerged. Both healers and doctors contributed to it. On the one hand, hybrid healers deliberately avoided an open confrontation with medical doctors. In so doing, they imitated postures, practices, and terminology firmly anchored in biomedicine. As for doctors, some endorsed nonrationalist and nonmaterialist vitalist notions; that is, the conviction that the functions of a living organism are regulated by a vital principle distinct from chemical and physical forces. In an article published in 1909 on the "question of quacks," Francisco Otero, a physician with a long, distinguished career at the Departamento Nacional de Higiene, pointed out that "by natural law, every individual has a connate inner drive to defend the integrity of his body, a sort of vital resistance against any event that conspires against physiological harmony."[80] Others—anarchists, socialists, and, some time later, in the thirties and forties, doctors who used to write in the health magazines *Vida Natural* and *Viva Cien Años*—passionately defended naturism and the benefits of exposure to the sun in the fight against tuberculosis.[81] In many healers' ads vitalist notions were also present. This world of ill-defined jurisdictions was also apparent in the way healers and doctors practiced. If in 1867 the medical journal *Revista*

Médico Quirúrgica reported that some doctors "declared they were quacks" in order to avoid paying professional matriculation fees, in the 1880s and 1890s it was said that certain quacks, after being pursued by the law, worked comfortably with professional doctors. In the late 1930s *Viva Cien Años* reported there were doctors who worked alongside "healers and quacks with a curious enthusiasm."[82]

Between 1870 and the late 1940s, the use of alternative antituberculosis treatments offered from outside the biomedical realm was widespread. According to opponents of these alternative treatments, they varied little over time. Judicial attempts to criminalize these practices ended up backlogging the legal system's administrative offices.[83] In 1876 it was said that Buenos Aires was "a paradise for quacks and clairvoyants." In 1890 an official publication pointed out that "pseudo-doctors, homeopathic doctors, healers, spiritists, mesmerizers, hands-on healers, and charlatans are having their heyday." In 1909 the Anales del Departamento Nacional de Higiene complained that "nowadays, suggestion and quackery are the modus vivendi in the modern city." In 1928, as part of his series of journalistic notes depicting urban life, its characters, and scenarios, Roberto Arlt published *El gremio de las curanderas y las Santeras* (which translates to "the guild of quack and Santería practitioner women"), a short story focused on healers and Santería practitioners. And in 1930 a headline in the newspaper *Crítica* read, "The city is packed with quacks and psychics."[84] Only the widespread use of antibiotics and the expansion of hospital services would bring about the decline of this mishmash of alternative and medical treatments that from the perspective of the tubercular were by and large complementary, not mutually exclusive. Only then did healers start to lose relevance in the history of tuberculosis, though not necessarily in the way people dealt with health problems in general.

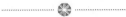

CHAPTER TWO

From Being Sick to Becoming a Patient

Institutional health care for tuberculars grew faster in the twentieth century than in the nineteenth. Yet it never managed either to treat the majority of people suffering from tuberculosis or to do away with alternative treatments, from home remedies to self-medication, hybrid healing, and quackery. Because of public awareness campaigns, individual counseling, and desperation, or simply because health care facilities were becoming more widely available, tuberculars became increasingly accustomed to and confident in medical institutions. After being diagnosed, many sick people, especially during the early stages of the illness, chose to ignore their condition and kept working and living as usual. Others sought treatment beyond home care, and one alternative was to delve into institutionalized care. There, in the medical institutions, people with tuberculosis became patients.

Of their own will, tuberculars were admitted to hospitals, visited dispensaries, or spent time in sanatoriums. These places provided a degree of hope, emotional support, and the possibility to leave behind the stigma of being a person with tuberculosis, someone with no place in a society of presumably healthy individuals. Furthermore, institutions relieved the family of the burden of having a contagious, feared sick person living in the household and demanding special attention. To varying degrees, institutionalized care restricted a patient's mobility, confining him or her to a world in which privacy and individual freedom took on new meanings. Tuberculosis hospitals, sanatoriums, and dispensaries effected a certain shift in the ideas and strategies surrounding health care. Former efforts intent on isolating the dangerously sick via indiscriminate quarantines and compulsory confinement at lazarettos were replaced by more modern initiatives aimed at watching over and controlling those who were already sick or groups of people believed likely to catch tuberculosis, instructing them in the hygienic self-government of their bodies. At these institutions, treatments attempted to teach patients hygienic, responsible, daily habits that would hopefully lead to their recovery and do away with the fear of tuberculosis patients as carriers of disease and agents of contagion. Most important, they were supposed to be trained in a sort of hygienic citizenship forged in routines designed by medical knowledge and aimed at modeling, reinventing, and managing the patients' bodies and souls.

At the end of the nineteenth century, the institutional network expanded thanks to institutionalized philanthropy, private charity, public welfare, and corporate and mutual help initiatives. This process changed who was in charge of taking care of tubercular patients. Relatives were somewhat, though not fully, displaced by the figures of the doctor, the nurse, and the dispensary health visitor, all of whom became more prevalent and influential. Access to these professionals and to health care institutions was not equitable; indeed, they were hardly able to meet the demands of the tubercular population at large. In the case of wealthy people with tuberculosis, home care and the country retreat to the large ranch *estancia*—many of which, in the twentieth century, had professional nurses on their staffs—supplemented medical attention at private and sophisticated sanatoriums as well as extended rest at health stations and luxury hotels in the Córdoba foothills or the Swiss Alps. For tuberculars from the middles classes and workers with stable occupations and incomes, treatment at private sanatoriums in the city or in the foothills meant a series of extra expenditures that were seldom covered by mutual help or prepaid health-care systems; if they were, it was for a short time. Frequently, these treatments ended up consuming the family's modest resources. In the case of poor tuberculars, free treatment at hospitals, dispensaries, and state-funded sanatoriums could ease the strain on the family budget, but available beds for internment were still very limited in number, and few had access to them. No wonder by the end of the 1920s tuberculars attempting to become patients and, in the process, moving from one hospital to another, were fairly common. Poverty-stricken tuberculars, the poorest of the poor, were quickly becoming a public burden; some of them were institutionalized alongside beggars and the insane.

The effectiveness of hospitals, dispensaries, and sanatoriums largely depended on the patient's condition when admitted. Only rarely did those with advanced, severe cases of tuberculosis survive. If a patient with a moderate case was in the early stages of the disease, recovery was not impossible. Evaluating the performance of these institutions before the arrival of antibiotics is not simple. However, most evidence indicates that, despite the expansion of a modest institutional infrastructure during the first decades of the twentieth century, the care provided at hospitals, sanatoriums, and dispensaries was quite limited in scope and never substantially altered the gradual decline in the overall tuberculosis mortality rate.

The Tubercular and the Urban Hospital

During much of the nineteenth century Buenos Aires hospitals were a sort of holding tank that performed an extensive, often vague spectrum of tasks geared toward surveying patients. Attempts to improve a patient's health were marginal, as were the success rates. At hospitals at that time, medical assistance was largely circumstantial, though people could find a palliative for poverty. To a great extent the hospital was a depository where terminal patients, indigents, and poor tuberculars were confined. In 1918 Emilio Coni spoke about his years working as a medical practitioner at the Hospital General de Hombres, which opened in the early 1870s. His account contains almost frightening images: "I had the chance to contemplate, in [the patients'] dark, humid and dreary rooms, a veritable antechamber of death, where tuberculars were lumped together with other sick people and devoured by consumption and swarms of flies. . . . Of the forty sick people in a single room, half had tuberculosis." He recalled the "disdain and indifference" with which doctors, nurses, and nuns treated people with tuberculosis, "like moribunds." Furthermore, other patients didn't hide their "feelings of revulsion and nausea at tuberculars' persistent coughing and full spittoons."[1]

Between 1880 and 1910 there was a marked change in how hospitals were organized and what went on inside them. Such modernized hospitals became increasingly important health care institutions for the urban poor. Some efforts, such as neighborhood aid wards and house calls, sought to decentralize the health care that had been provided by the city government since the end of the nineteenth century. Though these initiatives never became real alternatives for most of the sick, they did help to expand the medicalization process into the city neighborhoods. In terms of premises, many hospitals enlarged their wards, at times according to the guidelines used for European hospital architecture and at times by improvising low-cost, temporary solutions. These changes came about more slowly than planned owing to administrative problems and a lack of funding. There were more and more doctors, and many were now specialists, defining new hierarchies. If at one time physicians mostly saw patients in their hospital offices and if the sick were usually treated by recently graduated medical students in training, now doctors began to be more involved in the daily life of the hospital. Starting in the twentieth century, nursing became women's work and tended to be performed by secular practitioners rather than by nuns. Hospital services also changed. By that time hospitals were already providing specialized outpatient consultations, which were soon widely accepted by the public. Outpatient consultations facilitated a faster turnover of the sick with diseases, acute or not, that required shorter stays than chronically ill people. These changes solved neither the problem of the lack of beds in general wards nor the problem of how to treat those requiring isolation. The growing population of Buenos Aires, and all the sick people who didn't live in the city but went there for health care, aggravated the problem of scarcity of hospital resources.[2]

The experience of tuberculosis inpatients changed over time. In the nineteenth century, when they were still called consumptives, the treatment they received hardly differed from that of any other poverty-stricken patient. As a result of the effort to separate chronic, acute, and infectious patients, by the end of that century the first hospitals specifically designed for tuberculosis patients began to appear.

CONSUMPTIVES IN THE WORLD OF THE CHRONICALLY ILL

Like most sick and poor people in the last third of the nineteenth century, tuberculars were afraid of hospitals. This was partly because poor hygiene facilitated contagion and partly because of the fact that most of the sick were moribund by the time they arrived at the hospital. No wonder the hospital mortality rate was enough to scare most people away.[3] In 1875 only one-tenth of the people who died in the city had received hospital care, and, as the director of the Hospital San Roque pointed out in a report, many died within six hours of being admitted to the hospital.[4] Nevertheless, fear of hospitals didn't necessarily mean rejecting the possibility of medical care. In 1883 and 1884, as part of a program sponsored by the city government, the number of sick people visited by doctors at their homes increased fivefold. These patients were given free medication at these visits and treated in an environment that was less hostile, less dangerous, and less alienating than the hospital. There was also a steady increase in the number of patients who visited doctors at outpatient offices, which by the mid-1870s had opened in some hospitals.[5] And as early as the mid-1880s some doctors were warning about a lack of hospital beds, indicating that the medicalization of urban life was in the making.[6]

Nevertheless, despite patients' fears and the scarcity of beds, there were consumptives in Buenos Aires hospitals. In 1878, of a total of 322 deaths at the Hospital General de Hombres, 88 died of acute diseases, and the remaining 234 of "chronic, incurable diseases, mostly tuberculosis."[7] In the seventies and eighties, the tuberculosis mortality rate at the Hospital San Roque ranged between 25 percent and 50 percent.[8] A few tuberculosis patients, mostly those with less advanced cases, were sent to the countryside to facilitate their recovery.[9] But, as stated by a municipal officer in the late 1880s, most tubercular hospitals "alienate [patients] from all the things that could positively affect their condition—hygiene, location, good diet."[10] Tuberculars participated in the world of the chronically sick, the poor, and the indigent, a world in which a successful search for a bed was followed by a regime of relative seclusion. At hospitals, nuns ruled over—"tyrannically," according to the anarchist newspaper *La Protesta*—the lack of hygiene, the practically nonexistent medical supervision, and the prevailing promiscuity.[11] Because there were few institutions for them, the situation was even worse for women.

At general hospitals the presence of tubercular patients was problematic: they took up the few beds available for excessively long periods, and they increased hospitals' mortality rates. Typically they were at death's door when admitted, either because fear of the hospital prevented them from coming sooner or because the hospital would relieve relatives of having to pay for their burial.[12] Regardless of the cause, in 1889 the director of the Hospital Rawson attempted, without much success, to reduce the hospital's mortality rate by systematically isolating tuberculosis patients.[13]

HOSPITALS FOR PEOPLE WITH CONTAGIOUS DISEASES

Starting in 1892, when they were separated from the acute and chronically ill, tubercular patients and other patients with infectious diseases shared the isolation wards of the Casa de Aislamiento, which had become, in those years, the Hospital de Contagiosos Francisco J. Muñiz, the hospital for infectious diseases. This was to be a provisional measure until a specific building for tubercular patients could be built. However, it took longer to construct the new building than expected, and tubercular patients ended up passing their disease on to other patients, and vice versa. Lack of beds and overcrowding were problems, largely because the population grew faster than the hospital infrastructure.[14] In this context, the mortality rate at the Hospital Muñiz was still strikingly high: between 1891 and 1904, of a total of 5,490 tubercular patients—many of whom were already very sick by the time they were admitted to the hospital—3,101 died at the hospital.[15]

The effort to gather tubercular patients at the Hospital Muñiz was far from successful. Some patients, who knew that visits from relatives were forbidden, did everything they could to avoid being admitted to an institution that couldn't meet the demand for beds. On the other hand, the absence of a tuberculosis hospital caused many patients to seek care at general hospitals. Starting in 1882 certain hospitals were designated to provide care for tubercular patients, on the condition that they had wards that allowed for a "total isolation from other patients." Only the Hospital Francés created special wards for tubercular patients; the hospitals related to other foreign communities—Italian, German, Spanish, and British—simply refused to take in tuberculars. The Hospital Rivadavia, a hospital for women managed by the Sociedad de Beneficencia, designated one of its rooms for women with tuberculosis, but it was soon closed.[16] Many tubercular patients ended up doing what the chronically sick did: moving from one general hospital to the next, trying to get a bed, even if, as was often the case, it was in a hallway or a basement.[17] By the beginning of the twentieth century chronically ill patients took up one-third of the available beds in the city's seven hospitals; though the problem was undeniable, it wasn't as dramatic as in the 1880s.[18] This was not only a consequence of the modernization and expansion of the city's public health agency, the Asistencia Pública, but also of an increasing recognition that hospitals could no longer be a holding tank for poor, chronically ill people.

These new services, though, led to a new clientele, which resulted in new problems. Starting at the end of the nineteenth century, an attempt was made to regulate the number of people requesting beds by creating an official certificate of poverty. Given by Asistencia Pública, this certificate granted free access to hospitals and free medicine. To get the certificate, applicants had to present a form signed by the chief of police in their district or by the *vecino* presiding over the district commission for hygiene in the neighborhood where they lived. In 1899 around thirty-eight thousand people had poverty certificates, a number that many observers believed was inflated by somewhat "affluent people taking advantage" of the Asistencia Pública's free health-care services.[19]

Starting in 1902, therefore, two categories of poverty were established: the *pobres de solemnidad*, who received health care free of charge, and the *simplemente pobres*, who had to pay a certain fee because they were "able to work, had some income or received help from their families or others."[20] A sort of paradoxical scenario emerged. Convinced of the convenience of getting free benefits at the state's expense, however deficient, some were taking advantage of the system. At the same time, others considered the certificate of poverty insulting, rejecting it because they perceived this public document as evidence of diminished individual respectability.[21]

All these issues were relevant since tubercular patients ended up mixing with other chronically sick patients. Officials sought to isolate them, as they did with other people with infectious diseases and sick prostitutes.[22] Nevertheless, there were nowhere near enough beds available. That's why, in the twentieth century, the problem of the chronically sick was finally subsumed by the problem of tubercular patients. This development was a result of the massive presence of the disease, the scarcity of specific hospital resources, and the absence of effective therapies.

HOSPITALS FOR PEOPLE WITH TUBERCULOSIS

Of the 2,081 certified deaths due to tuberculosis in 1908, approximately 1,000 were reported to have taken place at a hospital.[23] Many of these deaths occurred at the Hospital Muñiz, which treated all kinds of infectious diseases as well as people with advanced tuberculosis. It had only one ward for women, which was constantly overcrowded as the demand for hospitalization increased; this problem continued into the 1920s, when the ward was expanded.[24] In 1918 more than 50 percent of tubercular patients admitted to the hospital died within twenty-four to forty-eight hours of admittance. As at the end of the nineteenth century, the high tuberculosis mortality rate accounted for the hospital's high mortality rate. According to the doctors who worked there, hospital wards had turned into "deposits for incurable people" and "antechambers of death."[25] Some years later, in 1925, the hospital had a total of three hundred beds and a few wards, which were apparently better maintained and equipped. That year the annual report of the city government, the Memoria Municipal, described the Hospital Muñiz in slightly less apocalyptic terms than before.[26]

In 1904, after almost seven years of negotiations with resistant neighbors, who "feared contagion" and called the initiative "inappropriate and without our permission," the Hospital Tornú was opened. Designed as an urban sanatorium for the rest cure—that is, a treatment for tuberculosis based on rest and isolation in a good, hygienic environment—this hospital was probably the first of its kind in Latin America. It could accommodate at least a hundred men with mild and early-stage tuberculosis. In 1911 two wards for women were opened, and in 1926 five new pavilions were built, providing a total of 320 beds for men and women in 20 wards with "rest galleries" and leisure rooms.[27] In the 1930s the number of beds doubled, and by the 1950s there were 1,100 beds.[28] But even the expansion of the building through the acquisition of new premises and the addition of new floors to the existing wards could not keep pace with the city's demographic growth and the increasing number of tuberculars who wanted to use the hospital. Some of those not admitted to Hospital Tornú went, in vain, to other hospitals trying to find a bed. Those who were admitted either had cases that were of interest to the doctors owing to random contingencies, or they had a "letter of recommendation from a local political boss."[29] In 1927 Hospital Tornú rejected six hundred applications for inpatient care and, years later, it was estimated that the city of Buenos Aires had only half the number of beds needed for tubercular patients.[30]

The shortage of beds was in part a result of limited infrastructure and increasing demand for hospital services by people who were not exactly poor. According to a city politician of the time, "[These people] don't hesitate to stop their cars in front of the hospital." And *Crítica*, a very popular newspaper, referred to individuals who were spending money on "frivolous and trivial things while doing everything possible to make sure they would receive health care free of charge."[31] On the other hand, it was common to reserve beds "for those who pay," particularly during periods of economic hardship like the thirties. It was also common for the hospital's support association, the Asociación Cooperadora, to collect a payment in advance in order to guarantee "the right to a little room," where the sick person received more and better attention. Those who couldn't pay "wandered from one neighborhood antituberculosis dispensary to another."[32] Thus, during the first half of the twentieth century tubercular patients posed the same kind of problem that chronically sick people, including consumptives, had in the nineteenth. Not until the fifties, when the disease was no longer killing people on such a large scale, did hospitals stop rejecting applications for admittance.[33]

Although the Hospital Tornú was designed to attend to patients with moderate cases of tuberculosis, by the 1910s it was also receiving people with advanced and terminal cases. In the thirties, this situation hadn't changed very much: over 70 percent of the inpatients died within ninety days. It's not surprising that one of them, interviewed by *Ahora*, declared, "You go to the hospital when you're finished."[34] Evidently, and as in the past, many sick people only considered going to the hospital when the disease was very advanced. This delay was attributable both to the scarcity of beds and to the effort to postpone cataclysmic effects produced by the institutional interment, not only on the individual level but also in terms of a patient's family, employment, and finances. In any case, the hospital recovery rate was quite low even in the 1940s. Admitted at the recently opened Hospital Nacional de Tuberculosis, which was providing services similar to those at the Hospital Tornú, Jorge S. describes a fairly gloomy scenario: "In the last semester, among the forty people admitted, only two have been discharged; three have gone to seek attention elsewhere; thirty died, and five remain alive."

In the 1950s the situation improved considerably, and the hospital mortality rate dropped to 15 percent.[35] But in the first decades of the twentieth century those rates were much higher, to a great extent because many patients, often admitted when at death's door, "asked to be discharged as soon as they perceived even a slight improvement, often one more apparent to them than to the doctor." The rush to get out was mostly motivated by concerns about work, "because many patients were parents, had families, and the fear of poverty lurks." In the end, these never-cured tubercular patients returned to the hospital "worse than before."[36] Two and three decades later this pattern was still noticeable. In 1935, of a total of 841 discharges, only 193 were registered as "clinically cured." In 1947 a lung specialist recognized that "if a tubercular patient, lacking economic support for his household, is forced to be hospitalized, the sick person will put off being admitted as long as he can and he will soon abandon the hospital to get back to work."[37]

In those years the widespread use of x-rays, a procedure usually performed on tuberculars as well as their families, and the more systematic analysis of sputum allowed for early detection of the disease. These advances heightened expectations for a cure, though they did not necessarily serve to cure more people.[38] Innovations such as pneumothorax (the induced presence of air in the pleural cavity to collapse the parts of the lung affected by tuberculosis) and thoracoplasties (a remodeling or reshaping of the thorax by removing some of the ribs so as to obliterate the affected pleural cavity) also gave some hope and demanded special wards. Surgical interventions were more common among less affluent people; they took the risk of complications and postsurgical infections because they needed to get back to work as soon as possible. But these innovations didn't solve the bed shortage or the lack of hospital equipment.

In 1938 more than two thousand tubercular patients were refused admission to the Hospital Tornú.[39] According to one congressman, the dimension of this unmet demand revealed that "sick people from all social classes were interested in going to the hospital."[40] An array of factors contributed to this "puzzling situation": the annulment of the poverty certificate in the 1920s; middle-class use of hospitals under certain circumstances; the positive perception of the services provided by some public hospitals; and the increasing complexity of the medical services available there, which were now more specialized and offered technology not found in most private medical offices.[41]

In the late 1940s, with the proved effectiveness of antibiotics, this tendency increased further.[42] As tuberculosis mortality declined faster than its morbidity, the problem was no longer dying patients, but the "chronically sick who can't be discharged." These people, who often lacked familial support, were too weak to go back to work, and releasing them presented the risk of spreading the disease.[43] By the late thirties the search for an inexpensive solution to avoid long periods of internment led doctors at the Hospital Tornú to set up two galleries, one for men and one for women, for what was then called "the daily rest cure." Designed for patients with moderate cases of tuberculosis who couldn't get a hospital bed, the treatment consisted of spending most of the day resting on a chaise lounge, eating three meals a day, and getting medical attention.[44] In addition, outpatient dispensaries were available, another resource which, starting in the early years of the hospital, aimed to alleviate the demand for beds. From the beginning these dispensaries were very popular, and their popularity increased over time: in 1909 they were visited approximately three thousand times and in 1951 close to twenty thousand. They provided accessible treatment that was less traumatic, if perhaps less effective, than being hospitalized. In any case, years later patients were asked to pay for their x-rays, which may well explain why many poor tuberculosis patients ended up abandoning treatments at dispensaries.[45]

In 1912 only men were admitted to the Hospital Tornú, and there were two foreigners for every native Argentine. Soon, women were also admitted and, in 1938, of a total of 1,221 patients, 956 were Argentines, 768 were women, and 453 men. In 1912 a quarter of the patients indicated that their permanent residence was out of town; in 1935 this number had risen to one-third, and in 1949 it was around one-half. In 1912, as in 1939, more than half of the patients admitted were under forty. This distribution reflects the impact of tuberculosis on the population of Buenos Aires during the first three decades of the century. However, by the end of the forties, the number of sick men under the age of thirty increased, though these patients did not, by and large, live in the city, where tuberculosis was declining. Instead, the bulk of these patients were residents of the increasingly industrial metropolitan area, where many migrants from the provinces were settling. In the provinces, particularly those in the northeast and northwest of the country, tuberculosis rates were as high as they had been in Buenos Aires twenty years earlier.[46]

Patients at the Hospital Tornú were mostly workers. In 1912 practically all were manual laborers and white-collar workers. In 1938, the most common jobs held by the 453 men admitted (more than 90 each) were day laborers and employees, referring to white-collar occupations; construction workers numbered more than 20. Of the 768 women, 550 were housewives; 46 were seamstresses; 37, domestic servants; and 36, factory workers.[47] By the late twenties there were more tubercular women at the hospital. Throughout the previous decade new wards were opened in order to do away with what, in 1909, was called "women's reluctance . . . to take their ills to public places."[48] In 1925 a special ward was opened, largely in order to receive pregnant women with tuberculosis who were "being rejected over and over by the hospitals, due to fear of contagion." Before the creation of this service, doctors advised women who were applying for a place in a maternity ward not to mention that "they have gone to the Hospital Tornú, because that single commentary would guarantee rejection."[49] The new maternity service, which was associated with another focused on breastfeeding, aimed at keeping pregnant women with tuberculosis in the hospital during much of their pregnancies so they could benefit from the rest cure. Naturally, this required convincing the mother, a responsibility most often met by health visitors and doctors working at the neighborhood antituberculosis dispensaries. After delivery, the newborn was given the BCG vaccine to avoid postpartum contagion. The newborn was also attended by a wet nurse from the hospital or elsewhere. When the child turned two, he or she was admitted to a preventive institute or given to a relative.[50]

At first, the Hospital Tornú had large wards. In the late twenties they were divided into smaller ones, and patients were distributed according to how advanced their condition was. This measure aimed at keeping those with mild cases of tuberculosis from witnessing the "demoralizing spectacles of advanced cases."[51] There were recreation and reading rooms as well as gardens around the hospital building, an attempt to reproduce the placid landscape surrounding a country sanatorium. The wards had galleries with huge windows with multicolored glass (mainly blue for its supposedly relaxing qualities) that were facing the northeast and southeast to provide sunlight and shelter from the wind.[52]

In addition to this infrastructure, there were detailed rules and routines. Once admitted, patients were given a set of cutlery, a dish, a vase, a cloak, blankets, clothes, a personal spittoon, and anything else necessary for personal hygiene. Patients also received a copy of regulations on how to behave at the hospital, stressing the obligation to "obediently heed the doctor's advice." One key aim was to model a patient who could control his or her coughing, rest for four or five hours a day, do light respiratory exercises and take walks, clean himself or herself almost obsessively, and be diet-conscious, particularly when it came to meat, eggs, and milk. The inpatients could be visited by relatives and friends twice a week, throw little parties, make use of a library

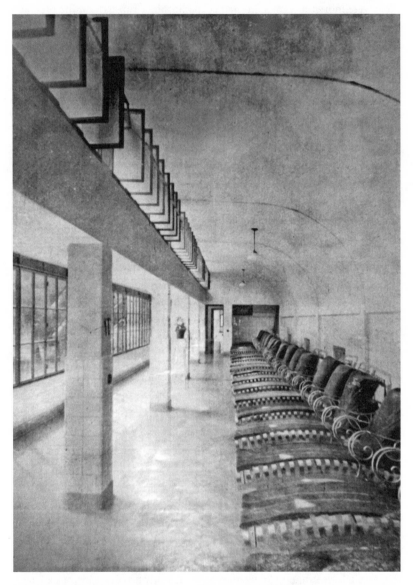

Gallery with chaise lounges and large windows at a tuberculosis hospital.
(*Resúmen de la memoria de la administración sanitaria correspondiente
al año 1926*, Buenos Aires: Talleres Gráficos Tuduri, 1927)

with a great many easy-to-read books, and even take music lessons. They had access to phonographs and, at the beginning of the century, were visited periodically by bands. Later they could enjoy listening to the radio and watching movies. All these resources were thought to constitute a sort of "needed psychotherapy" that, starting in the 1920s, was gaining recognition.[53] There were also religious services for those who wanted them. Smoking and alcohol as well as discussions about politics and religion were forbidden. Poor patients' families received aid through the dispensaries of the Liga Argentina contra la Tuberculosis, the most active nongovernmental organization involved in the antituberculosis efforts.[54] In the 1930s (although there had been similar efforts in previous decades) labor therapy was encouraged as a way of avoiding too much leisure and as a strategy for a gradual reintegration into the work world.[55] "Labor re-education wards," which aimed to train tuberculars in skills that demanded little physical effort, became popular among patients. Some doctors defended the wards, though indicating that, before acquiring new work skills, convalescent patients needed "occupational confidence so they wouldn't take just any job that crossed their paths." Others criticized the wards, believing that labor reintegration should be handled and controlled by neighborhood antituberculosis dispensaries.[56]

Tuberculosis in the Neighborhoods: The Dispensaries

The sick didn't reside in dispensaries, as they did in hospitals and sanatoriums; unlike doctors who examined tuberculars in their private offices, dispensary workers and health visitors tried to reshape patients' lives in the intimacy of their homes. Coni and Samuel Gache, two eminent early twentieth-century hygienists, conceived of the neighborhood antituberculosis dispensaries as multifunctional spaces that sought to offer prevention, education, cure, and care. Dispensaries were aimed at early diagnosis; accelerating admittance to hospitals for those who needed it; providing outpatient treatments, orientation, and support; and educating patients' relatives.[57] Compared to other treatment centers, dispensaries were fairly inexpensive, and they were chiefly designed to meet the needs of the poor. In moderate and mild cases of tuberculosis, it was understood that treatment had to be reinforced by home care. Once at the dispensary, the sick person was examined and a file was opened for his or her case. Then the hygienic conditions at the person's home and work environment were carefully reviewed; from then on, the tuberculosis patient and his family were supposedly under constant surveillance.[58]

The key figure at dispensaries was what would be later called the health visitor. At the beginning of the century the upbringing of antituberculosis visitors was mainly empirical, but by the 1920s women specifically trained for the job followed an agenda prepared beforehand by doctors.[59] In the 1900s the word *visitor* was usually used in its masculine form. *La Vanguardia* spoke of "visiting male nurses," and *La Semana Médica* indicated that visitors had to be "active, intelligent, empathic-seeming men, capable of speaking with some authority to the sick, men who take an interest in their physical and moral problems, becoming their confidants and friends if possible."[60] However, as in most paramedical professions, by the 1920s visitors were, judging from the pictures, middle-class women.[61] They were asked, as in the booklet entitled *Misión de la enfermera en la lucha antituberculosa* (which translates to "mission of the nurse in the battle against tuberculosis") to make use of their "sympathy, simplicity and feminine patience" in order to "become confidants of the submissive spontaneity and innocence of the poor."[62] The visitor's activity was mainly educational; she had to have an impact on "the patient's home, which was generally poorly ventilated due to ignorance and misconceptions." She had to bring to these homes "her easy, simple words in keeping with the humility of the patient's environment, and apply her femininity to a daily task that demanded sensitivity and delicacy."[63] As "civil sisters of charity," the visitor's mission was "to detect disease by meticulous inspection and collecting of minor data," "to investigate the environment where the tuberculosis patient lives," and to educate the family in "hygienic culture and daily habits to avoid contagion." She also facilitated access to medicines and taught home economics, from how to organize the family budget and prepare meals to how to behave at work and how husbands and wives should manage shared lives. Her purpose was to locate the person suspected of having tuberculosis rather than those already diagnosed with the illness.[64]

The first dispensaries opened at the beginning of the century.[65] Some were better equipped than others, though they all provided preventive, diagnostic, and treatment services as well as medicines, food, and even direct financial assistance. Dispensaries sent patients who needed inpatient care to hospitals and sanatoriums located in Buenos Aires and Córdoba with which they had agreements.[66] The services at dispensaries were free of charge and open to the public in mornings and afternoons. In the twenties, nine dispensaries depended directly or indirectly on the city government.[67] In 1938, 211,986 sick people visited dispensaries; 215,350 packages with eggs, milk, meat, and bread were handed out; and almost 24,000 homes were inspected by health visitors and 8,828 by doctors.[68] In 1950 the number of dispensaries run by the city government hadn't changed, but by then about 130,000 consultations were registered, revealing that tuberculosis was no longer as catastrophic as it had been.[69] Dispensaries were also run by civic, ethnic, and labor associations, as well as by neighborhood and charitable organizations. The most active dispensaries were managed by the Liga Argentina contra la Tuberculosis, the Comisión Villa Crespo contra la Tuberculosis, the Liga Israelita contra la Tuberculosis, the Mutualista Antituberculosa del Magisterio, the Asociación de Previsión Social de Correos y Telégrafos, and the Sociedad de Beneficencia de la Capital. All these private institutions joined the campaigns organized by the municipal and national governments and also developed their own preventive initiatives by means of films, conferences, brochures, and street signs. Their structure was similar to that of the city's dispensaries. Owing to a lack of economic stability, however, many of these private institutions were ephemeral.[70]

The dispensaries' effectiveness was suspect from the start. Some argued they weren't well equipped, especially in terms of x-ray apparatus. Others said there weren't enough dispensaries and that they were just palliatives for a defective network of hospitals and sanatoriums. They maintained that dispensaries cared for tuberculars who couldn't find beds at hospitals but had not been able to reach and help the tubercular poor. Nevertheless, according to a lung specialist writing in *La Semana Médica*, even if these treatments were not wholly effective, they still "served to attract the sick."[71] If discreetly, dispensaries managed to identify tuberculars and spread the antituberculosis hygienic code. A study from 1931 reported that 41 percent of the sick who resorted to dispensaries did so following a health visitor's advice, 31 percent on the recommendation of other patients, and 14 percent because of public health campaigns.[72] A few years before, in 1927, another study revealed that, of the 12,404 patients treated at the city dispensaries, 4,719 had tuberculosis. Of these, only 480 managed to be admitted to the Hospital Tornú and Hospital Muñiz, and most of those patients tried to follow the course of treatment indicated by the dispensary once they were released from the hospital.[73] That same year a city dispensary's annual summary of activities reported that 40 percent of the patients treated there had died, and only 18 percent could be considered cured.[74] Thirty years before, at the turn of the century, the statistics provided by another dispensary were similar: of every ten tuberculosis patients treated over a three-month period, four died, the condition of four remained the same or worsened, and only two improved.[75]

Since the scarcity of hospital beds impeded admitting patients, dispensaries played an important role in the medicalization of the city. Their relevance largely grew out of their specific agenda of preventing tuberculosis among children. This was a major concern partly because babies a few months old could catch tuberculosis and die, and partly because the figure of children was bound to eugenic notions of building the "Argentine race" of the future. Acting as itinerant arms of the dispensaries, health visitors had to exert their powers of persuasion on mothers in order to guarantee that children wouldn't catch the disease. It was in this context that dispensaries provided injections of the BCG vaccine; from 1925 to 1938 more than fifty-seven thousand children were vaccinated at hospitals, city health agencies, child health prevention centers, summer camps, and dispensaries.[76] If a family member was sick, dispensary visitors resorted to a practice called relocating the newborn, moving the child to a house where no one was sick. If the child was over two years old, he or she was admitted to a children's ward. If children showed signs of predisposition to the disease, efforts were made to strengthen their bodies: they were sent to summer camps for "weak children." At the beginning of the century these camps were established at the shore and in the countryside; starting in the thirties they were located in the foothills, where campers could benefit from hydrotherapy, a good diet, outdoor exercise, and excursions.[77]

Dispensaries brought the poor and working classes closer to certain therapies provided by professional medicine. In so doing, and as on other occasions, they unveiled the limitations of the antituberculosis discourse in the tuberculars' experiences with the disease. Thus, in 1941 a patient spoke ironically of the difficulties of "following medical advice, namely, treating the disease in its very early stage" when "plenty of workers have to live with [tuberculosis-like] symptoms because they can't do what hospitals and dispensaries recommend that they do in terms of health care."[78] Many of those who went to dispensaries had very advanced cases. By 1940 two-thirds of the people seeking health care at the dispensaries run by the Liga Argentina contra la Tuberculosis were "beyond treatment."[79] Here, the main issue was the so-called economic factor, that is, the fact that many who were sick put off visiting the dispensary on a regular basis and ignored the suggested treatments, mainly to avoid having to "quit a job, in the case of men, and [not being able to] care for children and home, in the case of women."[80] On the other hand, dispensaries' schedules usually coincided with the workday, which made it difficult for laborers to seek the care they offered. Not until 1937 did three dispensaries, all funded by the city government, stay open after 6 P.M.[81]

According to La Semana Médica, "onetime visitors and tuberculars coming to get the opinion of a specialist and then never coming back" were quite common. Once they knew their diagnosis, some tuberculars decided to move and take menial jobs in the countryside or small towns — the only rest cure avail-

able to the poor—or to move back to their original countries, as many Spaniards did. Others took every precaution to avoid the stigma of having tuberculosis: they gave a fake address at the dispensary or moved without leaving a
new one, which made it impossible for health visitors to find them.[82] Finally,
some resorted to the dispensary because there they received "different kinds
of treatment and help." According to one of the leaders of the antituberculosis movement in Buenos Aires, this strategy was fundamental to having an
impact on the population; he affirmed that French dispensaries, which only
provided a diagnosis and dispensed with advice, were not "in keeping with
our people's character." Food was the most important benefit offered at dispensaries. It was greatly sought after, and many took advantage of the lack of a
coordinated private-municipal-national effort by visiting several dispensaries
and managing to get more than one food package.[83]

Occasionally, dispensaries sought out tubercular patients at their workplaces. In the late thirties a team of health visitors was deployed to pinpoint
the causes of absenteeism in 1,271 workers. The report produced after this initiative indicated that 123 factories and a total of 30,700 workers were reached,
that after receiving the health visitor at his or her home only 258 workers
visited a dispensary and got examined, and that 40 percent of those examined learned they had tuberculosis. The report also established that this time
it wasn't workers' concerns over losing their jobs that caused them to neglect
the visitors' advice, but the "factory owners' reaction to the matter, manifesting a sheer indifference [and] a lack of understanding of the need and advisability of facilitating workers' health care at dispensaries."[84] Something similar happened when "unreachable mothers" resisted the health visitor's advice,
responding with "a sordid hostility" to the invitation to have their children
examined and, if necessary, treated at the dispensaries.[85]

Despite these tensions, limitations, and shortcomings, the presence of dispensaries in the city clearly reveals a steady process of medicalization. In Villa
Lugano, a neighborhood of over fifteen thousand inhabitants and, in the late
twenties, a modest network of health services, the people demanded an antituberculosis dispensary.[86] Even more revealing of the strength of the medicalization trends are the words of the anarchist activist Juana Rouco Buela, a
woman used to understanding daily life in ideological terms and, as might be
expected, reluctant to support initiatives originating in state, public welfare, or
philantropic institutions. In her memoirs she wrote, "We don't care about dispensaries until one of our relatives gets sick; then we do visit the dispensaries
run by the Liga Argentina contra la Tuberculosis, looking for relief. There,
health care is free of charge, you don't need to know the right people, and the

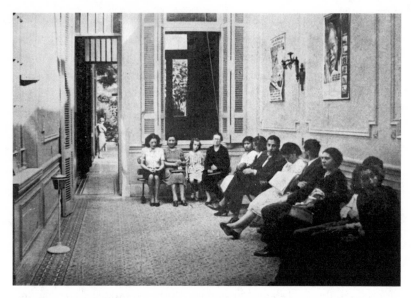

Waiting room at a neighborhood dispensary run by the Liga Argentina contra la Tuberculosis. (*Archivos Argentinos de Tisiología*, January–March 1940)

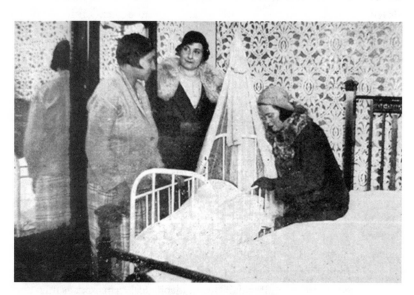

Neighborhood dispensary visitors at work in the homes of the poor. (*Archivos Argentinos de Tisiología*, October–December 1928)

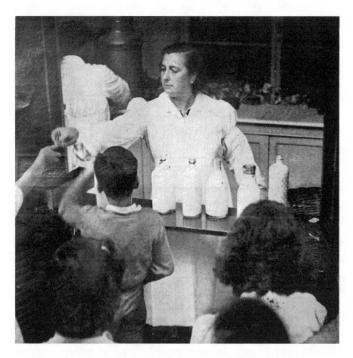

Children receiving food supplies at a neighborhood dispensary.
(Archivos Argentinos de Tisiología, October–December 1935)

doctor welcomes you with a smile on his face. My personal experience, taking my little son there weekly—who's now almost cured thanks to the dispensary treatments—has made me realize and understand the value of the great work carried out by the Liga.[87]

Rest Cures and Voluntary Exiles

In the 1870s Domingo Faustino Sarmiento, probably one of the most influential thinkers in nineteenth-century Argentina, stated that "the Córdoba foothills, like Switzerland in Europe, will soon become an indispensable complement to the cultivated, elegant life of Buenos Aires."[88] Sarmiento's prophecy was only partially realized, largely because the Buenos Aires elite continued to travel to Europe, but also because, starting in the 1880s, an increasing number of tuberculars began to visit the Córdoba foothills in order to undertake a rest cure. For some years the foothills were a common ground shared by tuberculars and wealthy families from Córdoba city on vacation. However, the *Manuel du voyageur: Baedeker de la république argentine* observed at the beginning of the century that "the marvels of the region are mainly enjoyed by people from Buenos Aires with chest diseases."[89] By the end of the 1920s some doctors deemed patients' presence "a chaotic, dangerous invasion of sick people" looking for "a promised land, an oasis to calm their fevers, strengthen their bodies and lighten their souls."[90]

Nonetheless, the Córdoba foothills were not the only place for rest cures. The seacoast; certain places in the provinces of Mendoza, La Rioja, and Jujuy; the open spaces of the Pampas; city suburbs; and even certain neighborhoods in Buenos Aires were deemed appropriate for the rest cure.[91] After all, the rest cure didn't require much infrastructure or luxury. It did call for cleanliness and a healthy diet. Rest cures combined outdoor living, medical supervision, and repose in what was thought to be a beneficial climate: cold, dry air for some; hot, dry air for others; warm, humid air for still others; or any combination of the above. Climatology, an active field of knowledge at the end of the nineteenth century, developed this logic.[92] By the beginning of the twentieth century, health care providers in these various climates were taking credit for successful treatments and, as might be expected, their failures were not publicized. Ultimately weather and geography were losing relevance in the rest therapies, further emphasizing the importance of repose and a good diet.[93] The question was particularly crucial to poor tuberculars. In 1909 Coni suggested that impoverished sick people "should seek a cure in the countryside, not far from the city where they live," in order to avoid the economic and emotional problems connected with moving to the mountains. This argument was still voiced and defended by highly respected lung specialists into the late thirties.[94]

Despite the reservations of hygienists and doctors, and regardless of the fact that most patients did not have access to the relatively luxurious rest cure, the Córdoba foothills were symbolically important to the sick, who for nearly half a century believed they would be cured in that healthy environment. People who could afford it traveled there, and those who could not dreamed of it. The importance of the foothills was not limited to the sick, however, as many considered spending a season in Córdoba as a preventive and restorative experience. In 1890, for example, this belief persuaded a young lawyer with early-stage tuberculosis to "travel to the foothills in order to follow carefully the recommendations in a book about the rest cure." Later, in the twenties, Tomás G., a bohemian young man from Buenos Aires with a very advanced case of tuberculosis, traveled to Córdoba "because he wanted to get cured." In 1940 Aron B., a self-employed worker who was only twenty years old, decided to take "a preventive trip, because [he was] afraid of developing tuberculosis," though he had not been diagnosed with the disease.[95] In any case, quite soon it was clear that for patients with early-stage tuberculosis the rest cure in the foothills could indeed have a significant impact. Not so for those with advanced cases of tuberculosis. For them, most of the time, the Córdoba experience was completely useless.

The celebration of the outdoors and its benefits in terms of health effected a transformation of much of the Córdoba foothills. By the beginning of the century a handful of "grand luxury" hotels were built to make "life [there] a prolongation of life in Buenos Aires," a place where the advantages of climate were accompanied by the refinements of civilization.[96] These fancy hotels were soon followed by varyingly equipped private and state-run sanatoriums, cheap hotels, improvised boardinghouses, houses with rooms for rent, and even shacks, all willing to take in the legions of tuberculars from Buenos Aires who kept coming until the 1950s.[97]

Private sanatoriums, so-called health station hotels, and clinics soon launched their own publicity campaigns. At the high end of these offerings the typical selling points were the quality of the care, the discipline, the comfort, transportation, recreation, music, availability of doctors and trained staff specialized in tuberculosis, and the benefits of the climate.[98] At the bottom, boardinghouses simply announced "the right hygienic environment required for the rest treatment," underlining the existence of "well-ventilated rooms and a good diet seasoned with fine oil and butter."[99] In addition to these alternatives there were other ventures, luxurious or not yet entirely in line with the basic tenets of rest cure, that sought only profit and were often accused of being focused on "making money from rather than treating tuberculosis."[100]

Given impetus by both locals and outsiders, places geared toward the rest cure came to populate the valleys of the Córdoba foothills, particularly the Valle de Punilla. Some people owned hotels and boardinghouses, others ran small stores, and still others, the majority, worked as cooks, laundresses, and staff members at the sanatoriums.[101] Most of the new residents came from Buenos Aires. Among them were tuberculars seeking the rest cure; doctors, themselves tuberculars, who wanted to improve their own health while continuing to work in their profession; and former tubercular patients who decided to stay, taking jobs that didn't require much physical effort or opening small businesses with the money obtained after selling what they had owned in Buenos Aires. In some cases, it was quite apparent that families were trying to avoid dealing with the uncomfortable presence of a tubercular relative still feared fragile. On occasions, these families even provided the sick with some amount of money to facilitate a certain degree of financial independence. This world is recalled by the lung specialist Santos Sarmiento, who worked as a doctor in the foothills for more than forty years. He states that 50 percent of the sick people who survived tuberculosis in Córdoba never went back to Buenos Aires. Delia G. agrees with this assessment. In the early forties she spent the summer at a camp run by the Casa de la Empleada at Cosquín, the town in the Valle de Punilla most affected by the tuberculosis phenomenon, and remembers that everyone who worked there, from the maids and drivers to the photographers and the cooks, was a former tubercular patient. Similarly, many staff members working at sanatoriums and boardinghouses were former tuberculars themselves who, besides being more sensitive to the patients' problems, were less afraid of contagion and familiar with the routines of the rest cure, such as taking someone's pulse and temperature, disinfecting rooms, and rubbing the patients' chest with balms. Since these job opportunities were limited, many former tubercular patients ended up living in poor conditions but stayed on in the hope that "Córdoba's magic" would keep them from relapsing.[102]

The rest cure at sanatoriums and boardinghouses in the foothills was an attempt to address widespread concern about tuberculosis as a public health issue. As a result of the growing antituberculosis discourse that fed fear of contagion and promoted an image of the sick as dangerous carriers of disease, concern about tuberculosis was growing at the beginning of the twentieth century. This discourse didn't encourage compulsory confinement but communicated much more subtle initiatives directed toward controlling the circulation of the tubercular. A rest cure meant choosing a voluntary system of internment: a tubercular patient sought recovery in the foothills, accepting that, from then on, his or her movements would be restricted in order to avoid passing the disease on to the healthy. This decision entailed a sort of self-exile in which the tubercular ceased to be a social threat and became a responsible, conscious, and largely self-controlled patient.

Exile in the Córdoba foothills meant not only a rest cure as inpatients at sanatoriums, but also the alternative of noninstitutionalized, unsupervised rest cures. Thanks to the supervision of doctors and nurses, sanatoriums taught patients to assimilate strict hygienic routines. Unsupervised cures depended on the tuberculars themselves, who were in charge of managing their treatment with greater autonomy. These patients would live at boardinghouses, hotels, and family houses, and periodically visit an antituberculosis dispensary or a doctor's office.

Internment at sanatoriums sought to make patients self-aware, and the routines there worked to transform the sick into systematically monitored children. In 1905 Coni noted that "in order to get cured, the sick must be enthusiastic and docilely follow good advice." Several decades later Juan José Vitón, a well-known lung specialist, depicted the sanatorium as a "school for the sick" where the physician was the great educator.[103] Not surprisingly, when entering a sanatorium a patient was forced to agree to the rules in writing and to accept the fact that every day at the sanatorium was meticulously planned in advance. The system privileged strict hygiene, diet, repose, a rigid schedule, programs and activities, and, above all, self-discipline.[104]

First and foremost, the hygienic cure was geared toward helping the patient incorporate certain daily habits that would allegedly restore health: punctilious personal hygiene, living in rooms with open doors both during the day and at night, taking plenty of fresh air, and using hand spittoons to avoid swallowing sputum or spitting it on the ground. The sick were in charge of filling out a daily personal record, what was called the observation bulletin. They were supposed to carefully record the variations in their cough, appetite, weight, and temperature. Patients also had to describe their state of mind, suggesting that the sanatorium endeavored not only to effect a physical recovery, but also to monitor "the cure of the soul," as Basia R. recalls.

By the end of the nineteenth century recommendations on diet for tuberculosis patients stressed that "they should eat not only to be satisfied, but fundamentally to rebuild their bodies." In fact, sanatoriums tended to overfeed patients. Patients regularly ate meals rich in fat, legumes, and carbohydrates. There was a fixation on eggs, cod liver oil, milk, and raw meat. Some diets included a little wine because of its nutritional value. Starting in the late twenties, though, sanatoriums stressed "refeeding, not overfeeding" the patient, acknowledging that a correct diet had very little to do with "eating until you burst."[105]

Finally, life at the sanatorium entailed regimented rest in beds, chairs located indoors, and chaise longues on roofed and open-air galleries, where patients could breathe fresh air. The goal was to provide a life without physical and intellectual fatigue. Initially, rest was considered a major source of restoration, so patients were encouraged to read simple books, play board games, listen to light music, and perhaps attend a lecture or see a movie. Daily life at the sanatorium was largely one of idleness, and by the beginning of the century this was being questioned. Now, depending on the specifics of a patient's case, rehabilitation included a "gradual exercise cure" and sometime later "the work cure." Both were meant to distract the sick and, fundamentally, to train patients for a productive future. Some tubercular patients began going for strolls, gardening, farming, bookbinding, making baskets, taking blood samples, and giving injections.[106]

The patient experience, then, was a voluntary banishment. In addition to allowing tuberculars to distance themselves from an urban life saturated with stigma, this self-imposed exile entailed, at least at the discursive level, a sort of subculture of isolation in which self-discipline, coercion, fear, and hope were entangled. As part of this context some doctors thought it advisable to group patients according to their "social status, intellectual level or profession" in an attempt to "alleviate withdrawal from the active life."[107] For this reason—and also because many sanatoriums were run by social, charitable, philanthropic, and corporate organizations—starting in the twenties there was no lack of internment institutions strictly for workers, army members, employees, university students, members of the Italian, Spanish, Japanese, and Jewish communities, public employees, priests, women, and children.[108]

People were free to enter and leave the sanatorium. Some people stayed for a few weeks, others for three or four months, and still others for a few years. Some patients suspended the rest cure because they couldn't tolerate it or because they had run out of money, or, in the case of rebellious patients, because they were expelled.[109] Others pretended to be sick even though they were practically cured; they stayed on at the sanatorium to avoid becoming highly suspect former tubercular patients in a world of supposedly healthy people. Among the cured patients, many decided to stay on "for the weather" in the foothills.[110] They wanted to regain strength, but they also believed their place was no longer in the city, among the healthy, but in the peaceful foothills, with their self-contained and voluntarily segregated life.

The Sanatorio Santa María was one of the most important sanatoriums in the country and probably the most decisive feature of the long-lasting association between the Córdoba foothills and supervised rest cure. Originally it was a private venture run by a doctor. By the beginning of the twentieth century, in a climate of serious economic problems, the sanatorium was bought by the state. Though some low- and middle-income people paid a small fee for special internment services, most were treated free of charge. Some were sent to the sanatorium by the usual way of professional referrals, that is, city doctors affiliated with neighborhood dispensaries or outpatient hospital wards who advised patients to seek a supervised rest cure. Others, a good many at certain times, got in thanks to recommendations from influential people.[111] In its first ten years the premises of the Sanatorio Santa María expanded considerably, and it had beds for eight hundred patients. In the following years this number climbed, reaching one thousand and, later, thirteen hundred patients. The sanatorium's large scale and certain features of its buildings were often criticized. Although the sanatorium included some features of the latest antituberculosis hospital architecture—for example, large windows and rounded corners to avoid the accumulation of dust—the premises consisted of a cluster of overly luxurious, expensive buildings several stories high with no elevators. The advantages of simple, inexpensive sanatoriums like some of those used in North America were ignored.[112]

For decades it was thought that tuberculosis patients simply did not get discharged from Sanatorio Santa María. The lung specialist Antonio Cetrángolo recalls the commotion among patients when one of them walked out of the sanatorium, cured.[113] There were several explanations for the sanatorium's poor performance. One blamed the patients themselves, who apparently failed to recover owing to their inability to incorporate discipline and the rest cure. A much more convincing explanation, quite widespread in the twenties and thirties, was that those admitted to the sanatorium had advanced cases of tuberculosis and benefited little from the rest cure. This was the view of many specialists. Rather than blaming the patients, they claimed that general practitioners didn't know how to diagnose the disease in its early stages and, what was worse, recommended rest cures for advanced cases.

Of the private institutions located in Cosquín, in the Valle de Punilla of the Córdoba foothills, Sanatorio Laënnec was probably the most expensive and sophisticated. It was founded in the 1920s by two doctors from Buenos Aires, one of whom had spent a season in a Swiss sanatorium, not as a doctor but as a patient. The sanatorium's clientele consisted of, according to Oscar F., the son of a nurse who worked there for over two decades, "tubercular patients with money, artists, night crawlers, and partygoers." The building's design was like that of the sanatoriums in the Alps. There was a section for men and a section for women, a capacity of 120 beds in single and double rooms equipped with metallic furniture and toilets. Along with permanent medical supervision, a service not found in most of these institutions, it offered first-class hotel services. In fact by the 1940s its cook was formerly *chef de cuisine* at the most distinguished hotel in Córdoba, and among its patrons were both wealthy people with tuberculosis and tourists looking for a healthy vacation in the foothills. The sanatorium had a pig farm, a dairy, a small apiary, and a stable with horses for riding. Known for a copious nursing staff, personalized examinations, and a strict admission policy that expelled patients if they didn't follow the rules,

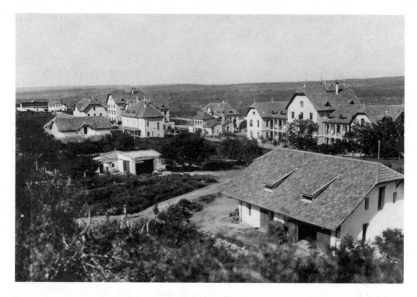

Panoramic view of the Sanatorio Santa María in the Córdoba foothills.
(Courtesy Eli Tedesco)

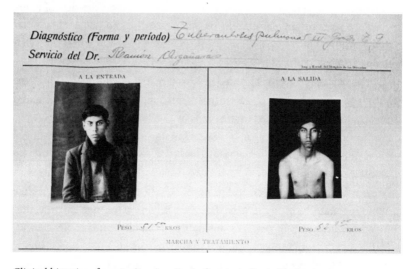

Clinical histories of sanatorium inpatients, Sanatorio Santa María, ca. 1920.
(Courtesy Eli Tedesco)

the place built a strong reputation over time. It also proved to be highly profitable: by the mid-1930s the two doctors who had founded it bought the land surrounding the sanatorium, which eventually they partitioned and sold, creating what would become one of the fanciest neighborhoods in Cosquín.

The sanatorium option had limited impact on the tubercular population. Very few could afford it, and the few sanatoriums that were free of charge couldn't take in all the applicants. Besides, by the late 1890s low-income people who dreamed of going to the Córdoba foothills were warned that such a trip might sink their families into poverty. In the early twentieth century these warnings were even more apparent, and the idea of supervised treatments for nonwealthy tuberculars in an institution far away from Buenos Aires had begun to decline. Instead, rest cures in affordable urban and suburban sanatoriums seemed on the way to becoming a more democratic choice.[114] Nevertheless, this never happened. The number of suburban sanatoriums never became significant, and the Córdoba enclaves remained the point of reference for those interested in a supervised rest cure.

One of the underlying aims of the sanatoriums was to radically transform the sick into hygienic, self-regulated citizens, capable of assimilating the rest cure's routines and rituals. Daily life at the sanatorium meant introspection and moderate reading and writing. The sick wrote about their health to their relatives and doctors. They corresponded with inpatients at neighboring sanatoriums, even with people, mostly of the opposite sex, whom they had never met: ads in magazines announced patients as well as healthy people interested in exchanging letters. Some patients even sent notes and stories to popular newspapers and magazines. A few wrote personal journals, chronicles, and novels.

One striking example of the achievements of supervised rest treatment and re-education was a magazine connected with the library at the Sanatorio Santa María. Originally a patients' initiative, but one that soon gained the support of doctors, the library was created in 1916. It started with some two hundred books, and within two years it had thirty-two hundred. Library members paid a small fee that authorized them, among other things, to elect an organizing committee that was discreetly supervised by the sanatorium's authorities. On the one hand, this initiative occurred at the same time as a vigorous movement to open public libraries in Buenos Aires neighborhoods. On the other, it reflected certain aspects of the rest cure, mainly its interest in re-educating the sick. By 1920 the library was endowed with a printing workshop where the magazine *Reflexiones* was published. In 1921 the subtitle was *Publicación Mensual de Arte, Ciencia y Literatura*—a monthly publication focused on the

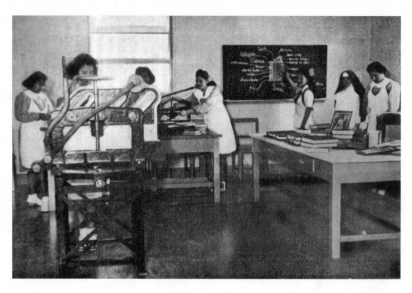

Sanatorium inpatients doing light manual work.
(*Archivos Argentinos de Tisiología*, January–March 1945)

arts, science, and literature. By the end of that year the name had changed
to *Publicación Mensual Editada por la Biblioteca Sarmiento, Dirigida, Admi-
nistrada y Confeccionada por los Enfermos en sus Talleres Propios de Reedu-
cación Profesional*, that is, a monthly publication edited by the Library Sarmiento, directed, managed, and produced by the sick working in professional
re-education workshops. The magazine was sold (for twenty cents) inside the
sanatorium only. It had ads for local pharmacies, private doctors, boardinghouses, hotels, and private sanatoriums, as well as for correspondence courses,
beverages, and clothing shops.

Men wrote most of the articles, which usually focused on the re-education
of the sick, life inside the sanatorium, and literary and emotional matters. The
re-education pieces were mainly informative and generally written by doctors
with occasional contributions by patients. The topics discussed included convalescent patients' reintegration into the work world, personal hygiene, rest
treatment routines, the negative effects of gambling and drinking on patients'
health, relationships between patients and doctors, and the social dimension
of tuberculosis. The articles that centered on life in the sanatorium reported
on patients' theater groups; lessons in arithmetic, spelling, and accounting;
picnics; parties in the countryside; and celebrations of national holidays and
labor day. Literary and personal articles included fragments of texts by famous
authors as well as stories and poems written by patients, which often explored

their inner worlds. Some articles praised the role played by the magazine, stating that "we humans need to communicate our joy, sadness, and pain, especially because as patients we live an isolated life; for us, the expressions, memories, and recollections of those who are no longer with us come during the nostalgic hours we spend reading, talking, writing."[115] Other articles took issue with what were labeled literary excesses. They criticized the "poor and plain writing" of those who "crave their lovers and let out the cries of the soul," those who were "moved to tears by the pain of others, repeating amorphous literature," those who, out of piety, "advised others what to do when dealing with a difficult love."[116] Although there was little talk of politics in *Reflexiones*, occasional reference was made to articles published in the socialist newspaper *La Vanguardia*, to the nurses' and sanatorium workers' union and its initiatives, and to the publications of the Liga Roja contra la Tuberculosis, suggesting the existence of some leftist sympathy among those who were editing the magazine.

The regimented cure was aimed at creating a sort of self-sufficient bubble or enclave. This led to a strong feeling of isolation that the sick tried to alleviate in various ways. Enrique T. remembers the importance of the "godmothers" and "spiritual girlfriends" with whom patients corresponded. In their letters, they didn't speak of health, but of aspirations and "the stuff of life. I greatly looked forward to receiving those letters. I wanted to receive answers to what I had written." Patients made use of these bridges to the outside world, accepting that their own lives existed only in the realm of voluntary exile. An article written by a patient in *Reflexiones* keenly condenses the author's heightened sense of self-awareness: "And I fled the world I loathed already, the people who feared me, and I was admitted to this sanatorium not in order to get cured—that would be like asking the sun to stop shining—but to never again see that merciless life that knocked me down, to learn to live with my pain until death tears me off the surface of the earth."[117]

UNSUPERVISED REST CURES

The foothills were also a place where tuberculars themselves, as opposed to an institution, could administer their time and recovery. Patients rented rooms in family homes and in houses that had been transformed into boardinghouses or into improvised clinics. A character in *El balcón hacia la muerte* (which translates to "a balcony overlooking death"), a partially autobiographical novel by Ulises Petit de Murat, is a man from Buenos Aires who makes his living as a hairdresser for patients in boardinghouses and sanatoriums. Tired of doctors, he decides to leave the big city and move, along with his family, to the

Córdoba foothills in order to improve his health by means of alternative thera-pies, herbs, balms, and hearty stews.[118] He is one of the many tuberculars to choose "the free, unsupervised cure," a common practice in Europe and the United States. Unlike the hairdresser in the novel, though, most of the people who went to the foothills looking for an unsupervised cure wanted to receive treatments provided by professional medical practitioners. Alberto T. and his family arrived in the foothills immediately after his father was diagnosed with tuberculosis; they sold everything they had in Buenos Aires, traveled by train to Córdoba, and rented a room with a kitchen and bathroom in Cosquín. While the mother worked at a hotel, the father regularly visited the antituber-culosis dispensary. A similar story is told by Gerardo B. When he found out his wife was sick, he closed his shop in Buenos Aires and moved to Cosquín. There, they bought a small house and undertook a free cure. But it wasn't working, and Gerardo's wife was admitted to the Hospital Sanatorio Domingo Funes, a women's sanatorium, where she died two years later.

Based on herbs and balms or professional medicine or a combination of the two, free cures required a level of self-discipline that not everybody had. In 1899 *La Semana Médica* commented, concernedly, that the repose supposedly sought by tuberculars who had come to the foothills for the summer usually turned into "a shindig of sick people dancing, smoking, drinking until dawn in after-hours pubs and . . . [followed] the next morning with long and dan-gerous horseback rides."[119] By the beginning of the century, when some health stations were becoming towns and even small cities in which, consequently, the pace of daily life was changing, Francisco Súnico, a doctor who wrote a meticulous study of the impact of tuberculosis on the Córdoba foothills, warned of the existence of a "chaotic social life." According to him, "Local women acquiesced extremely easily to the sexual petitions of the sick," and "sex, sensuality, and the vices of people from Buenos Aires" had reached the foothills. In fact, in a study in 1919 based on interviews with 232 tuberculars practicing unsupervised cure, only 16 said they were actually keeping up with its basic rules. Two decades later, when Amílcar F. was trying to recover his health in a Cosquín sanatorium, the social environment of the unsupervised cures was quite similar, and his memory is filled with images of what he calls "unhealthy disorder where nobody controls or disciplines the sick."

Despite criticism, the foothills were considered a laudable possibility. Here, relative isolation and exclusion were not compulsively demanded of patients by law in the name of public health, but were the result of their own decision. Two texts illustrate this point of view. One of them focused on the so-called sanitary village, an imaginary, almost utopian setting meant to guide patients who were trying to decide among the antituberculosis initiatives encouraged by the state. The other account consisted of a sort of militant narrative about the experience of tuberculars pursuing a rest cure in a boardinghouse in Cosquín. In both cases the Córdoba enclave appears as the place where very specific communities of people with tuberculosis are supposed to find effective assistance, emotional support, and a clear agenda of what tuberculars could and couldn't do.

The sanitary village expresses the possibility of retreating to the foothills with one's family. In an article published in 1921 in *Reflexiones*, Genaro Sisto, a doctor at the Sanatorio Santa María, imagined "a small settlement, just 300 or 400 little houses with two, three or four ample rooms each. [The houses would be] well ventilated, full of sunlight and surrounded by forest. . . . [They would be] very simple, easy to clean, cheerful, comfortable . . . and in keeping with the hygienic code." Tuberculars and their families would live in these "inexpensive homes." From Sisto's point of view, family warmth would replace the "unhelpful" environment of hospital wards and sanatoriums, and the sick would be attended to by their relatives. Full of "dedication and love," this family environment would provide an "antituberculosis education" that would in the end prevent "passing the disease on due to the patient's carelessness." Medical supervision would rule over the village, which would have a solarium, private doctors' offices, disinfection equipment, a farm, a school, gardens, a gym, a library, and common spaces for leisure and conversation.[120]

The sanitary village would attract low-income people with early-stage tuberculosis, those who could still be helped by the rest cure. According to Sisto, the cost would be close to that of a sanatorium or a hospital, but the benefits much greater: it would not be necessary to pay "mercenary nurses," and, importantly, it would optimize the rest cure by providing the "moral tranquility" that comes with having family close by. The sanitary village represented a community of convalescent patients that did not break up the family, an unfortunate side effect of most rest cures.

The premise of the sanitary village was that tuberculosis needn't be fatal. The challenge was to make the voluntary retreat happen at the right time, so it would not be seen as a last resort. The idea of the sanitary village could be read as one of the many evidences of the low-income tubercular in a process of transformation into a sick person who is conscious of both the threat he or she imposed as an agent of contagion as well as the self-imposed boundaries of their life. The peculiarity of the sanitary village lies in its communal nature. The goal, wrote Sisto, was to achieve "a life in common, gratifying and hygienic," though austere and as isolated from the outside world as possible.

However, the village was only a proposition. The only actual occurence that resembled it was realized by the sick people who moved to the foothills with their families and rented rooms or, if they could afford it, bought single-family homes in Cosquín and surrounding towns. These people survived on strictly limited resources, eating whatever food they could obtain, occasionally visiting dispensaries or a doctor's office, all in the—indeed—pure air and healthy climate of the foothills.

If the sanitary village epitomizes the free rest cure in the company of one's family, the boardinghouses and inexpensive hotels were the setting for the individual exile in the foothills. This theme appears in *El balcón hacia la muerte* by Petit de Murat, *Ester Primavera* by Roberto Arlt, and *Boquitas pintadas* by Manuel Puig, probably the best explorations in Argentine literature of the passions and daily habits of the rest cure in the foothills.[121] In no way didactic, these narratives have very little in common with *Cosquín: Falsedad y verdad*, by Marcelo Castelli, published in 1954. *Cosquín: Falsedad y verdad* reads as an exhaustive list of what a person with tuberculosis must do to control his or her disease and stop being a threat to society. Castelli was once a medical school student. He was diagnosed with tuberculosis and immediately decided to undertake a rest cure in the Córdoba foothills. Later, he became a resident of Cosquín and married a woman with tuberculosis, with whom he had two daughters. The couple managed to bring their disease under control, and, once cured, they made a living running a boardinghouse for people with tuberculosis.

Cosquín: Falsedad y verdad offers a detailed, laudatory, even romanticized account of the world of the boardinghouse. The characters are tuberculars conversing about the disease. Though not a medical doctor, one of them skillfully articulates the biomedical discourse on tuberculosis. By quoting revered lung specialists, this boardinghouse resident recommends that his peers rigorously follow the catalog of daily habits indicated by the rest cure; he informs them about the breakthroughs in medical treatments for tuberculosis and educates them on all sorts of issues regarding what he judges to be disposable and nonscientific cures.[122] The enlightened tubercular, undoubtedly the kind of person Castelli would have wanted to be, speaks didactically to the other residents and lectures his potential readers as potential sick people and weakened city dwellers. In the book, vulnerable urbanites are repeatedly invited to "get out of the city and come to the foothills before it's too late." They should "dare to live the way we live here, getting plenty of rest and eating a healthy diet, breathing this pure golden air."[123] To the upset tubercular who has been "banished from society, the bosom of the family, and the joy of friends," the enlightened tubercular offers a warm community of voluntary exiles. Supposedly everyone is equal in this community: having tuberculosis apparently allows people to disregard their particular pasts. In the foothills, everybody enjoys the benefits of good weather, everybody is seeking rest, everybody becomes part of the meticulous plan for daily moral re-education. This re-education is aimed at preventing relapses, reforming the sick, and turning them into hygienic individuals capable of self-regulating and, crucially, into people who refuse to be agents of hazardous contagion. The goal is to remodel the sick person's soul, to prepare the ground to create a new self out of suffering from tuberculosis. The idea is to mold the former tuberculosis patient into a person who has learned to control the disease, which may have left forever or may be lurking and reappear when least expected. Here, the relative geographical isolation of the foothills merged with an educational effort focused on self-control.

Castelli's pedagogical account describes the crucial features of the ideal tubercular boardinghouse resident and patient, the one who has managed to forge a new identity. This is the tubercular "who has started over again; who, with a certain measure of sacrifice, intelligence and willpower, has begun a meaningful life in the foothills." Castelli also writes that "the sick person must muster courage, discipline, obedience, and sacrifice; he must know that today, tomorrow, and his entire life and salvation depend on the kind of caring he gives for his body." He advises "the tubercular to be conscious that he does not belong to society; he must, instead, belong to his body and to his disease; he must devote himself to his body, and follow the rules of good sense and moderation."[124]

Castelli's praises for and almost militant devotion to a pragmatic exile in the Córdoba foothills leads him to call boardinghouses and sanatoriums second homes. This depiction contrasts with the images displayed in the works of Thomas Mann, Camilo José Cela, and Petit de Murat, in which, in the geography of voluntary exclusion, leisure is portrayed as vice. In these novels, the rest cure brings forth a slow-moving world in which the aspiration to health dissolves into an immense sea of death. Gradually, the tubercular surrenders to this self-disciplined life in exile, marked by the blurry passage of the disease. In Castelli's work, on the contrary, life at the rest cure retreat is good enough, and there's no reason to long for anything else. It's a microcosm with its own morals, rules, and habits in which one can forget the outside world.

Removed from the world, the rest cure enclave is organized around disease. This scenario allows Castelli to explore physiology, aesthetics, ethics, politics, love, friendship, time, and, naturally, life and death. In his sentimental narrative Castelli depicts the boardinghouse as a community of sick people with the ability to provide both assistance and emotional support to one another. The tubercular patients have chosen to live in exile and have no intention of leaving. They are very different from Hans Castorp, the main character of Mann's *The Magic Mountain*. Castorp is a young engineer from Hamburg who is visiting his cousin at a sanatorium in Davos, Switzerland. While there, he gets lost in the overwhelming and omnipotent passing of time on the mountain, loses connection with outside life, and grows convinced that he too should live in the sanatorium bubble. In the end, he realizes that real life lies far from the mountain, "down the mountain," where freedom reigns in a world of uncertainties and dangers that deserve to be lived. Castelli's tuberculars, meanwhile, have bought one-way tickets. After leaving everything behind in the city, they find, in the foothills, the "magic casket" that will finally "bring life back."[125] Castelli's patients have accepted their exclusion; they don't waste their time questioning a culture that has given their lives new meaning. They're looking for a cure, but they know they must be banished because they are contagious. By choosing this sort of ostracism or exile, they cease to be a threat to society.

Castelli's world pretends to be an autonomous place of healing where the sick are aware of their obligations. These are self-conscious, disciplined tuberculars with an identity marked by civic and medical responsibilities aimed at answering to the urgency of avoiding contagion. Inpatients at sanatoriums, where rest therapy routines were usually supervised by professionals, were also encouraged to be self-aware. But Castelli's boardinghouse tuberculars were solely responsible for complying with the rest cure's regime. Hence, people with tuberculosis engaged in an unsupervised rest cure at boardinghouses—not sanatorium inpatients—were, according to Castelli, the culmination of the hygienic re-education of the tubercular sick.

In *Cosquín: Falsedad y verdad*, the rest cure and the voluntary banishment it requires seem like a fairly affordable option. However, by the late 1940s and early 1950s, when the author wrote and published the book, it was already becoming apparent that the complex world that had emerged in the last third of the nineteenth century around antituberculosis rest cures in the foothills was beginning to wane. In less than a decade, the advent of antibiotics, which were consumed by an increasing number of people with tuberculosis, challenged the economy and the society created around the rest cure. The sanatoriums and boardinghouses in the Córdoba foothills, like those in the Alps, started losing their clientele. Very soon these places had to choose between going out of business or becoming hotels. This is probably why, along with a narrative focused on the unrivaled advantages of Cosquín in terms of weather, geography, and social environment, Castelli advances a complementary notion: restorative, restful vacations for the healthy. And he stresses the fact that healthy people needn't fear contagion, since they can share the foothills with sick or formerly sick people who have learned to manage their disease and have become hygienic citizens.[126]

Castelli's book captures this period of transition at the Córdoba tuberculosis enclaves. It was in this era that Juan Domingo Perón's first administration began to encourage tourism on a mass scale, helping labor unions and civic and private associations transform former sanatoriums and boardinghouses into tourism hotels for their constituencies.[127] By the early 1960s the city of Cosquín began to promote itself as an attractive mountain resort with plenty of fresh air. Over the next few years, thanks to the efforts of residents, doctors, sick people, and former patients who were active in some twenty civic organizations, it emerged as the national capital of folk music. Folk music was certainly a way to rid the area of the stigma of tuberculosis. By the end of the 1960s, when the connection between folk music and Cosquín was firmly established, Puig adopted this setting to portray, once again, the world of tuberculosis. But his *Boquitas pintadas*, which combines features of the experimental novel with pop narrative, kitsch, and intentional tackiness, has very little in common with the pedagogical, picturesque, and sentimental account that, only fifteen years earlier, Castelli offered in his *Cosquín: Falsedad y Verdad*.

CHAPTER THREE

Unruly and Well-Adjusted Patients

Regardless of economic status, people with tuberculosis could either accept their diagnosis with resignation or choose to fight for a cure. If the tubercular wasn't overly pessimistic, therapy often began at home and entailed self-medication; visits to the pharmacist; and treatments offered by professional doctors at hospitals, clinics, and neighborhood medical wards. Treatment might also include visiting healers, herbalists, or quacks. There was no pre-established course of action: every person with tuberculosis did it his or her own way, and every instance meant very different experiences. However, as the twentieth century progressed, more and more people chose to visit doctors, though the health care infrastructure was never able to meet the ever-increasing demand. At the institutions run by professional doctors, the tubercular became a patient and circulated in a sphere where the doctor tried to control everything. An uneven relationship developed in which the person with tuberculosis was decidedly subordinated to the medical professional.

There is abundant evidence between the 1880s and the 1950s of this unequal relationship and of how subordination was perceived and reinforced by medical doctors. By the end of the 1920s, for instance, a book entitled *Lo que todo tuberculoso debe saber*, written by Juan José Vitón, a professor at the Universidad de Buenos Aires Medical School, laid out the roles of doctor and patient: "Each fact must be analyzed from a physiological point of view, and the patient must confide everything he observes to his doctor—his *baquiano* [specialist] and guide. The sick person must never jump into the muddy waters of interpretation; he must trust his doctor completely. Indeed, his doctor is the true guide in this journey where the 'pilgrim of health' cannot be trusted to identify the proper roads, as he might ignore the true and exact interpretations of what he sees, feels, or thinks is happening." Later in the book Vitón offers a word of advice: "To become healthy, the sick person must contribute to organizing a 'fight plan' by submitting unconditionally to the orders of the one in charge, whose every suggestion must be seen as an obligation. The guide is, thus, also a dictator, though a generous and kind one, since all he wants for himself is to triumph by curing his patient."[1]

This rigid division of roles was part of a broader picture that, well into the forties, was laden with uncertainties about biomedical treatments for tuberculosis. The uncertainty is more than apparent in Ulises Petit de Murat's *El balcón hacia la muerte*. At the doctor's office, in response to the doctor's recommendation of a specific therapy, the patient cynically says, "Who will demonstrate the lack of usefulness of what you're giving me?"[2] This sense of uncertainty also appears in the recollections of Elma M., who grew up in a boardinghouse for tubercular patients in the Córdoba foothills: "Many times the doctors were not sure if a remedy could actually cure us; they tested the remedies on the sick people who had been abandoned by their families. They used them as guinea pigs." Nevertheless, some doctors not only assumed these uncertainties, but also warned about their sociocultural effects. In the 1940s the lung specialist Antonio Cetrángolo spoke of "fooling the person with tuberculosis." He estimated that "every five years, what I call the tide phenomenon takes place—that is, the irruption of a new medication that, with the aid of the press, stirs up hope but only for a little while."[3]

In this context, every tuberculosis treatment—from tonics, serums, vaccines, and surgery to rest, good diet, and fresh air—was part of an uneasy scenario involving doctors' natural inclination to offer patients solutions, explanations of how the recommended therapies had won public favor, and the enduring hope of those suffering from the disease. Patients' reactions varied greatly, from adaptation to acceptance, resignation, and protest. This tangle of reactions and perspectives was particularly evident at sanatoriums and hospitals. Some patients in these institutions tried to follow the doctor's advice as closely as possible. Others attempted to devise alternative therapeutical methods, resisted treatments they felt were not trustworthy, rejected those that went against what they perceived to be their individual liberties, and demanded the right to try treatments that hadn't been approved by doctors or health authorities.

Though their choices and agency were certainly limited, some patients were able to negotiate, confront, and engage in subtle battles with the medical profession. Their strategies included abandoning treatment, devising schemes to accelerate or delay their internment in a hospital or sanatorium, and writing letters filled with petitions.[4] There were occasional collective protests, but most of the time they were lodged by individuals. Unlike the sick workers who hid their disease for fear of getting fired, inpatients had little to lose. In fact, the hospitalized patients' willingness to participate in collective action inspired a tuberculosis specialist to speak of a certain "gang spirit." These patients were capable of negotiating with and confronting doctors and managers of health care facilities; they shared their demands and often ended up organizing patients' coordinating committees that lasted for some time. Protest usually started as petitions addressed to the doctor in charge of the ward; if the request was denied, the claim was sent to the hospital's director. On occasion verbal petitions were reinforced by public protests or by lobbying the offices of congressmen and ministers of the national government.[5]

Generally, collective protests and individual requests involved similar issues: the question of food and order at inpatient institutions and the right to receive certain treatments. Collective protests at the hospitals didn't go unnoticed by the press. The potential popularity of this sort of story was obvious, and each media outlet sought the tone and the topics most suited to its agenda. The positions of the newspapers and magazines covering the conflicts tended to stress not only their compassion and support for the patients, but also issues such as individual rights in the broader context of social reform and enhanced notions of social citizenship. Interestingly, media coverage was largely the result of patients themselves methodically supplying firsthand information about the conflicts. The information was included in letters and notes signed by individuals, groups of patients, or patients' coordinating committees. Indeed, the media's sources were often reports written by patients who had been journalists before being admitted to the hospital or former patients who had spent some time at a hospital or sanatorium and now worked for a newspaper or magazine. Regardless of the source, once these stories were published the patients' demands entered the public realm.

The Food Question

At the hospitals Tornú and Muñiz (in Buenos Aires), as well as at the Sanatorio Santa María (in Cosquín in the Córdoba foothills), petitions related to food started appearing early in the twentieth century. In 1920, for instance, a letter signed by hundreds of patients at the Sanatorio Santa María was addressed to the minister of international and religious affairs, whose jurisdiction included regional hospitals, asylums, and sanatoriums. The letter stated that "medical science indicates that the recovery of tubercular patients and their useful integration into society depend on a regime of healthy, plentiful nourishment; however, at this sanatorium the food available leaves much to be desired: it's bad, insufficient, and indigestible." Ten years later, in 1930, five hundred patients at the same sanatorium left their wards to protest in front of a director's office, shouting, "We're starving to death," and "We want to eat." They claimed food was scarce, bad, and harmful to the body, despite the "veritable army of employees working in the kitchen, the abundant resources, and the availability of quality food." In 1934 the newspaper *La Montaña*, published in Cosquín, reported that "patients lack proper nourishment," and the "petitions, hunger strikes, and press campaigns supported by reporters and very renowned journalists have been useless."[6]

Inpatients often received packages of food from their families or money to buy food from local grocers in order to, as some put it, avoid hunger. In their protests the patients described the typical menu in language that stressed the meagerness of the food at the internment facilities as opposed to the benefits such institutions were supposed to provide: "For lunch, hot soup and hard bread; flour cooked in hot water with no salt, full of dust and weevils; overcooked meat. For dinner, hot water soup with pieces of raw cabbage, poorly cooked, hard broad beans, tough and poorly stewed donkey meat." Fifteen years later, in 1934, another petition called the vegetable stew a "repugnant hodgepodge," the *puchero*, or meat stew, an "amorphous mass," the bread "scarce and hard," and milk and beefsteaks as "forever absent." Patients were even more indignant when they corroborated that "doctors and nuns take the best food from the pantry."[7]

In response to this diet, some patients threatened not to eat or to eat as little as possible. In the early 1920s such pressure gained them access to the daily food inspection. By then, a report written by a specialist seemed to endorse the "new science of nutrition" and indicated that the problem was not a lack of resources, but the need for a personalized diet designed for each patient according to his or her sex, weight, and size. However, it was impossible to put this idea into practice, first, because personalized diets in a kitchen that prepared more than one thousand meals several times a day—as the kitchen at the Sanatorio Santa María did—required a sophisticated logistical organization. But this scale of operation underlined other problems as well: the total number of patients was just over six hundred, but the kitchen was preparing one thousand meals, many more than were necessary. This was because it not only fed an enormous auxiliary staff but also allowed some of the employees to take food home. Two scenes were not unusual: employees leaving the sanatorium with a "little bag of food" under their arms, and patients just "picking at" the food on their plates. In a tone both critical and ironic, the socialist newspaper *La Vanguardia*, published in Buenos Aires, pointed out in March 1924 that "at the Sanatorio Santa María the patient who doesn't eat soup is waiting for stew, and the one who doesn't eat stew is saving room for veal parmesan." Both scenes reveal that there was no lack of resources, but rather the absence—dating from the 1910s—of a well-defined budget that led to an ineffective use of available funds. By the end of the 1920s the sanatorium administration made an effort to rationalize expenses, a policy that caused patients to protest once again against what they perceived as a new period of food shortages.[8]

Sometimes problems at the sanatoriums were bound up with administrative issues or provincial politics. In May 1922 a patients' strike not only resulted in an improvement in the food situation but also established that former patients would have priority when it came to filling vacancies on the health-care staffs, a demand in keeping with what was then called the work cure, a way of helping patients on their way to recovery to reinsert themselves in the work world. The patients' triumph became an opportunity for the sanatorium's director to consolidate his power. He decided to replace nurses active in the union with recovered or nearly recovered patients. The strategy worked well: the director won the support of the patients and exasperated the unionized staff. It also seriously affected the quality of health care that required trained and skillful nursing personnel. A few months later, in early October 1922, employees of the union of national public hospitals and asylums went on strike. At the Sanatorio Santa María the conflict was followed by the dismissal of 130 workers. The director said this measure was owing to cuts in the budget, even though the institution's massive hiring policy had caused some newspapers and magazines to say, ironically, "Pretty soon the sanatorium will have more staff members than patients." The union argued that the dismissals had to take seniority into account. Within a few weeks the conflict had evolved into a totally politicized issue. In the end, it became clear that what really mattered was the fact that the director hired new staff members as political favors. Indeed, this was part of a strategy designed by the Unión Cívica Radical, a major political party, to gain political control of the district. As an electoral stratagem, this wasn't particularly original. It revealed how health institutions could be useful to local, clientelistic politics. The Partido Demócrata de Córdoba vehemently denounced the move, stating that the sanatorium was being used to "transform the province of Córdoba into a bastion of the Unión Cívica Radical." There was some truth to this assertion, since the *radicales* in charge of the operation (the director of the sanatorium and his secretary, a former congressional candidate), were doing everything possible to win easy votes by offering jobs in the public sector—those of the recently hired sanatorium employees—while getting rid of workers in the union movement.[9]

A group of patients expressed their sympathy with the fired workers by refusing to eat. Some did so out of a sense of social justice and others because they were starting to feel the undesired effects of an untrained nursing staff. *La Vanguardia*, which had enthusiastically covered the conflict and supported the union, reported that "while the scabs are overwhelmed by the weight of their work, the patients . . . whose moral and physical state is getting worse . . . protest and scream that they don't want these new nurses, and refuse to eat until the competent staff returns, that is, the striking workers."

By the end of 1922 it was evident that the Unión Cívica Radical's political apparatus had managed to build a strong base of support among patients, who could, after all, become voters. Indeed, the party's efforts in this direction began in the first months of 1922 and bore fruit the following year. Two specific examples illustrate the dynamic between patients, on the one hand, and the party and the sanatorium's director, on the other. One April day the director invited eighty patients to the party celebrating the opening of the local Unión Cívica Radical headquarters, an occasion on which drinks, food, and fun abounded. On the way to the party, though, the patients had to stop by the local registrar's office to officially change their addresses so they would be eligible to vote in local elections. In early August, in an attempt to exchange political loyalties for amusement and pleasure—two scarce resources at the sanatorium—the director allowed a group of female patients and male nurses to go to Cosquín on an outing. By the last week of October an observer of the conflict reported that most patients didn't support the dismissed workers anymore, not only because of the special favors granted them by the director, but also because of the unmistakable improvements in the food served, thanks to special funds allocated by the national government, which was in the hands of the Unión Cívica Radical.[10]

Doctors, too, discussed the issue of food and, more generally, the nutrition of the tubercular inpatients. Some of them insisted that "the food is great" and maintained that the patients' complaints were "political conspiracies." Others pointed out that "for those who are not millionaires, . . . food—a crucial component of the sanatorium rest cure—has been nothing but a solemn mystification." The memoirs of the tuberculosis specialist Cetrángolo, who, in the 1920s, was in charge of one of the wards at the Sanatorio Santa María, offer a balanced perspective of these contradictory explanations and interpretations. In his book he acknowledges that the food was really bad during some periods and had probably caused intestinal problems in hundreds of tubercular patients. But he also states that in the early forties, when he wrote his memoirs, the notion of the ideal antituberculosis diet was no longer based on recommending that the patient "eat good beefsteaks," formerly a firm, well-established belief among both doctors and people with tuberculosis.[11]

In the life of tubercular inpatients the issue of food unquestionably went beyond the ingestion of nutrients. Except at critical moments, the diet for inpatients was largely similar to the diet of nontubercular workers and employees, and most patients were of those social backgrounds. Therefore, it is difficult to explain the dynamic of patients' demands as a result of the quantity and quality of the available food. Furthermore, similar demands were made at the private sanatoriums, where the patients received a great deal of attention and a diet comparable to that of luxury hotels. In a broad sense, then, the problem seems to have been related to the very experience of being an inpatient. Imposed rest turned the food issue into a way to express the patients' personal drama. In the world of internment, with so many routines and so much spare time, many patients experienced intense loneliness and longing for the world outside, as well as enduring daily struggles with the staff and burning anxiety about recovery. One witness of a food conflict added to these reasons the "arrogance of the inpatient who thinks he's the owner of the place and wants to give orders, change the rules, and even threaten."[12]

In addition to tedious routines and alleged arrogance, the inpatients' perception of the rights they had already acquired was a relevant factor in these conflicts. On the one hand, tuberculars spoke as responsible patients of the importance of strengthening their bodies by closely heeding the recommendations of doctors: among them, a diet meant "to fatten themselves up" or the generalized belief that, when it came to the rest cure, "the true medicine is the restaurant and the pantry." On the other hand, patients demanded that the sanatorium provide them with a kind of service that would help them regain their lost health, a quality of service they thought they weren't getting owing to the incompetence, negligence, and arbitrariness of the hospital's administrators. In any case, according to the memories of staff members, doctors, and patients, the hunger strikes did not seem to have gone very far, despite the dramatic and threatening language they employed. Urbano C., who worked at the Sanatorio Santa María in the 1940s and witnessed many of these conflicts, recalls that "patients were on strike, but they ate anyway. What they didn't eat was the soup, [which] they often threw down the stairs and out the windows.

The truth is that they knew that, despite all that, food was still coming to the wards. And patients would always have their way and get something to eat. The hunger strike was not really a strike; it was staged for effect." As a strategy, it seems to have tried to underline the absurdity of the need to rely on such measures precisely at an institution whose treatments were largely based on the benefits of good diet.

The Question of Order

At hospitals and particularly at sanatoriums the question of order was crucial. In the early 1920s some tubercular patients spoke of the Sanatorio Santa María as a "mansion of horrors" and "a place of violation and arbitrariness" that by no means met the basic requisites of an "institution of health."[13] Ten years later *La Montaña* condemned frequent military actions at the establishment, where "bribes and favoritism prevail, as well as other things that have transformed [the sanatorium] into a campaign tent. It's like a model prison, or a lazaretto where dangerous people are set apart."[14]

The complaints were not untimely, considering that the sanatorium authorities had recently reacted to tubercular patients' protests with measures that ranged from subtle punishment to overt police intervention. Common practices included retaining patients' personal mail, controlling communication between patients in different wards, refusing to hear petitions and complaints, and prohibiting visits to the library. Patients were forbidden to go to parties or go out for a ride, and they were forced to stay in bed and deprived of dessert. Occasionally, according to a report published in *La Voz del Interior*, a Córdoba city newspaper, the authorities also used corporal punishment.[15]

At times, the arbitrariness frequently denounced by patients was related to religion. Inpatients at the hospitals in Buenos Aires and at the Sanatorio Santa María refused to exchange their atheist convictions for gentler care from the Sisters of Charity, whose power in those institutions was diminishing but still present. They protested when the nuns attempted to oblige them to pray, get married in a religious ceremony, or vote for candidates close to the Church.[16] Their claims against such actions included letters to newspapers, which cited their right to use the hospital unconditionally. On occasion some of the patients involved in protests were eventually expelled from the hospital, which is why *Idea Hospitalaria*, the hospital workers' newspaper, spoke of a "religious dictatorship."[17] Undoubtedly, these conflicts were another chapter in the long struggle for the patient's soul, one in which the traditional power of the Sisters of Charity clashed with the efforts of many doctors and political sectors to run the hospital's daily operations without depending on nuns and relying instead on professional, secular nurses, both men and women.

Rape occurred at sanatoriums and hospitals. Sexual intercourse between tuberculars and staff members was a fact of life at inpatient institutions; after all, each party had plenty of reasons to be interested in these encounters, from pleasure to obtaining better care. Rape, however, was a different matter. When forced sex ended in pregnancy, the veil of secrecy was swept away and the issue often became public. In 1920, for example, a patient was locked in a room at the Sanatorio Santa María because, according to some doctors, she had gone insane. The patients' version was different; they claimed she was locked away to hide her pregnancy. The woman was finally expelled from the sanatorium, and one of her relatives reported that the director was responsible for the whole affair, including the pregnancy.[18]

Hospital authorities deployed a series of strategies in response to the massive protests: one entailed stigmatizing the patients involved, often by means of a xenophobic discourse. In the early 1920s a sanatorium's administrators stated that some patients' demands were orchestrated by foreigners, particularly Russians or Spaniards, two national groups that, among the many stereotypes that surrounded them, were recurrently associated with Bolshevism and anarchism, respectively. The tubercular patients denied this publicly, pointing out that the members of the patients' coordinating commission were "all Argentines, with only one Englishman." In 1924 a prestigious tuberculosis specialist suggested that, in order to avoid overpopulating the hospitals, Argentine tubercular patients should have priority. In a collective letter the inmates replied that "though we are not doctors, we are, unfortunately, sick, and we know enough to say that [such a measure] would only feed the fire." In another letter, a very detailed one which articulated a history of the conflict, the patients stated that clashes with the hospitals' "internal police" worsened after "some inmates were insulted" when staff used in a highly pejorative way the term *gallegos* to refer to Spanish immigrants. This time it was not the stereotype of Spaniards as anarchists but the belief, present in some medical circles, that the region of Galicia, in Spain, was ridding itself of tuberculars or people predisposed to tuberculosis by sending massive numbers of them to Argentina.[19]

Another classic way of stigmatizing was by calling the protesting patients extremists, radicals, or revolutionaries. In 1920 a journalist covering a conflictive week at the Sanatorio Santa María asked one of its leaders about her political views. The woman curtly replied, "I've been labeled a revolutionary, but I'm a liberal, a follower of our founding fathers Sarmiento, Mitre, Rivadavia, and

Alberdi."[20] Two years later the authorities were warned about "committing the cowardly mistake of considering some poor hungry people with tuberculosis bandits." The comparison was not irrelevant considering the troubled political scene in 1922, when confrontations in faraway Patagonia between rural sheep ranch workers and the military were making headlines in the national press. In any case, it was common for the authorities to use terms like "politically harmful elements" or "tubercular patients with socialist ideas who scream phrases like 'long live anarchy!'" In at least one public statement, the inpatients denied they had an organized socialist group. However, *La Vanguardia*'s careful coverage of several sanatorium conflicts, and the existence in Cosquín of the Liga Roja contra la Tuberculosis, suggest a close relation between some inpatients and local socialist and anarchist groups.[21] In the late 1930s it was said that many conflicts involving both patients and staff at the Córdoba sanatoriums had been organized by the local communist newspaper *La Chispa*, and the same connection was reported by the newspaper *Los Principios* published in Córdoba city in the early 1940s.[22] During the first Peronist administration, the minister of public health, Ramón Carrillo, wrote to President Juan Domingo Perón about the visit of the famous American dancer Josephine Baker, "I must let you know that [Miss Baker] will end up creating a veritable insurrection among the tubercular patients in the hospital, where all it takes is half a word of discomfort or external support to activate the communist cells at the institution, something that would never happen with mental patients or lepers."[23]

Hospital authorities regularly expelled protest leaders.[24] When the director of the Sanatorio Santa María called in police units in charge of imposing order, the patient leaders ended up in a cell at the Cosquín police station. Though men in uniform were seldom instructed to intervene, their mere presence was disruptive and intimidating. "Last night," an inpatient wrote in a letter to a newspaper, "they patrolled the premises around the ward on foot and horseback, making so much noise that it was impossible to sleep. We are very troubled by these events. Now I have a higher fever than I have had since my name was put on the list of critical patients."[25]

Occasionally, policemen disguised as inpatients infiltrated hospitals and sanatoriums in order to obtain information about the organized protests.[26] In 1920, in its coverage of the conflicts at a Córdoba sanatorium, *La Vanguardia* included a series of photographs in which the morose figures of tubercular inpatients contrasted with a picture of two cops on horseback and guards armed with guns and clubs. The ironic headline read, "New treatment for tuberculosis: armed sentries."[27] In 1932, after another conflict, *La Montaña* spoke ironically about the incapacity of hospital authorities to deal with patients' uprisings. The title of the article was "Men armed with Mauser rifles to tranquilize tubercular patients at the sanatorium."[28]

In the mid-1920s, when the protests were particularly frequent, the authorities decided to create an internal police force; its presence contributed to producing an extremely tense atmosphere. In July of 1924 patients started playing soccer during hours when it was not permitted. A guard tried to stop them, and what followed was a violent exchange of words and even a physical struggle that ended with several inmates being detained by the police and others wounded. The patients responded by marching in protest and demanding the release of the detained tuberculars. The police intimidated them by shooting in the air. Some time later the patients threatened to desert the sanatorium, and 250 of them headed to Cosquín's police station in a "solemn and silent" march. On that occasion the director of the sanatorium was able to stop the picketing and restore calm by demanding the immediate release of the detainees and promising to curb the powers of the sanatorium's police force. However, the patients' triumph didn't last long. Two months later, once they were identified, the "mutinous leaders" were formally asked to leave the sanatorium; if they refused, they would be driven out by force. The expelled patients decided to camp out in Cosquín's central square. A commission of people living in the area supported them by holding town fairs and sending petitions to the National Congress. After a couple of weeks and despite the precarious state of the tuberculars, who had been camping out on the plaza, the protesters were finally dispersed. Some went back to Buenos Aires, while others were admitted to tuberculosis and general hospitals.[29] In 1930 another mass protest ended similarly.[30]

An explosive combination of three factors largely explains the persistence of collective conflicts at the Sanatorio Santa María during the 1920s and the early 1930s: first, the large size of the sanatorium, unusual for mountain hospitals; second, poor management; and, finally, according to the medical press, the "abominable meddling of politics in the therapeutic process of rest, hygiene, order, and discipline."[31] By that time it was abundantly clear that for many years the sanatorium had been the site of a great deal of local politicking. Indeed, the politicization of the sanatorium had become impossible to hide. It was evident in the admission process, during which patients were cross-examined about their political views; it was also evident in the careers of many local politicians, who had started out in medical or administrative positions at the sanatorium and gone on to hold powerful positions in the local party or the provincial legislature.[32]

Nonetheless, such conflicts were not the rule during the first half of the twentieth century: sanatoriums and hospitals did not turn into battlegrounds where patients relentlessly struggled or resisted doctors and staff. There were long periods of tranquility during which patients seem to have accepted, with varying degrees of enthusiasm, resignation, hope, and submission, inpatient treatments based on rest, multiple therapies, re-education, and relative isolation.

At the sanatorium the relationships between patients, doctors, and nurses were colored by many expectations. Attachments were formed in a context of both intensive daily contact and inevitable tension. For the doctors and nurses, working at the sanatorium was an opportunity to display not only professional competence and commitment, but also ambiguous or even contradictory feelings and attitudes such as compassion, negligence, and abuse of authority. For the sick, the sanatorium experience could either accentuate patients' desire to believe in what biomedicine and medical doctors could do to help or it could reveal how their private lives were becoming the object of rules that threatened their adulthood and independence.

A somewhat ironic article published in *Reflexiones*, the magazine written by inpatients at the Sanatorio Santa María, recounted a typical week in the life of a patient. It touched on the issue of re-education and pointed out how easily the rest therapy routines could be broken or ignored, while listing everything a patient was not allowed to do. The title of the article was "Diary of an Inpatient": it enumerated harmful habits and behavior such as "smoking, drinking, having sexual encounters with other patients, going to nightclubs, and gambling, particularly playing cards for money."[33] Many of these transgressions were relatively easy to engage in, since the careful monitoring of inpatients at the sanatorium required a cadre of doctors and nurses that far exceeded the available staff. In the 1920s, for instance, patients at Sanatorio Santa María saw their doctors only once every three or four months, partly because each professional was in charge of two hundred or three hundred patients.[34] It was not uncommon for some inmates to consider internment a form of custody rather than a healing process and hence to break the rest therapy rules as a way of enjoying what little time they had left. From the perspective of many patients, the hygienic prohibitions—particularly those against alcohol and sex—meant foregoing something exciting and vital. Drinking was a social occasion. Sometimes people drank at the sanatorium, hiding the alcohol they managed to smuggle in with the complicity of staff members. At other times they escaped from the building for a few hours to drink at local bars. Relationships between patients and between patients and staff members were also an opportunity to break the rules. In 1923 *La Vanguardia* reported in a quite moralistic tone that the women's ward at the Sanatorio Santa María had become a "house of seduction, where the sexual excitement of the young female patients is aroused, leading them to . . . depraved lives." Similarly, at the frequent parties in the town of Cosquín, "women patients and staff members [ended up] doing whatever they wanted, drinking champagne, eating, and dancing tango."[35]

Whether real or imaginary, all of these stories of love and sex were occasions for chatting and gossip; the experiences or fantasies around them were marvelous ways of fighting boredom and the passing of time, which was perceived, usually, as a sort of never-ending compulsory Sunday rest. It was also a way of finding something other than death and the slow spread of disease to talk about. Indeed, for those who actually had affairs, they must have been a way to show, both to themselves and to others, that tuberculosis didn't render them unsuited to love and sex. Love affairs probably offered them a means to be individuals in a world whose discourses and re-educational routines tended to equalize all patients. Daily life at the sanatorium gave rise to some odd characters who ignored certain social distinctions that mattered in the outside world but not in the sanatorium. There were those who were able to walk around; those who were convinced they were controlling the disease; those with a positive or negative saliva examination; those who denied their condition; and those who were endlessly optimistic and insisted that their bloody saliva was a problem with their throat, not their lungs. There were also the long-suffering patients; the stoics; the escapists who concentrated on looking for pleasure in almost every opportunity; those who tormented others by commenting on or predicting not their own fate, but that of their neighbors. There were the *pitucos engominados*—the stylish ones who used hair gel; the loafers; those who "stayed in their pajamas all day"; and "the ladies who wear makeup."[36]

The language used to articulate these varyingly transgressive conducts, as well as many individual and collective protests, was informed by ambiguous ways of referring to the doctor–patient relationship and an almost desperate criticism of the internment experience. In 1930 a story published in *La Montaña* called it a "regime of oppression and immorality."[37] In the patients' view, along with the issues of food and order, there were also moral issues. To them, eating badly or thinking one was eating badly, knowing one's mail had been read by sanatorium personnel, not being able to go for a walk, learning that "rebellious [patients] who can't adapt to the medical prescription" were discharged more quickly, and not finding anyone sensible to talk to about their complaints were simply the logical consequences of an "administrative, scientific and moral disaster."[38] They argued for "respecting the sick" and accused the doctors of being incapable of understanding the "psychology of a person with tuberculosis." They stated that those who had decided to move to the foothills to be inpatients "had found only moral decline fed by wrongdoing that was much sicker than patients' lungs."[39] Undoubtedly, patients stressed the denial of their integrity and respectability—a recurrent feature in the functioning of any isolationist institution—so forcefully because, after all, they had voluntarily chosen to become inmates.

In terms of the particular psychology of people with tuberculosis, many doctors agreed in the early 1940s that it was indeed very complex and deserved much more attention than it had received in previous decades.[40] Finally, regarding the immorality that characterized many institutions during certain periods, a story from 1954 about life at a boardinghouse for tuberculars in Cosquín, where unsupervised rest treatment was practiced, reveals what some viewed as the shortcomings of institutional internment. The narrator, a former tubercular, exalts the healing qualities of a restful and ordered life in the foothills while criticizing the sanatorium system, which supposedly re-educated patients in questions of diet and hygiene. In *Cosquín: Falsedad y verdad*, the world of hotels, boardinghouses, and family homes is depicted as utopian and harmonious, a place where tuberculars learn to live with their disease by putting into practice medical recommendations and self-discipline, and, most important, by not falling into the immorality and abuses common at inpatient institutions like sanatoriums.[41]

Biomedical Uncertainties and the Right to Try Out Treatments

Advances in modern bacteriology aroused enthusiasm in doctors and scientists searching for specific, effective treatments for tuberculosis. In 1890, after isolating the bacillus, Robert Koch attempted to find a treatment by using tuberculin, a lymph resulting from filtering bacillary cultures. In 1903 the Italian scientist Edoardo Maragliano injected human beings with a vaccine made from dead bacillus. During the first two decades of the twentieth century other vaccines were developed by Henri Vallé in France, Hideyo Noguchi in Japan, Friedrich Loffler in Germany, and Alessandro Bruschettini in Italy. Via different techniques, ranging from heat to chlorine, they all attempted to destroy the tuberculosis bacillus. Others, like Friedrich Friedmann, created vaccines from strains of bacteria taken from tubercular animals that were not virulent in humans. Emil von Behring, Koch, and Fred Neufeld worked on vaccines made from living bacilli taken from virulent human and bovine strains that were then attenuated through chemical and physical processes. The Spanish scientist Jaime Ferrán i Clúa created a preventive vaccine that attempted to immunize against the bacteria he believed later transformed into Koch's bacillus. These serums and many others, as well as curative and preventive vaccines, gave rise to intense debate within European scientific circles. Developed by Albert Calmette and Camille Guerin, what is now the widely accepted BCG vaccine was also part of this atmosphere of debate. In fact, starting in the 1920s and continuing well into the 1940s, this vaccine was received with open hostility in some countries and with great enthusiasm in others. Even into the 1950s it was regarded with some skepticism.

Academic circles in Buenos Aires published these developments and debates in the pages of medical journals and occasionally did clinical research on the effectiveness of vaccines and serums. In 1941 some of the successes and failures of this process, which had been underway since the beginning of the twentieth century, appeared in an article in *La Semana Médica* in which the author, Daniel Priano, discussed the fruitless efforts of biomedicine to find an effective vaccine. Priano commented on and criticized many of these efforts, among them the BCG vaccine.[42] He also mentioned the Friedmann vaccine but did not elaborate on it. Curiously, this vaccine was one of the few that stirred debate beyond the specialized journals and even gave rise to a peculiar discussion in the Congress. The case involved Augusto Bunge, a medical doctor and socialist congressman who was ardently committed to an initiative he called the Tuberculosis Elimination Law. His proposed law would have not only mandated the Friedmann vaccine for all children, but also punished adults who failed to give it to their children.

In addition to writing a 550-page academic work defending the vaccine discovered by Friedmann twenty-five years earlier—a subject of great debate in European academic circles—Bunge published a number of articles in daily newspapers with enormous readerships. In both his academic and popular writings he accused those who opposed his bill of being professionals involved in the lucrative "tuberculosis business." In the National Congress his defense of his proposal, which runs to more than 150 pages in the records of legislative debates, emphasized the vaccine's effectiveness as well as the responsibility of congressmen to make accountable decisions about the "social problem of tuberculosis." Some legislators and many doctors, the prestigious Antonio Cetrángolo among them, questioned not only what they considered an excessive involvement of political power in areas beyond its expertise, but also the idea of making mandatory a treatment whose benefits were far from obvious and infallible. Laureano Fierro, a physician, also publicly questioned the effectiveness of the vaccine and was later sued by Bunge for not respecting his "legislative rights and prerogatives." The courts rejected Bunge's suit, and, in less than a year, the legislator's enthusiasm for mandating the vaccine declined and faded from the public scene.[43]

Interestingly, if Priano's article mentioned the Friedmann case only in passing, it blatantly ignored the Villar serum and the Pueyo vaccine. These two cases demonstrate how long periods of scientific uncertainty can become tightly bound to social and cultural questions that go far beyond biomedicine. The Villar serum was produced in Buenos Aires at the beginning of the twentieth century and the Pueyo vaccine in the late thirties and early forties. Both treatments made headlines in newspapers and magazines of the day and goaded tubercular patients to demand access to treatments that had been written off in medical circles.

THE VILLAR SERUM

From the end of the nineteenth century, Carlos Villar, an experienced clinical and research physiologist, had been working on what he called "a serum that permitted organic rehabilitation by means of nutrition and significant weight gain, physical vigor, and vital capacity."[44] Villar held an important position at the Hospital Militar, where he had treated more than fifty patients with his serum, some of whom, according to his accounts, enjoyed astonishing results. His method was celebrated by his colleagues, and soon what had been just a rumor around the hospital became a news story. On March 24, 1901, the newspaper La Nación published an article about the serum, and within a short time the rest of the major print media followed suit. Newspaper articles generally had a mediating tone that attempted to effect a responsible assessment of the scientific novelty. El País announced that a doctor would report on the novelty in order to provide "information aimed at putting an end to indifference and disbelief."[45] El Diario requested "strict control" over Villar's serum, invited fifteen prestigious medical doctors to voice their opinions on the issue, and during the first two weeks of May alone published seven articles on the topic. La Prensa reported that it had created its own "examining commission" of "distinguished professionals," and Caras y Caretas stated that, though it wouldn't "pass judgment on the subject," it wished "the invention great success," emphasizing that it was a "brilliant attempt."[46]

Antonio Piñero led the professional criticism of Villar's discovery. He was one of the doctors El Diario had called on to evaluate the new serum. Piñero objected to the fact that Villar had kept his theories and the chemical composition of the serum a secret. He also opposed the way in which he had used newspapers to spread his findings rather than allowing his peers and the scientific press to assess them. Piñero was the first to point out, correctly, that the solution proposed by Villar was not a serum. Once Piñero had stated his reservations clearly and publicly, he changed focus and used the Villar case to relaunch his career as a doctor involved in political affairs. Starting with his second article, his journalistic contributions to *El Diario* emphasized the inability of the authorities at the Departamento Nacional de Higiene to control how and when the serum would be offered to the public. Although harsh and direct, Piñero never placed Villar in the large group of untrained scientists taking part in the frantic race to discover the cure for tuberculosis. He spoke of the Military Hospital doctor as a "righteous, impassioned and sincere man," a tone shared by other newspapers. *La Nación* considered Villar a serious, accomplished man, and *El País* called him a gentleman.[47]

The issue quickly became a hot topic in the press. Indeed, only this could explain the meeting between Villar and President Julio Roca on April 30, 1901, and Roca's subsequent statements clarifying that there would be no government involvement in the issue since only professionals were qualified to decide on the effectiveness of the treatment.[48] Days later Villar presented his discovery in a series of conferences at the Asociación Médica Argentina. At the first conference, held on May 13, a crowd was forced to wait outside the building because they did not have invitations. Among those denied entry were sick people who had already taken the serum at Villar's private office, which had just opened downtown, as well as people interested in getting the vaccine and poor tubercular patients who had been getting it for free.[49] Ignoring the demands of the tubercular patients and others in the crowd, the president of the association justified their exclusion by arguing that this was a strictly medical issue, and the presence of unqualified individuals was unnecessary.[50]

After the conference a commission of doctors started testing Villar's findings. They concluded that it wasn't a "specific remedy," that its "healing value was null," and that its application "could be dangerous" because it "delayed the application of a rational treatment."[51] When the commission's report was published, *El País* pointed out that "many unfortunate individuals" were convinced that the commission's opinion was just the work of "envious professionals" reacting to an "astonishing discovery." According to the newspaper article, "many [of those] unfortunate individuals" were tubercular patients who got the serum in a dozen private doctors' offices that weren't run by Villar, revealing that some doctors were determined to use and profit from the new product. It also indicated that some tubercular patients were unwilling to miss their chance to try a new treatment.[52] Villar wrote a public reply to the doctors' verdict, but none of the newspapers in Buenos Aires published it. Choosing not to engage in a prolonged fight, Villar retreated to his private medical office, where he continued to examine people with tuberculosis, giving his treatment to those who wanted it and training his son—himself a former tubercular who supposedly had recovered thanks to the treatment—in the preparation and application of what he wrongly called a serum.

In a detailed study published in 1936 Enrique de Cires reported that Villar's son had been distributing the concoction in city hospitals during the 1920s. This was a common practice for handling treatments whose performance was questioned by health authorities yet whose use had not been made illegal. At the Hospital Pirovano, where he worked as a doctor, de Cires had not only been giving the Villar serum to many of his patients, but had also managed to identify its chemical composition. He had the treatment approved by the Departamento Nacional de Higiene, not as a serum, since it didn't actually immunize, but rather as a therapy. In fact, Villar's treatment was built on the basis of nineteenth-century antituberculosis and reinvigorating diets and anticipated, in a quite original way, what in the 1930s—that is, in the time of de Cires, not of Villar—would be called proteinotherapy, a treatment based on ingesting large doses of protein in order to "repair lung tissues."[53]

In its own way, the Villar serum brought to the fore two issues the Pueyo vaccine would raise four decades later: the role of the press in the development of supposedly effective healing or preventive treatments and the reaction of tubercular patients trying to get these treatments. In the Villar case, the issue caught the public eye but, for many reasons, didn't become a public issue. First, because the press, still quite traditional, simply set out to inform readers about the advance; it made no deliberate attempt to produce a journalistic story about it, profit from it, or act as a means to celebrate treatments criticized by the medicoscientific establishment while airing doubts and reservations about biomedicine. And second, because in spite of the repeated failures in the field of antituberculosis treatments, the demands of the sick didn't become a collective voice capable of using the press to exercise pressure and to facilitate access to the Villar serum.

THE PUEYO VACCINE

The absence of a cure for tuberculosis in the first half of the twentieth century encouraged tuberculars to embrace any sort of therapy, even when its effectiveness was dubious. Both doctors, who were interested in overcoming the impotence they felt, and the sick, driven by the hope of recovery, could fall into this peculiar enthusiasm. Information about treatments circulated in the semipublic world of hospitals and medical wards as well as in the much more private world of doctors' offices. Some remedies were only fleeting presences in the arsenal of tuberculosis treatments suggested by the medical profession. Others lasted longer.

The problem arose when one of these treatments produced headlines in the press and was closely covered for months. The impact of such reporting on the public varied according to each medium's reaction to a treatment, and a story that produced headlines in one newspaper or weekly magazine might be barely mentioned or totally ignored by others. In truth, the treatments—and, along with them, the sick—became news when they provided stories that suited a certain journalistic style. That was the case of the Pueyo vaccine, an incident in the history of tuberculosis in Buenos Aires in which the resistance of the academic establishment to a new therapy that came from outside recognized medical circles not only became bound up in modern journalism—which acted as a public voice for the demands and expectations of the tuberculars—but also revealed the limited but real role of the sick in looking for effective cures.

Jesús Pueyo started working as an amateur biology researcher in 1929. In 1932 he got a job as an assistant in the laboratory of the bacteriology department at the Universidad de Buenos Aires medical school. There, he worked on developing a tuberculosis vaccine. First, he experimented on animals and later on people. He tried, repeatedly and in vain, to get some kind of official and academic recognition of his just-discovered vaccine. At the same time, many tuberculars were becoming interested in trying Pueyo's vaccine. News of its existence leaked from the laboratory and was well received by people with tuberculosis, many of whom were always willing to try promising new treatments. Among doctors, the reception was mixed. Some considered the vaccine a hopeful attempt to find an effective cure, an attempt that deserved serious attention. Other doctors were more cautious, requesting more information. Still others were suspicious and rejected it from the start. At the laboratory where Pueyo worked, the necessary evaluations were being put off, he averred, because of his marginal position in the world of researchers fighting tuberculosis. The delays, he said, were hindering access to the vaccine. "Convinced by the insistent offers of journalism," Pueyo decided to go public with his discovery.[54] Some magazines and newspapers, particularly those that were decidedly modern by the 1940s, made Pueyo's vaccine a hot story. The newspaper *Crítica* and the biweekly *Ahora*, both with enormous print runs and a very large audience, were decisive in their efforts at turning the vaccine into a public issue. Between 1940 and 1942 *Crítica* printed more than eighty articles on the case, including two-page stories, big headlines, interviews, and photographs. *Ahora* reported on the case seventy times, and its sophisticated graphic coverage included reproductions of tuberculars' letters, x-ray images, pictures of Pueyo in the laboratory and at the editorial offices, drawings of the bacillus, and photographs of patients at hospitals presenting petitions to the authorities and demonstrating in the street. *Ahora* used pictures to build the news, and every issue presented the reader with a shocking visual story followed by big headlines and short texts.

Undoubtedly, the Pueyo vaccine had all the ingredients for a juicy story. It voiced the anxiety of people with tuberculosis, questioned the authority of high-ranking doctors, and fed the curiosity of an audience used to reading both scientific and pseudoscientific articles. Indeed, both *Crítica* and *Ahora* subtly intertwined the coveted cure for tuberculosis, the common person's potential access to it, and the story of the humble microbiology lab assistant who, despite the attacks of the medical establishment, was determined to save desperate people with tuberculosis. Pueyo's figure was never presented to the audience as a quack or a healer who offered alternative cures to the poor and the ignorant. On the contrary, pictured in the lab surrounded by microscopes, pipettes, and test tubes, he was described as being a worthy researcher, devoted to his work, and unfairly ignored by the medical establishment.[55]

Pueyo's own public presentation always underlined his condition as both a hardworking scientist to whom the media had turned in order to inform the people and a researcher not involved in any sensationalistic yellow journalism campaign. In 1942, when the affair had ended, Pueyo published a book with his version of the facts. It was a compilation of letters he had sent to doctors and government officials who refused to seriously consider his findings. In each of the letters, which were written over the course of three years, Pueyo represented himself as a member of the scientific community fighting against a marginalization orchestrated by the interests of the "medical bureaucracy." The book, published by Editorial Científica, was probably financed by Pueyo himself. In it, he emphasized that his vaccine was not a panacea, like the treatments offered by charlatans and quacks. And while he criticized what he regarded as the unfair and unyielding resistance of certain powerful figures in academic circles and in public health agencies, Pueyo stressed again and again the enthusiastic support he had received from prestigious doctors active in the clinical care of people with tuberculosis. Regarding the press that followed him so closely, Pueyo said, "I only use it to let the people know about the current research." He claimed it was an "instrument for progress and a spur against academic paralysis." Not without craftiness, he distanced himself from *Ahora* and *Crítica*. He said he let these media and the people "do the talking," while he delivered papers to the "most competent personalities so they can then make their verdict with due seriousness and serenity."[56]

Crítica and *Ahora* transformed the medical establishment's rejection of Pueyo into his main virtue. The "modern Argentine Pasteur," as *Ahora* called him in its issue of December 27, 1940, quickly saw that his professional biography could be seen as an example of what could happen to a scientist who had chosen not to be corrupted by power. When interviewed by a magazine that had a poor opinion of his credentials, Pueyo didn't hesitate to state that his exclusion from reputable academic circles was the price he had to pay for "not accepting the scientific patronage" of powerful interests.[57] In his view his career was a clear example of the struggle against a lack of resources and bureaucratic obstacles, two barriers that ordinary people, "people without contacts," often had to face.[58] Considering this portrait, it wasn't hard for *Crítica* and *Ahora* to conclude that Pueyo embodied science as it should be: removed from lavish funding and luxuriously equipped labs and firmly committed to people's needs.

The reaction of the medical establishment changed over time. In 1936 Pueyo started making available his treatment to doctors who had patients with tuberculosis. Moreover, many eminent local doctors sent him patients who quite soon reported remarkable improvements, at least according to an article in *Ahora* dated 1941, at the peak of the controversy, but committed to giving readers a retrospective renderings of the events.[59] This state of affairs started to change, however, when the vaccine became a public issue, largely owing to the print media. From then on, doctors took an increasingly negative stance. In 1938 an article published in *La Doble Cruz*, the magazine of the Liga Argentina contra la Tuberculosis, spoke of the "great experience and seriousness" of the many people who are looking for effective treatments as well as of the "opportunism and lack of credentials" of others.[60] In 1941 *Viva Cien Años*, a health magazine, offered readers the opinions of professors, doctors, and government officials in a style that purposely contrasted with *Ahora* and *Crítica*. Some of these figures voiced their reservations by speaking in the name of the patients whose "hopes are resuscitated by this press campaign; they think there's a life raft they can cling to, but when it sinks, it will bring down with it their dreams, and this, in the end, is very dangerous to their weakened spirits and bodies." Others questioned Pueyo for having flagrantly broken academic rules and scientific ethics. They said, "The author of a discovery must" prove his findings "with scientific evidence. A vaccine is not something spiritual that must be accepted as a dogma. It's something material, with a given physical reality; thus, in order to believe in the vaccine, it is necessary to know it. And, until now, the information given about its composition has not been adequate."[61]

Once the issue had gone public, the vaccine's effectiveness, and particularly its harmlessness, entered the purview of the Departamento Nacional de Higiene. In order to reach his verdict, the director of the department invited Pueyo to do the necessary testing at the department's laboratory. The results were a long time in coming, however. Along with *Ahora* and *Crítica*, Pueyo blamed the delay on a bureaucracy that kept slowing down his work. Meanwhile, government officials accused Pueyo of keeping the composition of the vaccine a secret and of not showing up at the laboratory where he was to test it.[62] The minister of internal affairs, a politician, tried to restart the dialogue. He received Pueyo in January of 1941 and issued a resolution authorizing the application of the treatment to two hundred people with tuberculosis and three hundred animals. The tests never took place, however, because the director of the Departamento Nacional de Higiene and the director of the Instituto Bacteriológico, a confirmed opponent of the vaccine and its discoverer, imposed conditions Pueyo found unacceptable.

In reaction to these postponements, tubercular patients rallied. For some, "media buzz" was to blame for the agitation of the sick and the general public.[63] The coverage in *Crítica* and *Ahora* and the delays in the paperwork required for studying the innocuousness and effectiveness of the vaccine only served to heighten the despair of people with tuberculosis. In November 1940 *Crítica* reproduced a pamphlet signed by tubercular patients inviting the people to support them in the fight to get the vaccine. It warned the casual reader that "anybody, you or one of your relatives," could be "the victim of this calamity."[64] In December the newspaper reported on a march of sick people in Plaza de Mayo, in front of the seat of the national government.[65] In early 1941 headlines in *Ahora* ominously declared, "A revolt of people with tuberculosis [is] about to break out across the nation." In the same issue, an article entitled "Doctors accused of conspiring against science" placed the Pueyo vaccine case in the realm of science and official medicine.[66] By then, pamphlets and manifestos were circulating in tuberculosis medical wards, hospitals, and sanatoriums. One of those pamphlets hailed the "humanitarian decree signed by the Minister of Internal Affairs," who by then was more open-minded than the heads of the Departamento Nacional de Higiene; the last line of the pamphlet read, "Pueyo has vanquished, and he will continue to vanquish. Time is up for the octopuses who suck the people's blood."[67]

Occupying a third of a page, a manifesto reproduced in *Ahora* voiced the agenda of the tubercular activists: "To the people of the Argentine Republic!!! The time has come to take to the street and demand what we deserve, what no man can take away from us. The medical professionals and defenders of official science conspire against us and against Pueyo, and they are willing to do everything they can to keep our nation from getting the tuberculosis vaccine that its discoverer has offered, free of charge, to the national government." The manifesto questioned "the attitude of those professionals who make a living from their patients: an attitude that was publicly unmasked by Pueyo, who [in several letters] has clearly established that doctors seek to preserve their economic interests and their plentiful State funding." It called for action: "The people have already chosen their way in this notable crusade. . . . It's just a matter of time before we leave hospitals, leave the beds where our lives are consumed, and undertake a caravan through the city streets towards the government house and . . . request and demand before our government that justice be done and the people receive the vaccine." The manifesto ended by saying, "Enough! The world will soon know how a people sick and tired rallies behind the man who made the antituberculosis vaccine possible, the man who unmasked the philistines at the sacred temple of medicine. With Pueyo and for Pueyo. Against the capitalist bureaucracy of medicine!!!"[68]

Contrary to the arrogance of the powerful figures of official medicine, Pueyo embodied the figure of the humble bacteriologist who had not only given out his cure for free but had also exposed those who profited from the disease. The therapy the tubercular patients were defending was not part of the home medicine tradition. Neither were they seeking access to the solutions offered by alternative or popular medicines. They were, rather, reaffirming their right to try a treatment that was on the margins of academic science. Their indignation was not untimely, considering that the vaccine's harmlessness had already been proven. On these grounds, a tubercular patient stated, "If a remedy is not harmful, even if its benefits are still unknown, the logical thing to do would be to give it to the people who want it. Especially in the field of tuberculosis, where so far nothing really effective has been found, despite the fuss over the preventive merits of the Calmette Guerin vaccine, whose obstinate enemies include eminences such as León Taxier, at the Children's Hospital in Paris, Professor Otolenghi in Rome, Doctors Tucunouva and Larinouva in Moscow, and Doctor Olbretch from Brussels."[69]

By then, it was evident that *Crítica* and *Ahora* had become enmeshed in the tuberculars' movement. *Ahora*'s editorial office became a sort of general headquarters where patient activists gathered to plan future actions. Like *La*

Prensa, which at the beginning of the century had provided welfare services to the poor in one of its buildings—a peculiar philanthropic act by a very traditional newspaper—*Ahora* backed the advocates of the vaccine and their demands for social justice. In a style cultivated by *Crítica* in the 1930s, *Ahora* established itself as a publication sensitive to the dramas of the needy. It even offered a mailing address at which doctors and sick people who were interested in the treatment could reach Pueyo.[70]

Largely because of the commotion created by the tuberculosis patients and the actions of Pueyo himself, the minister of internal affairs ordered that tests to establish the harmlessness and effectiveness of the vaccine be accelerated. Meanwhile, Uruguayan health authorities had already certified its innocuousness, and the authorities in Brazil, Peru, Bolivia, and Chile were studying it as well. This news started to circulate in Buenos Aires at the same time that the Departamento Nacional de Higiene affirmed its opposition to the medication, pointing out, among other things, that Pueyo had not performed the appropriate tests at the appropriate time. In response to this, tuberculosis patients wrote dozens of letters to the Comisión de Higiene y Asistencia Médico-social at the National Congress and again took to the streets.[71] In early winter 1941 tubercular patients in Buenos Aires and other parts of the country marched to the National Congress shouting, "We want the Pueyo vaccine!" The photographic coverage of the protest in *Ahora*, which reproduced enlarged copies of images from other events during the first part of the year, depicted a morose scene: sick people wrapped in hospital blankets and their sullen relatives, skinny mothers carrying their children. There were signs identifying neighborhood and regional associations that supported Pueyo, and many banners with a large *V* in reference to the vaccine. There were also confrontations. The police intervened, and some patients were detained.[72]

Nevertheless, the Departamento Nacional de Higiene didn't change its policy. Indeed, the minister, who early on had been receptive to the demands of the patients, sided with the medical establishment, as did the National Congress, largely owing to the initiative of a legislator who happened to be a doctor. In this context, Pueyo was fined and sued for malpractice, which led to a spontaneous outpouring of contributions sent by sick people to the *Ahora* editorial office. In less than forty-eight hours, twice the sum of the fine had been raised. Pueyo didn't accept the help, and this reinforced his virtuousness and humility in the eyes of the public, demonstrating once again a position diametrically opposed to that of doctors interested in profiting from people's ill health. The trial and the fine didn't go far because Pueyo had distributed his treatment free of charge with the permission of the Ministry of Internal

Affairs. Furthermore, he had also distributed it to doctors who had requested it, doctors with patients eager to test whether the vaccine could restore their health.[73]

On July 11, 1941, Pueyo accepted the official resolution, and from then on patients' activism declined, as did media attention to the controversy. At the end of the year, in reporting that Uruguay had recognized the vaccine's innocuousness and that Brazil was using it on an experimental basis at several hospitals, *Crítica* continued to point out how irrationally Argentine authorities had dealt with the issue.[74] In any case, the issue continued to appear in the newspapers, usually in the form of warnings to the public of fake Pueyo vaccines for sale. Tubercular patients and their relatives, and even some doctors, apparently were still interested in trying out the treatment in spite of the official condemnation of it. Oscar O. vividly recalls how he got the injection in the early 1940s: "I was admitted to the hospital. When I met a doctor who administered it for ten pesos at his private office I decided to go ahead and try it, without mentioning anything to my doctors at the hospital. The doctor was very kind; he gave me hope and convinced me that the cure was effective." According to Ricardo H., a tubercular patient who arrived in the Córdoba foothills to pursue a rest cure in the mid-1940s—at which point the Pueyo affair had ceased to be a public issue—the vaccine was still circulating because "people suffering from the disease were willing to try anything that might save them." The tuberculosis expert Santos Sarmiento, who had a long career as a doctor in Cosquín involved in public and private sanatoriums and his own practice, recalls trying to dissuade patients who were demanding the Pueyo vaccine: "Time and again I explained to them that 'it's nothing but water, it won't do you any harm or any good.' But they didn't care at all."

Explaining why people behaved as they did is not easy. At least to a certain extent tubercular patients didn't care if the vaccine was soundly effective because they were eager to believe in the possibility of a cure at a moment when biomedicine could offer them only uncertainties. With that predicament, the patients forged a common identity around their illness, the threat of death, and the belief that the new treatment was harmless and perhaps capable of curing them. The obstacles set up by the medical establishment and the public health authorities impeded easy access to the vaccine and hence encouraged further collective action. Though the battle to legalize the vaccine had been lost, patients continued to believe in its innocuousness and possible effectiveness. There's something of this tight web of belief, biomedical uncertainties, and therapeutic novelties in the way Pedro R., who survived the disease, recalls his experience with the vaccine. At the age of eighty, some sixty years after being vaccinated, he is still convinced that of all the treatments he tried—and his is a clear case of a tubercular who, in fact, tried cures originating both in the realm of biomedicine and outside of it—the "unfairly persecuted Pueyo vaccine" was the one that helped him most. And he took the treatment despite the opposition of a doctor whom he still respects enormously and remembers with a high degree of veneration.

Benito S., a tubercular patient actively engaged in the Pueyista protest, explained in an interview published by *Ahora* in the midst of the dispute the reasons for the conflict as well as the tubercular patients' point of view: "It's painful to see the intolerance of many doctors. They interpret any sympathy for Pueyo and his vaccine as a categorical rejection of them and their methods. Unable to grasp the spiritual drama we experience, all they do is repress the irrepressible joy that the possibility of an immediate cure with a new therapeutic method has brought to the sick." Benito had trouble understanding why certain doctors avoided "speaking of the vaccine" and "when they were forced to do so, owing to the legitimate and inalienable right of the sick person, they diminished its importance . . . even when they had never studied it."[75] Directors of hospitals and sanatoriums showed an even more hostile attitude. Most of the time, they ended up discharging the activists' leaders as well as tubercular patients who had received the vaccine. At the Hospital Muñiz women interested in Pueyo's treatment were often punished by being sent to the solarium; there, their condition worsened, and many eventually left the hospital. In other cases, the punishment was expulsion from the institution. In 1942 an inpatient at the Hospital Central de Tuberculosos recounted his experience with the vaccine: "Following my doctor's advice, I was admitted to the hospital on August 29, 1940 . . . ; once there, I was prescribed a thorax x-ray, calcium injections every other day, and salycilate injections." After realizing that "my health hadn't improved" and reading about the Pueyo vaccine in the newspaper, he said, "I decided to take it" at a doctor's private office. "Of course, that day I asked for permission to leave the hospital without saying where I was going. After the first injection, the change in my health was radical: the fever decreased, the expectoration disappeared, and I gained weight." When the director found out that one of the inpatients had received the Pueyo treatment, he called him to his office, scolded him, and asked him "not to say anything to the other patients. . . . [In my case, he told me] he would study the situation and, if the test went well, he would definitively investigate the cure more carefully. In the beginning, I believed him, but it was soon clear that the last thing he wanted to do was study the effects of the vaccine: he never came to my bed again. No more thorax x-rays were taken, nor was my sputum analyzed; he even stopped saying hello." He concluded, "I was discharged from the hospital . . . or, more precisely, I was put out on the street by a police officer on January 2, 1941. I was not cured, . . . but I had improved so much, both physically and morally, that I felt like a new man and, what's more important. . . . I had recovered the will to live."[76]

In the sanatoriums and boardinghouses in Cosquín, Pueyo's treatment was also greeted with hostility from many doctors, though there were exceptions. Oscar F., the son of a nurse who worked for several decades at one of the most expensive sanatoriums in Cosquín, recalls that on an occasion in which Pueyo was visiting sanatoriums in the foothills the doctors didn't allow him into the building. And even when the dispute ended, the Pueyo vaccine, or versions of it, was circulating among tuberculars anyway, probably as a small-scale, informal business developed by those who continued to see in it a lucrative opportunity. For some tuberculars the price of the vaccine was almost prohibitive. Jorge G. remembers that "the Pueyo vaccine cost [him] an arm and a leg." For Gerardo B., who must have been in a better economic position, getting the treatment didn't seem to be a problem: "A young guy who had recovered from tuberculosis made a living injecting the vaccine at people's houses."

Patient activism was barely covered by the *La Nación*, *La Prensa*, *La Razón*, or *La Vanguardia*. This editorial decision was made largely out of the deep respect the people running these newspapers had for well-established science and medicine. *La Vanguardia*'s indifference to the Pueyo case is particularly striking. In the twenties the paper had covered the conflicts over food and order at the sanatoriums and hospitals in Buenos Aires and the Córdoba foothills, explaining it as part of a broader problem related to the health of the working classes. In an austere, didactic style that did not play on the reader's sympathy, *La Vanguardia*'s coverage of these conflicts was quite traditional; it spoke of the "people's causes" but in a quite traditional journalistic style that contrasted with the refurbished and brisk one modern newspapers like *Crítica* and *El Mundo*, for example, had been cultivating since the 1920s. In the late 1930s and early 1940s, during the Pueyo affair, *La Vanguardia* did not cover tubercular patients' protests for their "right" to access to the treatment. Perhaps this was partly owing to the considerable number of medical doctors in the leadership of the Socialist Party. After all, Pueyo and his vaccine circulated on the margins of academic medicine and questioned the legitimacy of a "medical class" of which many eminent socialists were part.

Ahora and *Crítica*, meanwhile, were central in turning the Pueyo vaccine into a public issue. Echoing the demands of common people who regularly faced the arbitrariness of power, particularly, in this case, in the sphere of medicine, these newspapers are fine examples of the so-called new journalism. This sort of journalism was modern and featured many illustrations, photographs, and large headlines that were provocative and intriguing; it informed, offered opinions, and dialogued with readers. In their coverage of events surrounding the Pueyo vaccine, *Ahora* and *Crítica* sometimes ended up situating themselves at the center of their journalistic narratives, relegating the sick and their activism to a secondary role.

The Pueyo vaccine is one of many examples of developments that promised effective cures during the first half of the twentieth century. Usually, the discussion of these advances was confined to academic circles, and its impact on the daily mass media was minimal. However, in the case of the Pueyo vaccine the debate was public; it was a dispute between the medical establishment and a scientist outside that establishment. Pueyo's credentials were questioned over and over again, and Pueyo, supported by *Ahora* and *Crítica*, refused to be treated like someone outside the scientific community. In this struggle, which was greatly affected by modern journalism, academic medicine's hostility toward the treatment increased as Pueyo's findings were celebrated by modern newspapers and magazines and, more important, by the many patients interested in receiving a treatment that filled them with hope in times of biomedical uncertainty.

The individual and collective transgressions and demands of patients—including drinking alcohol, escaping from sanatoriums, going out dancing, writing petitions, striking, and marching to get a vaccine—indicate the considerable gaps in the power and authority that marked the relationship between doctors and patients. Such gaps allowed for an array of behaviors and situations rich in duplicity and complicity, hegemony and subversion, control and resistance, socialization and difference. In this context, many sick people discovered not only their capacity to exert influence, either individual or collective, over the public sphere, but also what some of them deemed a "legitimate and inalienable right."[77] This discovery was not in keeping with the image doctors like Juan José Vitón, the author of *Lo que todo tuberculoso debe saber*, had of their patients; like others, he considered sick people ignorant of "the true and exact interpretations of what they see, feel or think is happening."[78]

The newfound ability to exert pressure on the public sphere also evidences the role of health and disease in the complex process of broadening social citizenship. It manifests what in the first decades of the twentieth century in many nations was called "the right to health." Demands related to this right were, in general, sporadic. In the first half of the century questions of disease

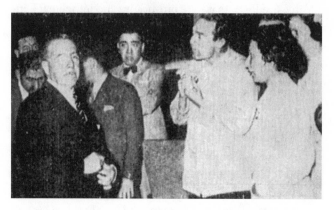

Tuberculars lobbying government officials and Congress for easy access to the Pueyo vaccine. (*Ahora*, August 1941)

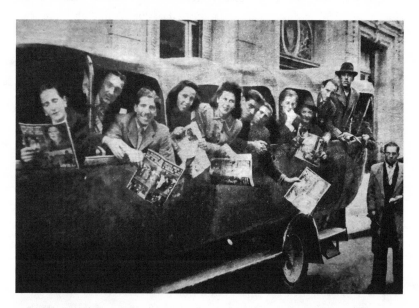

Tuberculars campaigning from a bus sponsored by the magazine *Ahora*. (*Ahora*, May 1941)

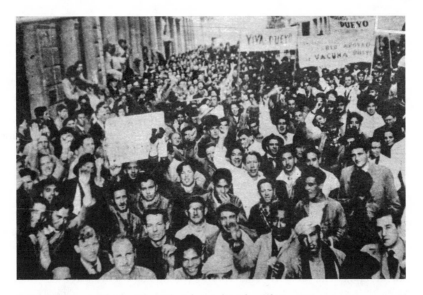

A street demonstration by tuberculars demanding the right to access to treatment based on the Pueyo vaccine. (*Ahora*, December 1941)

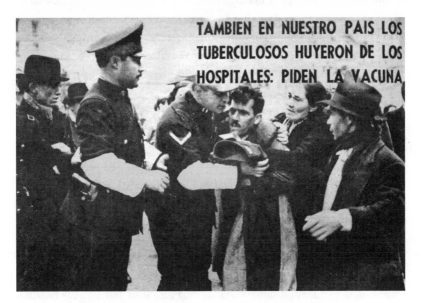

Tuberculars negotiating with the police on Plaza Congreso, in front of the House of Representatives. The headline reads, "Also in our country tubercular patients are escaping from hospitals. They are requesting the Pueyo vaccine!" (*Ahora*, December 1941)

and public health infrastructure, from potable water and sewage systems to hospitals, were not crucial to the agenda of organized labor, and neither were they the primary impetus behind social movements. Only in conjunction with other issues, for example, a shorter workday or better working conditions; or when connected with the charitable efforts of ethnic and worker mutual associations; or when a certain pathology was connected to certain jobs did questions of health and disease become central. Beyond these situations, the limited, if real, importance of tubercular patients—or people afraid of becoming such patients—hardly served to turn them into influential and decisive actors capable of generating or modeling the incipient public health policies before and during the first Peronist administration.

Demands focused specifically on tuberculosis and originating in the workplace were exceptional as well. Only the bakery workers undertook initiatives, including strikes, in which tuberculosis treatment featured on the list of demands along with more hygienic working conditions, a shorter workday, and the issue of nighttime work.[79] Generally, the unions—whether led by anarchist, anarcho-syndicalist, socialist, or communists groups—and the Círculos de Obreros Católicos spoke of tuberculosis but did not take specific measures. This was largely because it was hard to sustain an explicit connection between the disease and working conditions. There were, though, individual lawsuits that considered tuberculosis a work-related malady. Though the number of such lawsuits was small at the beginning of the century, it grew in the thirties and forties. Often well-grounded and supported by doctors and lawyers, some of these cases became important in the ongoing effort to see tuberculosis as a workplace disease that, as such, had to be protected by laws governing accidents in the workplace.[80]

In the long, uncertain wait for an effective cure, patients accepted or confronted the therapies available, whether they originated within the medical establishment, in the realm of scientists with questionable credentials, or with healers, herborists, quacks, and practitioners of home medicine. Regardless of the origin of the treatment, patients were moved by the desire to defeat tuberculosis or, at least, to believe it was possible to do so. Their individual and collective actions reveal not only the complexity of relationships between doctors who wanted to cure and tuberculars looking for cures, but also the fact that any therapy—from vaccines to the rest cure—served to express a complex set of social and cultural problems that went beyond the medical establishment's perception of the effectiveness or harmlessness of a treatment.

.... ✾ ....

CHAPTER FOUR

The Fight against Tuberculosis and the Culture of Hygiene

Starting at the end of the nineteenth century and especially during the first half of the twentieth, changes in the health-care infrastructure, as well as in tuberculosis morbidity and mortality rates, were accompanied by an emergent secular catechism of hygiene. Printed material such as books, brochures, and pamphlets and, starting in the 1920s, radio broadcasts prescribed, with varying degrees of enthusiasm, how to live a healthy life.[1] Many of these prescriptions became fundamental to material and moral life in the contemporary city. The scope of the prescriptions was broad: they touched on sports and free time, sexuality and child rearing, dress and eating habits, school routines, the layout of the workplace, the organization of households, and the use of public spaces.

Medical doctors were central in introducing these ideas, norms, and behaviors, which, once a part of people's daily lives, were supposed to lead to the "indirect prevention" of tuberculosis. In 1940 a brochure published by the Centro de Investigaciones Tisiológicas said it was indispensable to carry out a coherent and ongoing hygienic education project that made use of the printed media and the radio, mailings, and signs on trolleys, buses, and trains. It was hoped this strategy would make it possible to publicize a clear message that would "surprise the subjects we want to educate." The message would "go after them and seek their attention."[2] The use of modern advertising and communication strategies to convey hygienic behavior as a means of preventing contagion was nothing new. Similar efforts had been made, if somewhat less assertively, at the turn of the century, when the discourse of fear and defensive hygiene dominated a social agenda designed to fight epidemics. These communication strategies had also been used in the 1920s, when modern advertising reinforced the prevailing discourse on a healthy life and positive hygiene in order to introduce other, more general ideas of social harmony and social consensus as well as social justice and citizenship.

By the beginning of the twentieth century, campaigns against tuberculosis were recurrent and commonplace. They used signs, posters, brochures, and pamphlets that, according to the campaigns' organizers, were easy for everyone to understand. Sometimes, different languages were employed in order to reach the growing immigrant population. Just like campaigns against alcohol, venereal diseases, and flies, these messages aimed at informing and educating the public; they sought to capture attention and used quasi-religious and quasi-military metaphors such as "Catechism against Tuberculosis" and "War against Tuberculosis." In 1901 and 1902 alone, hundred of thousands of such ads were posted in trains, factories, mutual aid societies, hospitals, workers' centers, churches, and schools.[3] Other communication strategies were also employed. Conferences on tuberculosis prevention were frequent, both in the exclusive halls of the Sociedad Rural and in the modest, plebeian headquarters of ethnic associations. And there were a certain number of real communication novelties, such as printing "instructions on how to avoid the tuberculosis contagion" on matchboxes, on the back of pharmacy prescriptions, and on municipal poverty certificates. At elementary schools, "postal stamp antituberculosis campaigns" were greatly encouraged. The public's attention was sought through various contests that gave prizes to the healthiest child or to the best design for personal spittoons or to the most original propaganda strategy. Antituberculosis advertisements began to appear more frequently in films, newspapers, and popular magazines.[4] And there was even a proposal, which did not materialize until much later, to establish a Museum of Hygiene.

These communication efforts combined the ideas of modern hygiene and consumerism. In the 1930s people of all classes were consuming more and more products that were advertised as being somehow connected to notions of tuberculosis and hygiene: hygienic soaps, water heaters that encouraged frequent showers "even in the winter," over-the-counter syrups that promised physical and emotional strength. Some advertisements reminded potential readers about the need for a vacuum cleaner, "if one was to really fight the most dangerous microbes." Radio broadcasts often equated health and beauty and attempted to create a hygienic awareness aimed at "improving the national race" by an array of means, from a good diet to appropriate and healthy conduct.

Early on, the effective communication of habits that were believed to decrease the risk of tuberculosis contagion made use of modern marketing strategies. Such communication became an essential part of the debate around, as well as the design and actual practice of, what was then called the fight against tuberculosis, that is, a set of specific initiatives that attempted to control the disease. To a great extent in the history of that fight continuity prevailed over change; biomedical uncertainties and the lack of an effective treatment were realities throughout the period, when the decline in the tuberculosis mortality rate was slow and often difficult to notice. In any case, most of this drop took place before the late 1940s. The arrival and use of antibiotics significantly accelerated the declining trend; by then, in Buenos Aires, the problem had shifted from tuberculosis mortality to the problem of those getting the disease and being in need of medical attention. Up until then, the fight against tuberculosis was steeped in a feeling of powerlessness. There was a clear antituberculosis rhetoric, one which was at times very articulate and informed. Designed first by hygienists and later by tuberculosis specialists, many ambitious initiatives were in the works by the beginning of twentieth century, and they frequently gained ground through reformulations in the following decades. These initiatives lasted for almost five decades. They were marked by persistent demands to increase the role of the state in health care, to receive more funding in order to accelerate the growth of hospital infrastructure, to create compulsory antituberculosis insurance, and to improve hygienic education as a preventive measure against the disease. Only some of these initiatives gave rise to specific public policies; discussions and discourses about tuberculosis do not necessarily mean that specific policies were formulated, implemented, or, much less, affected the lives of the sick or those who feared getting sick.

Because of the ongoing lack of clear medical solutions, a certain feeling of inertia surrounded the tuberculosis issue. This sentiment is expressed in an article entitled "Organización de la lucha social contra la tuberculosis," written by Gregorio Aráoz Alfaro in 1936. In the article Aráoz Alfaro, a distinguished hygienist, tuberculosis specialist, and major player in the Argentine antituberculosis movement, states that he was repeating something he'd said ten years earlier at the First Pan-American Congress on Tuberculosis, held in the city of Córdoba, Argentina, in 1927. On that occasion he addressed an audience of experts and state public health officials: "In the last decades, overall mortality has declined gradually, mortality due to infectious disease has declined considerably . . . , yet the tuberculosis mortality rate has stayed the same. . . . All the past efforts to combat this modern calamity have come to nothing . . . ;

we're standing just where we were before. . . . [We are faced with] a lack of social legislation and efficient health infrastructure, a lack of means, a lack of a comprehensive plan and real fighting methods."[5]

Tuberculosis as a Public Matter

Tuberculosis was probably the most talked about disease in the first decades of the twentieth century. It was also an important part of an agenda in which issues of hygiene, urban environment, and social welfare were discussed in the broader context of an imprecise ideology of the public. This ideology aimed at seeking to lay the groundwork for a new social state responsible for the protection and well-being of the population. Ambitious and reformist, this ideology of the public invoked the figures of social solidarity, order, and the enhancement of certain social rights. It also created institutions and experts who would produce an array of specific policies geared toward moving beyond private charity and limiting the power of religious institutions.

In the last third of the nineteenth century, the consolidation of key public institutions was well underway. By then, a modernization process characterized by mass immigration, rapid urbanization, and incipient albeit modest industrial development had substantially shaped a social question that focused on two sets of problems. On the one hand, conflicts between capital and labor, growing labor organization, and the elite's responses—either in a reformist key, assuming that social conflicts should be solved through laws and a regulating state, or in a repressive style, dealing with such conflicts as social threats that must be brutally suppressed. On the other hand was the issue of hygiene and disease in the city, especially after the yellow fever epidemic of 1871, a watershed in the history of modern Buenos Aires. In dealing with this second problem, the reformist agenda and the ideology of the public were more consistent than they were when it came to the workers' question. To a large extent, turn-of-the-century hygiene reformism, with all its nuances, tended to cope with infectious diseases and tuberculosis by treating them like social maladies. It connected them with other social problems and emphasized the need to do something to avoid them.

As early as 1868 José Antonio Wilde stated that "people's health rests on instruction, morality, nutrition, fresh air, sanitary precautions, public welfare, public charity, work and even free amusement; in the end, anything that may be needed by each and every one of the people living in the city."[6] Though the hygienist discourse of people like Wilde changed somewhat over time to reflect the changes taking place in the urban world, the core of this discourse remained the same: it deemed the city an artifact and social fabric in which fear of contagion, the morality and living conditions of the urban masses, and concerns about faulty city infrastructure were closely associated. By the early twentieth century, sewage and potable water systems had made it possible to control infecto-contagious epidemic cycles—though not tuberculosis—and so the discourses of hygiene began to emphasize the problems of poverty and the need for a network of health care institutions.

This urban reformist agenda was well received by an array of political groups, from liberals to conservatives, from social Catholics to socialists. Even anarchists enthusiastically participated in certain aspects of the hygienist program. All political groups championed and defended the modern ideal of hygiene, although some disagreed on how to carry out projects, others doubted its actual effect on people's daily lives, and still others had quite diverse readings of its preventive and disciplinary dimensions. Nonetheless, this loose consensus was facilitated by the combination of a series of factors that allowed vague concerns about hygiene voiced before 1870 to become a modern program for urban intervention. Starting at the turn of the century and for the next fifty years concerns about a fast growing city made possible a rough definition of collective and social medicine based on advances in modern bacteriology, statistics, the growth of state-run institutions focused on questions of public health, and the increasingly important role of the medical profession in public affairs as well as in individual private lives. This medicine of the modern urban world came into being as a politico-medical endeavor in which the state was seen as the key manager of a dense medicalization web based on sanitary city infrastructure, institutions of care and assistance, and specific public health campaigns.

The transformation of tuberculosis into a public issue began in the last third of the nineteenth century and the first years of the twentieth. During this period, conservative governments facilitated the creation and consolidation of a modest administrative bureaucracy. Working at the Departamento Nacional de Higiene and the Asistencia Pública Municipal, some medical doctors—the *higienistas*—took the lead in this process. They were not a homogeneous group. Some explained their new technico-bureaucratic agenda and position in terms of what was then called, in the French tradition, "social solidarism"; others believed that health care as a social issue should be considered an individual right; and still others deemed the problem of tuberculosis part of a broader effort to forge the national race. These differences usually evaporated, however, when it came to the role of the state and its officials. And all agreed they should play an active role as builders of what were increasingly discussed as public health matters. After all, carrying out public health initiatives called for the technical skill of a new professional group that was, in the process, attempting to define its own sphere of influence. These professionals regarded themselves as being knowledgeable and proactive and tried to be independent of the pressures of social and political groups. In fact, higienistas were a professional group that, on the one hand, acted and presented itself to society as doing work that was superior to that of notables, that is, those in control of the conservative republic's quite exclusionary political system. At the same time, as a group they believed they should abstain from representative politics in order to become more efficient and effectively fulfill their enlightened promises.

In this context, the emerging medico-administrative bureaucracy created the modest basis for a relatively autonomous, state-run antituberculosis health care network. Congress doesn't seem to have played a decisive role in this process; legislation on the issue was very limited. Though the topic of tuberculosis was often heard in turn-of-the-century congressional debates, it was usually discussed in the context of other problems like the fight against epidemics, housing for the working classes, Sunday as a mandatory day off, urban hygiene, the eight-hour workday, child and women's labor, and immigration. Only rarely did tuberculosis lead to specific debates; one such debate resulted in the passing of bills aimed at accelerating the creation and, later, the nationalization of the Sanatorio Santa María in the Córdoba foothills.[7] Certain opinions about the issue of tuberculosis were voiced at this time: economic losses due to tuberculosis mortality; the need to democratize the rest cure in sanatoriums, since it had been "effective for the rich, and should be used on the poor"; the advisability of coordinating public and private initiatives in the fight against tuberculosis; and the idea that state intervention on the issue of tuberculosis was part of "a State socialism that would necessarily come to be."[8] The positions and actions of the national and municipal governments were not very different. If on the labor question the government oscillated between reform and repression, the presidents of the republic did espouse the ideology of the public, in which tuberculosis was considered a social issue. Though they were never overly negligent or overly proactive, the conservatives acknowledged tuberculosis as a public issue and took specific, if modest, initiatives, mostly in reaction to pressure exerted by the higienistas lobby. In a message to Congress in 1906 President Amancio Figueroa Alcorta voiced the conservative stance on the tuberculosis issue; he pointed out not only the overcrowding of city hospitals, but also their inability to care for the sick, whom "the State has the duty to protect in order to protect the interests of society as a whole."[9]

The administrations of the Unión Cívica Radical, which took control of the national government after winning the presidential election in 1916 (the first in which all adult Argentinian males were entitled to vote) didn't effect major changes; nevertheless, tuberculosis gained recognition as an unavoidable component of the social question. Policy innovations were the result of a decidedly interventionist discourse that emphasized the state's social responsibilities. In 1917 Aráoz Alfaro supported the idea that the state should intervene in the problem of tuberculosis. Such intervention would ultimately peak during the first Perón administration, between 1943 and 1955, though it was already in the making and indeed partially in effect before the 1940s. Aráoz Alfaro advocated relegating "private charity organizations to a secondary role in the health care of the population, giving them an important, yet temporary, role in handling catastrophes, public calamities, and major unforeseen disasters; [there is a need to organize] an effective and permanent State-based social welfare system. The State has the undeniable obligation to meet people's general needs, even though popular collaboration and initiatives should be welcome."[10]

In this era the state was recognized as a key arbitrator in conflicts between workers and bosses and as a decisive agent in the promotion of a reformist agenda aimed at achieving modest progressive change and social justice. This notion of the state was shared not only by the many factions of the workers' movement, where the discourse of revolutionary change had lost the strength it had had at the turn of the century, but also by the political forces that helped to buttress the parliamentary system and political democracy that followed electoral reform in 1912.

Organized labor deemed tuberculosis to be evidence of unrest and of the need for change. Socialists made tuberculosis part of a more ambitious project aimed at gradually taking over state-run agencies in order to put them at the service of workers. Anarcho-syndicalists considered tuberculosis further proof of the importance of consolidating their control over workplaces in order to fight capitalism. However, except for the bakers' union, organized labor's demands in relation to tuberculosis were sporadic; regardless of their ideology or political affiliation, unions rarely encouraged or initiated specific actions related to the disease. They did speak about tuberculosis, but only in general terms: as a consequence of social injustice and overwork or as a topic connected with other problems, such as the struggle for reducing the workday, the need for better working conditions, and union and ethnic initiatives geared toward providing mutual aid and health care.

In Congress the question of tuberculosis was often discussed in the context of debates brought to the floor by the executive power and by an array of socialist, social Catholic, liberal, radical, and conservative congressmen, many of whom happened to be medical doctors. The debates, as well as the positions represented, were well informed; their tone betrayed a moderate reformist leaning indicative of how most legislators, regardless of their political affiliation or ideology, approached the problem. Owing to the consensus on the need to further the fight against tuberculosis, the debates lacked the ideological bent and passion that marked other congressional deliberations in those years. It was common at that time for socialists to call social Catholics activists of capitalism, for social Catholics to call socialists zealous collectivizing-revolutionaries, and for radicals to try to differentiate themselves from both the conservatives and the socialists. This was not the case when it came to turning the rhetoric against tuberculosis into concrete policies. Though the debates were relatively friendly, their practical results were modest and totally consistent with a Congress that rarely managed to transform initiatives and proposals into specific bills. From 1916 to 1930 Congress was trapped in a sort of paralysis that kept it from using legislation as an effective instrument for advancing a political agenda of social reform. The stasis was attributable partly to the increasing intensity of inter- and intrapartisan conflicts and partly to the Congress's inability to channel increasingly fragmentary social demands.[11]

The bills brought before Congress during this period were not very different from those brought during the period of the conservative republic. Such bills spoke of "the need for the State to intervene in the struggle against the social calamity of tuberculosis"; they called the "defense of people's health" a "primordial function of the State" and the fight against tuberculosis an "essential government duty"; they cited the problem of "pecuniary losses." Legislators stated that "private action is not enough to tackle the problem" because "the fight against tuberculosis must be a collective endeavor, and the State must regard the individual as part of a single social body." Tuberculosis epitomized "the whole social question," and the solving of the tuberculosis problem required "structural changes," although smaller initiatives were "also necessarily useful."[12] Some of these bills were very ambitious, others modest and limited. Specific debated measures included, for example, creating a Comisión Nacional Antituberculosa as a centralized agency in charge of the fight against tuberculosis; prohibiting night work in bakeries; financing the antituberculosis efforts of both state-run and private institutions; setting up a compulsory national health insurance plan for hygiene and tuberculosis prevention; creating institutes to produce preventive and curative serums; training specialists; coordinating the hygienic antituberculosis education of society as a whole; and building urban and mountain sanatoriums and hospitals, anti-tuberculosis wards for children, and summer camps for weak children.[13] One of these initiatives, the compulsory health insurance against tuberculosis as a joint effort of the state, capital, and labor, channeled a recurring and ambitious preoccupation of tuberculosis specialists, most of them well positioned in state agencies and antituberculosis organizations.[14] However, despite all these efforts, the intense discussions about the disease led to the passage of only a few minor bills, mostly those aimed at funding very specific projects or, as with Law 11338, prohibiting night work at bakeries.

During the decade after the military coup in 1930, the state was further consolidated and, along with it, the medical bureaucracy. By then, the need to give the nationwide fight against tuberculosis a clear direction—a goal that had been discussed in the previous decade—was central. In terms of city government, the department of the Lucha Antituberculosa Municipal was established.[15]

In 1930 organized labor was unified in the Confederación General del Trabajo (CGT). At the CGT, syndicalists, socialists, and communists reaffirmed the already dominant agenda that, gradually and through negotiations, sought to improve working and living conditions. Two strategies were developed regarding issues of disease and health. On the one hand, negotiating salaries, regulating the workday, building public housing, guaranteeing paid vacations, and public health insurance were seen as indirect ways of intervening in these issues. On the other, some unions began setting up *mutualidades*, mutual aid institutions supported by workers and employers that provided members with health care, hospital services, and medicine. These efforts began in the thirties and became more pronounced during the first Perón administration.[16]

The obstacles to turning the topics discussed in Congress into specific bills—a problem that had been so apparent during the previous period—didn't vanish, but the debates lost some of their rhetorical luster. Nonetheless, in the late 1930s, during the Agustín P. Justo and Roberto M. Ortiz administrations, there were some legislative achievements. Although it took time to turn them into real actions, more effective legal instruments were coming into being as the question of tuberculosis was becoming nationalized. In 1935 and 1938 legislation mandated the expansion of the Hospital Tornú in Buenos Aires and the building of eighteen new hospitals in the country. It also established twelve flatlands sanatoriums on the Pampa plains. Also in 1935 a law awarded federal funding to the Liga Argentina contra la Tuberculosis in order to create the Instituto de la Tuberculosis, and in 1938 the Comisión Nacional contra la Tuberculosis was created by law, expanding the health care infrastructure in

Buenos Aires and the provinces. The law defined a management structure involving national, provincial, and city governments; it allocated federal funds to encourage the activities of antituberculosis organizations and considered the urgent need to provide worker's insurance against tuberculosis.

A few years earlier, in 1933, the president presented to Congress a welfare bill, one of whose articles stated, "Every Argentine . . . has the right to . . . be recognized by public authorities in the case of extreme need caused by disease." In 1935 a decree issued by executive power supported the "Crusade against Tuberculosis"; another decree, in 1936, urged that tuberculosis be included in a new, expanded list of work-related diseases if a causal connection could be established between a certain job or workplace and the onset of the disease.[17]

Although both the executive branch and Congress based their initiatives and actions on notions formulated in previous decades, they were not only a continuation of past measures and thinking but also signified a more apparent and more articulated resolution to build a social-minded state. President Justo synthesized this shift in a speech in 1935 in which he emphasized that "people's health, in the broadest sense, is the primordial mission of the public powers because all social efforts must be geared toward the welfare of the population. [In the fight against tuberculosis] it's essential to develop unified, extensive action, to take good care of the human being while still at the mother's bosom, and from there onward never to abandon him, not even in death. . . . Take the individual and society, the city and the metropolis, the entire republic, and make them healthy, keep them from evils and make them happier."[18]

Via a number of laws and decrees, the first Peronist administrations put into practice on a new scale many ideas about health care that had been talked about in Congress since the beginning of the century. The executive became a frequent source of bills that were speedily passed by Congress. There was a clear intention to fight tuberculosis throughout the country, beyond coastal Buenos Aires, where there were areas in great need of dispensaries, hospitals, and sanatoriums. In 1947 the *Plan Analítico de Salud Pública* indicated that Buenos Aires had enough hospital beds and that investment should be focused on the provinces, where many of the sick sought care at city hospitals.[19] Generally speaking, the Peronist public health plan focused on early diagnosis, treatment, and follow-up, as well as on the reintegration of cured former patients into working life.

New state-run agencies were the means to enact these projects, many of which were formulated in the past—but were never brought to fruition—by legislators of many ideological backgrounds, including socialism, liberalism, and Catholic nationalism. Although these projects entailed a sustained effort to centralize health care, a single, state-run and universal health care system never developed. Another important feature of the period was the substantial broadening of the hospital network, especially in the provinces. The enactment of the Segundo Plan Quinquenal, in 1952, curbed this expansion significantly, owing not only to the then-apparent limitations of the Peronist project when it came to economic growth and a far-reaching welfare system, but also to the resistance of the organized medical profession, trade union–affiliated health care organizations, mutual associations, and charitable organizations to a fully socialized or state-run health care system.

On social policy matters the Peronist project displayed an emphatic discourse that conceived of health care as a universal, egalitarian right to which everyone should have access. But in reality things were somewhat different. In fact, the Peronist social state produced a very uneven and relatively ineffective health care network based on potentially universal state-run public health institutions, on the one hand, and a large number of fragmentary and differentiated workers' associations, on the other. These associations, some of which had been active since the 1930s while others were created after 1945 with the support of the Peronist administration, gave renewed relevance to health care matters; received substantial financial support from the state; politicized the associationist link as never before; and accelerated the stagnation and decline of traditional mutual associations. In the end, they consolidated themselves as key players in a nonuniversal health care system—the Obras Sociales—run by unions with strong backing by the state.

In the forties and fifties, as a result of the attractive job opportunities resulting from import substitution, many Argentines moved to the litoral region, mainly to Buenos Aires and the metropolitan area. Accordingly, tuberculosis in Buenos Aires, which by then was no longer a major cause of death in the city, came to be associated with domestic migrants confronting urban and industrial life. Their level of tuberculosis immunity was much lower than that of city dwellers. In this new context, the demands on an already insufficient health care system substantially increased, and by the beginning of the 1950s the system also faced the challenge of providing access to antibiotics. By this time, the problem was not one of people dying of tuberculosis but one of sick people who needed access to effective therapy. And access was not equal for everybody. Although the Peronist social state expanded access to health care as never before, it was not able to universalize it. At times the state lacked the political will to advance this agenda. At other times state initiatives were perceived as a threat to trade unions' role in health care, and, furthermore, unionized workers who did have access to health services were frequently indifferent to the egalitarian, universalist principles proclaimed, but never really put into effect, by the Peronist social state. Instead, they willingly participated in a system based on unequal access to the established right to health care and social citizenship.[20]

The Making of a Professional Group and the Antituberculosis Campaign

The initiatives aimed at controlling tuberculosis between 1870 and 1950 were the work of an ideologically heterogeneous group of doctors, including hygienists, public health doctors, and, later, tuberculosis specialists, all of whom combined their humanitarian ideals with attempts at reordering, aiding, monitoring, and reforming Buenos Aires society. Some of them built their professional careers through extended periods, often in full-time positions, of involvement in the new national and municipal agencies focused on tuberculosis. Some combined their private practices with part-time, frequently nonpaid, work at the hospital. If working full-time at a hospital was the way some doctors made a living, for others a part-time position at a hospital, sanatorium, or neighborhood dispensary was a means of gaining the respect of colleagues, confirming their credentials to potential private patients, and demonstrating a true professional commitment to serving society.

Because of the lack of an effective therapy and the social dimensions of tuberculosis, the work of these doctors was defined both in professional terms and in terms of politics and morality. In this context, the figure of the *médico social*, or socially concerned doctor, often emerged in connection with the figure of the *médico político*, facilitating some doctors' path toward becoming mayors, governors, congressmen, senators, or national or municipal cabinet members. The expansion, growth, and bureaucratization of a state-run health-care network made most of these doctors key members of a technico-professional group that was associated with city and national governments. Many of them were able to keep their positions and survived successive political administrations.

The Departamento Nacional de Higiene was established in 1880 and the Asistencia Pública Municipal in 1883. At that time, the city government had already indicated the need to create a commission specifically concentrated on the fight against tuberculosis.[21] By the end of the century, there was talk of "disinfection and prophylaxis to prevent tuberculosis contagion" and of efforts "to separate tuberculosis inpatients from other patients," because the inpatients were crowding not just those wards reserved for infectious diseases but all hospital wards. In the early twentieth century, certain projects that had been in the works for two decades began to materialize: first, the creation of institutions like the Hospital Tornú in Buenos Aires and the Sanatario Santa María in the Córdoba foothills, both specifically focused on the treatment of tuberculosis. Starting in 1910 tuberculosis treatment expanded steadily; out-patient treatment became available at the Hospital Tornú, and neighborhood antituberculosis dispensaries were opened. In the twenties, the Asistencia Pública Municipal opened a specific division, the Dirección de la Lucha Anti-tuberculosa Municipal, which until well into the 1940s fostered the growth of an antituberculosis network with inpatient hospitals, outpatient services, sanatoriums, neighborhood dispensaries, a maternity ward for women with tuberculosis, a service for "relocating the newborns" of tubercular mothers, BCG vaccination, summer camps by the sea, and urban prevention wards for weak children and "pretubercular children." On the national level, in the 1930s the Departamento Nacional de Higiene created a department specifically focused on tuberculosis prevention.[22]

All these initiatives were part of a hygiene reformism that, before and after the electoral reform, aimed at including vast social sectors by enhancing the meaning of social citizenship. It was a slow process, not only in terms of expansion and consolidation of health care institutions but also vis-à-vis the growing social acceptance of medicine. At the forefront was a group of doctors with strong convictions about what role the state ought to play. Drawing from the hygienist tradition of the 1880s and 1890s, which had been vaguely concerned with the fight against tuberculosis and hence could be easily assimilated into general hygienist efforts, in the first decades of the twentieth century these doctors managed to articulate a number of more specific initiatives. Although their efforts didn't do away with tuberculosis, they did spread, with relative success, a new hygienist "catechism" against contagion. At the municipal level, they also helped to consolidate for the first time a specialized medical bureaucracy.

Municipal reformism, which included national government initiatives, paved the way for this process, both at the beginning of the century and in the period between the world wars. The city government had to articulate the interests of the national state, those of an array of local economic forces, and the mostly consumer-oriented demands of the city residents. The antituberculosis welfare bureaucracy was born and developed in this context. Its doctors played a decisive role in creating, directing, and consolidating new municipal and national departments specifically focused on the fight against the disease. Working in these departments, they were able to define a relatively autonomous field of expertise. And as a professional group they weren't only meeting the demands of the state that employed them, but also legitimizing their field as a necessary medical specialization capable of meeting society's new health care requirements.

Once the topic of tuberculosis was on the public agenda, associations of experts on phthisiology came into being. This process did not involve the standard pattern in which the creation of training schools is followed by creation of local, provincial, and national associations, and ultimately, passage of a bill that defined the legal credentials necessary for a certain practice as well as its prerogatives.[23] In this case, it wasn't until the 1920s, after several decades during which the fight against tuberculosis had been led by hygienist doctors in state agencies, that phthisiology emerged as a medical specialization. In 1918 the Asociación de Médicos del Hospital Tornú was created; in 1925 the association was accepted into the Asociación Médica Argentina and renamed Sociedad Argentina de Tisiología. The *Archivos Argentinos de Tisiología* began to be published, and phthisiology became a more central component of the curriculum at the Universidad de Buenos Aires Medical School. Starting at the beginning of the century, several efforts failed to create a *cátedra*, a sort of university chair in the Argentine higher education system, focused on tuberculosis. However, by the mid-1920s and 1930s this project was well on its way and, by the beginning of the 1940s—after an alternative approach that would have included phthisiology as a topic in the existing general medicine courses was ruled out—the Cátedra de Patología y Clínica de la Tuberculosis was created. From the beginning, the cátedra published its *Anales*, one of several medical journals specializing in lung diseases. The Medical School included a postgraduate program for doctors specializing in phthisiology, and in 1940 the Medical School's board of directors stated that all students interested in participating in this program had to have medical degrees. The specialization program took two years; in the 1940s between forty and fifty doctors signed up every year, and half received postgraduate degrees in phthisiology.[24]

By the end of 1940 the Colegio de Médicos Tisiólogos Universitarios was founded and in 1941 the Sociedad de Tisiología del Hospital Nacional Central as well as the Sociedad de Médicos de Estaciones y Sanatorios de Montaña.[25] These organizations were the work not of specialists in tuberculosis, but of graduates of the university specialization program. The associations sought official recognition for the specialist in phthisiology degree in order to gain social prestige and recognition in the market of specialized medical services, chiefly in relation to other doctors who were treating tubercular patients even though they were not specialists.[26] Such aspirations were present long before the colegio was established. For example, in 1924 a bill in Congress aimed to contain not only quacks, but also what were called medical charlatans, that is, medical doctors who, in popular newspapers and magazines, claimed to be "specialists in social diseases" such as tuberculosis and syphilis, a strange combination considering that these two pathologies are quite different: one respiratory; the other, venereal.[27]

But the desires of the associations went unfulfilled, and it proved very difficult to monopolize the right to treat tuberculosis. A number of reasons account for the difficulty, among them the lack of an effective cure, the frequently not very clear symptomatology associated with the disease, the immense number of infected people, and the relative scarcity of specialists in phthisiology. Besides, in addition to phthisiologists who sought to monopolize specialized tuberculosis care, there were other doctors concerned with broader issues of public health who maintained that "a formidable bureaucracy is connected with diseases not in order to fight them, but in order to make a living out of them, [and of these diseases] tuberculosis is the leader." The main argument of public health doctors was that only certain specific bills were being brought before Congress, bills that, instead of fighting the root problem, sought to create employment and positions at state-run health care agencies.[28]

Tuberculosis, then, enabled the growth of a group of phthisiology specialists in a quite peculiar way. Though they emerged at the end of the nineteenth century, it was not until the twenties and thirties did they develop their own professional associations. On the other hand, as a result of their presence in state agencies, they played a central role in making tuberculosis a public health issue. Until the mid-1920s tuberculosis specialists didn't speak as a specialized professional group simply because such a group didn't exist. In spite of that, and because the fight against tuberculosis involved vast sectors of society and had become politicized as a substantive part of the extensive and still imprecise social question, these doctors succeeded in articulating, with a certain degree of autonomy, discourses and initiatives not only from within state agencies and institutions but also from an array of civil society organizations.

The Argentine League against Tuberculosis

Many doctors who ultimately became part of the bureaucracy that led state efforts against tuberculosis came from antituberculosis associations. Having one foot in the state and the other in those organizations, this group attempted to define the best way to fight the disease. The most important association was the Liga Argentina contra la Tuberculosis. Created in 1901, the league proposed to replicate locally the work of its North American counterpart, that is, a private institution that occasionally received state funding. From the beginning it endeavored to build consensus on the urgent need to fight the disease. This agenda became increasingly important after 1935, when the first antituberculosis crusade was presented to the public as an "effort involving us all, regardless of philosophical and political differences."[29]

The league was financed by contributions from its members and by the state, though the government grants were smaller than those given to traditional charities such as the Sociedad de Beneficencia. Close ties with politicians and important bureaucrats often opened access to the state's typographical workshops, allowing free printing of booklets and magazines; to the national post office, allowing free distribution of antituberculosis materials; and to some control over the funds raised in special national or municipal lotteries.[30] The league's unstable finances led it to pursue a number of initiatives, such as the Fight against Tuberculosis Week, periodic public fundraising days, the selling of antituberculosis stamps, and the aforementioned crusade against tuberculosis. All these endeavors aimed at both collecting money from the public and spreading the hygienic antituberculosis code.[31]

The league attempted to exert influence on the state and society by creating public awareness. It was fairly successful in this goal, owing to the participation of doctors who were also appointed to national and municipal public health agencies. The professional trajectories of Aráoz Alfaro, Rodolfo Vaccarezza, Alberto Zwanck, and Juan Cafferata illustrate the double role played by such doctors, building and later working at state facilities while tirelessly promoting antituberculosis initiatives within civil society. The league made antituberculosis education a top priority. Along with specific campaigns, at the beginning of the century it supported journals and magazines like *La Revista de la Tuberculosis*, *La Lucha Antituberculosa*, and *La Alianza de Higiene Social*, and, in the 1930s, *La Doble Cruz*. The league created and financially supported institutions that attended to the needs of poor people afflicted with tuberculosis. Later on these initiatives became the model for similar efforts developed by the state and by ethnic and workers' mutual associations. By the beginning of the century the league was working to found sanatoriums deemed crucial to the rest cure in the foothills. However, it soon became evident that mountain sanatoriums were hardly a real alternative for the thousands of working-class and disadvantaged patients. The league began to focus instead on increasing the number of beds at existing hospitals and on creating and supporting sanatoriums in the countryside, near Buenos Aires, as well as antituberculosis neighborhood dispensaries and special wards for the so-called children predisposed to tuberculosis. Along with the Sociedad Argentina de Tisiología, the league also insisted on the need to coordinate efforts among antituberculosis associations, and in 1936 the Federación Antituberculosa Argentina was created. Its main purpose, which went unmet, was to manage more efficiently the resources of some twenty private ethnic, labor, and professional institutions.[32]

The league was the longest lasting and most influential point of reference for the civil society organizations in the fight against tuberculosis. Starting in the second decade of the century and well into the 1940s there were other initiatives, though they were less long-lived and had a much narrower scope. Mainly the efforts of neighborhood organizations, mutual associations, and even doctors working on their own, they included the Asociación de Ayuda al Niño Débil de Nueva Pompeya, the Liga Israelita contra la Tuberculosis, the Liga Anglo Americana Antituberculosa, the Liga Antituberculosa del Ferrocarril Central Argentino, the Mutualidad Antituberculosa del Personal Civil del Ministerio de Marina, and the Servicios Médicos de la Mutualidad del Magisterio. Other, more ideological groups included the Liga Obrera contra la Tuberculosis and the Liga Roja contra la Tuberculosis, both of which emphasized a radical, class-based interpretation of tuberculosis and offered an alternative to the league's hygiene reformism. These two associations considered tuberculosis an evil that grew out of capitalism and would be eradicated only through profound social change. However, this point of view didn't prevent them from supporting the recommendations and actions carried out by the league and state-run agencies active in the tuberculosis cause. While in ideological terms they stressed the broader issues of exploitation and sought to create a society without "social evil and disease," in practice their initiatives were another way to spread the antituberculosis hygiene code championed by more reformist and less radical organizations. It was in this context that they promoted the creation, without much success, of a Federación de Organizaciones Antituberculosas as "an autonomous organization in charge of directing and orienting the sanitary campaign with state funds."[33]

The Antituberculosis Crusade of 1935

A key event in the history of the fight against tuberculosis in Buenos Aires was the Cruzada Nacional contra la Tuberculosis of 1935. The crusade, which lasted several months, encompassed many of the achievements and failures that characterized six decades of striving related to a major public health problem. According to a plan that never materialized, Buenos Aires was to be the site of a series of campaigns that would later be taken to the provinces. The crusade's organizational structure consisted of an honorary commission along with several other commissions and subcommissions. The president of Argentina presided over the honorary commission; other members included the vice president, several ministers, the mayor of Buenos Aires, the police chief, influential senators and congressmen, religious authorities, diplomats, military leaders, university authorities, and delegates from industrial, business, financial, athletic, and student organizations.

The crusade's objectives could not have been more explicit. On the one hand, it attempted to develop a "permanent popular education campaign" and to recruit a large number of new members who, according to the organizers, would become a sort of "living propaganda." On the other, it intended to raise funds to finish the construction of the Instituto Nacional de la Tuberculosis, a twelve-hundred-bed hospital project started in 1924 but never completed. It soon became evident, though, that the crusade was not meeting expectations, especially in terms of fundraising. As for the educational goals, the campaign's promotional and awareness efforts were very bold and certainly much more ambitious than in any previous campaign. "Everybody was aware of the Crusade," said one of its proud directors. Campaign statistics seem to support this claim: 423,000 posters and banners wallpapered the city; 156,000 signs in public transportation venues; 1,200 billboards in strategic locations; 312,000 brochures with drawings for children at school; 250,000 crusade rosettes and ribbons; and just under 5 million stamps sold for ten or twenty cents.[34] Along with these impressive statistics there were a number of initiatives that made use of what were then called "modern ways of spreading news among the masses." Crusade reports offered detailed accounts of these efforts; some examples illustrate the ambitiousness of the strategy. Everyone listed in the city phone book received the crusade's magazine at home. Without previous announcement, during intermissions of plays and movies, actors informed audiences about tuberculosis prevention. At school, teachers read children stories in which tuberculosis was depicted as Enemy No. 1 and the ferocious wolf. Buildings were covered with posters. Big fabric signs hung in train stations and, downtown, passersby could read news about tuberculosis in brand new neon lights. Every now and then a trolley car was transformed into a big sign. The radio broadcast shows about health reported on the crusade daily and repeatedly announced recommendations to prevent contagion. Newspapers and magazines gave extensive coverage. Troops of ladies and girls sold the crusade's rosettes in the foyers of movie theaters and department stores. More than two hundred conferences were held at factories and workshops, with titles like "Words to the workers" and "Conferences for popular awareness of tuberculosis." Many public collection boxes invited passersby to contribute to the campaign. At soccer fields loudspeakers announced antituberculosis recommendations, urging people to "make our country great by taking care of one's health." Parishes organized conferences and distributed brochures to their members. Famous athletes made public their support for the campaign. Department stores had window displays whose theme was the fight against tuberculosis. One of them combined the modern hygienic optimism of the 1920s and 1930s with the unyielding conviction of medieval knights waging war to conquer the Promised Land. Carved in wood, the effigy of the Crusader against Tuberculosis, complete with sword, helmet, and shield, was designed to capture the attention of both children and adults, encouraging them to join an army of civilians determined to conquer another holy land, the land of health that the prophets of hygiene were promising and announcing.[35]

In terms of money raised, the crusade's outcome was less spectacular. The meticulous accounts included in the report of the crusade demonstrated great care at a time when business scandals were often making headlines.[36] An analysis of the fundraising indicates that the campaign was indeed popular, with numerous small donations that in total constituted the bulk of contributions. Once again, the traditional Argentine elite reaffirmed its enduring tendency to participate in public philanthropy and charity — in fact, many members of the elite sat on the honorary commission as well as other commissions — without investing any of their own money. This time the elite's participation was not restricted to women; both sexes used their political influence to raise money from the state and to involve some of its agencies in the crusade. In any case, the actual monetary contributions they made were insignificant.

Businessmen took part in the campaign through the Unión Industrial Argentina. Taking into account the damage tuberculosis was doing to the workforce, the crusade invited businessmen and factory owners to consider the need to create a social insurance funded by the state, workers, and businessmen. In the eyes of its organizers, the crusade had to be instrumental in overcoming social, political, ideological, and religious differences. According to Rodolfo Vacarezza, the president of the crusade, the goal was to have Argentine society declare its "determination to promote the well-being of workers, whether out of generosity, as a clever way of adapting to new times, or out of demagogical inclinations." Workers were interpellated through the Socialist Party but more as consumers of the antituberculosis credo than as active propagators of it. By the mid-1930s anarcho-syndicalism was in decline, and the Socialist Party was growing in the railways workers' union, which actively participated in the crusade. Unions that had many communist members and a recent history of serious labor conflicts—such the carpenter, metal-lurgical, textile, and construction workers' unions—didn't explicitly support the campaign, though the last three had used Monsignor Miguel de Andrea, a fervent advocate of the crusade, as a mediator in their negotiations with the bosses. Sixteen smaller unions endorsed the campaign, among them the Unión de Obreros Municipales, which represented city government workers, and the Asociación de Empleados de Farmacia, which represented pharmacy employees.

The campaign was a national undertaking that stressed the idea of unity. It was presented to the public as an "enterprise [for] all of us, regardless of philo-sophical and political tendency." Three examples evidence this pursuit of con-sensus. First, the membership of the honorary commission, which, in addition to President Agustín P. Justo and Mayor Mariano de Vedia y Mitre, brought together strikingly divergent characters: the archbishop of Buenos Aires, Luis Copello, and the head rabbi of Argentina, David Mahler; the socialist sena-tor Mario Bravo and the former president of the nationalist and philofascist Liga Patriótica Argentina Manuel Carlés; Senator Lisandro de la Torre, who was later assassinated as a result of his investigation into the meat processing business, and the president of the Cattle Exchange Market, Roberto Dowdall; the president of the Jockey Club, Manuel Alzaga Unzué, and the president of the grocery store owners' association, Manuel Entenza. Second, the opening speeches: in his, Monsignor de Andrea called on "every man who has ideals [not to look at] our differences, but instead observe our similarities [which are] fundamental and permanent; . . . from now on, for the good of the coun-try, let us be more tolerant, more Argentine, more Christian"; the following speaker, the socialist Alfredo Palacios, celebrated the "profound feeling of so-cial justice" expressed by the "admirable Christian" who had spoken before him. And finally, when one of the crusade leaders insisted that "nobody can say this fight is my doing, the work of my profession, my group, my party, my class, or my religion; rather, it must be considered the work of the people and the government, it's the work of us all, work from which nobody is ex-cluded."[37]

Consensus, the Hygiene Code, and the Fight against Tuberculosis

In addition to specific legislation and health services connected to an institu-tional health care and prevention network, the so-called fight against tuber-culosis involved spreading certain hygienic, healthy, and morally respectable lifestyles. It is hardly possible, perhaps impossible, to assess the fight's impact in either the short term or the midterm. It never managed to significantly speed up the already slowly declining rate of tuberculosis mortality. Nor did its new, expanded health services reach most sick people. Until the mid-1940s, before the arrival of antibiotics, initiatives to combat tuberculosis were persistently connected with a feeling of powerlessness and a lack of effective biomedical solutions and strategies.

Nevertheless, the antituberculosis efforts had an undeniable impact on daily life in Buenos Aires. The informal group of doctors who led it, in their capacity as members either of public agencies or of the Liga Argentina contra la Tuberculosis, succeeded in designing an ambitious agenda that was supported, if moderately, by very different political sectors. These sectors emphasized certain aspects of the fight and downplayed others, and their explanations of the deep social causes of tuberculosis in modern society differed. However, they all tended to agree that tuberculosis was a social disease and hence that it was necessary to improve living conditions. In the meantime, education in hygiene had to gain ground rapidly, and the supply of and access to health-care services had to expand. Not unexpectedly, some tensions and conflicts existed, owing to differing perspectives on certain issues, for example, between social Catholics and reformist socialists. But these differences were usually limited to specific issues and were never clearly articulated in legislative projects or policy. Usually the disparities were dissolved in or contained by the actions and discourses of the medical group who, though ideologically heterogeneous, shared an agenda of professional intervention and entailed more similarity than difference. At the core of this agenda was the effort to spread the catalogue of hygienic habits and conducts that supposedly served to avoid contagion. If the fight against tuberculosis was marked by powerlessness when it came to accelerating the decline in tuberculosis mortality and morbidity, the widespread acceptance of the habits it advocated—by common people as well as by diverse ideological sectors—reveals that, even if the results were not exactly what had been intended, the effort was still relatively successful.

Like many other processes that marked modern life, the spread of this hygienic, antituberculosis culture involved social mimicry, learning, novelty, tradition, and coercion. It defined not only behaviors that were believed to be clean and healthy, but also those regarded as filthy and antihygienic. It entailed a specific strategy to prevent the disease as well as a detailed list of everyday habits and moralizing prescriptions. In relatively few years, many of these prescriptions, save for those that were simply impossible to carry out, turned into material and moral requirements of modern urban life.

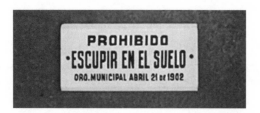

Signs like this one indicating that spitting on the floor is prohibited were usually posted in bars, subway stations, movie theater halls, and public spaces. Spitting was illegal under a municipal ordinance of 1902. (Courtesy Ana Laura Martin)

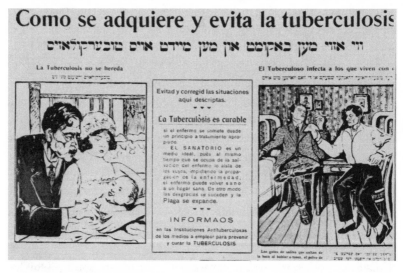

Poster in Yiddish and Spanish, ca. 1930, published by the Liga Israelita Argentina contra la Tuberculosis. It is titled "How to get and avoid TB." (Courtesy Biblioteca Hebrea Argentina Macabi)

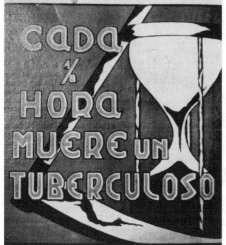

A street poster circulated by the antituberculosis agency of the Buenos Aires city government. It emphasizes specific measures for preventing tuberculosis: "Every half hour a tubercular dies. Early treatment and an x-ray examination of the sick person's relatives could have prevented it." (*Archivos Argentinos de Tisiología*, 1939)

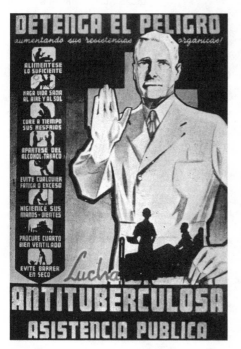

A street poster circulated by the antituberculosis agency of the Buenos Aires city government. It emphasizes general measures—mainly associated with lifestyles—and aims to build individual immunities: "Stop the danger. Strengthen your organic resistances! Eat well; Have a healthy life outdoors; Take good care of your colds; Do not smoke and drink; Avoid any kind of fatigue and excesses; Keep your hands and teeth clean; Have your room ventilated; Sweep floors with wet mops." (*Archivos Argentinos de Tisiología*, 1939)

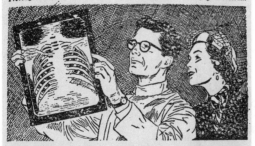

Prevéngase · vaya Ud. mismo y lleve a sus hijos a hacerse una radiografía del tórax.

PROTEJASE CONTRA LA TUBERCULOSIS

● Si la tuberculosis se descubre a tiempo, *puede curarse.* Vea a su médico para hacerse una radiografía de los pulmones. Esta es la mejor manera de descubrir la tuberculosis aun antes de que se presenten los síntomas.

SQUIBB

PRODUCTOS FARMACÉUTICOS
DESDE 1858

A Squib laboratory advertisement encouraging the reader to visit a doctor and get an x-ray: "TB is curable and a radiograph is the best way, even before the symptoms become apparent, to discover if one has TB." (*La Razón*, ca. 1940)

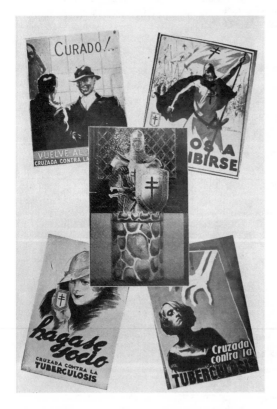

Posters for indoor and outdoor display during the antituberculosis campaign of 1935. Center and bottom left: Two of them invite the viewer to become a member of the Liga Argentina contra la Tuberculosis. (Liga Argentina contra la Tuberculosis, *Memoria de la Primera Cruzada contra la Tuberculosis*, Buenos Aires, 1936)

The effort to spread these new hygienic modes of conduct was felt at the beginning of the twentieth century, when the discourse of fear and defensive hygiene was a crucial resource in the fight against epidemics. It was also present in the 1920s, 1930s, and 1940s, when positive hygiene and prevention ultimately prevailed.

The reception and assimilation of these messages—a sort of antituberculosis and hygienic code—was far from uniform and absolute. It became part of much broader expectations of a new idea of respectability encouraged by organized workers. It was also an individual pursuit of those concerned with social betterment and mobility as opposed to a more ambitious collective project. The code's recommended habits—some of them moralizing, some associated with good taste, some clearly disciplinary, some simply in keeping with the new hygiene rationale—bore meanings that were not necessarily in line with the intentions of the medical group behind the fight against tuberculosis. Occasionally, efforts encouraged by other groups—Catholics, socialists, anarchists, communists—sought to connect individual and family behaviors to ideology. Depending on the case, this entailed further moralizing of the disciplinary contents of the hygienic code or questioning the habits it advocated as instruments being used to perpetuate an unjust social system. Nevertheless, the habits of common people vis-à-vis their hygiene were usually informed not much by ideology but by material limitations and the subjective assimilation of notions and explanations articulated by resilient traditions, as well as domestic and popular translations of modern bacteriology.

None of these accomplishments came as quickly or as effectively as hoped. Indeed, many doctors, some very active in the fight against tuberculosis, warned about the limitations of spreading the hygiene code. In 1940, a few years after the resounding antituberculosis crusade of 1935, Roque Izzo and Florencio Escardó indicated that, in addition to being "general and positive," future campaigns must "emphasize food, housing, and periodical health exams." These doctors discarded spectacular and sporadic strategies which, though well intended, had a limited impact on common people's education in hygiene. Indeed, such strategies were as ineffective as the "hygiene sermons one hears on the radio, which are invitations to change the radio station as fast as you can," or the "amazingly tedious conferences of major figures" whose impact on the audience was negligible. These doctors encouraged going after the targeted audience. They said it was "necessary to have these ideas and sanitary rules accepted just as the brand of a product is imposed on the market."[38] When Izzo and Escardó thought about spreading the hygienic code by using the emerging and increasingly systematized resources of advertising, the culture of antituberculosis hygiene started to become a very respectable value shared by the middle and working classes, including unionized workers associated with the ongoing import-substitution industrialization process. Starting in the 1940s, and more intensely during the first Peronist administration, all of these social groups embraced some aspects of the hygiene culture as part of a newly established right to health and health care, a right in which individual and state responsibility largely complemented each other.

CHAPTER FIVE

The Obsession with Contagion

Tuberculosis contagion entailed not only a preventative and prescriptive discourse on daily norms in the city, but also the notion that if one acted properly the disease could be avoided. In the mid-1930s the magazine published by the Liga Argentina contra la Tuberculosis, *La Doble Cruz*, called the struggle against the disease "an exacting effort" to forge "a widespread awareness that reaches all classes, starting with the most learned but including the least educated working classes, providing a precise idea of how tuberculosis gets its start and how it can be partially or wholly avoided."[1]

The message had to reach everyone because, to a greater or lesser extent, everyone was a potential victim of the disease. Antituberculosis preaching became yet another of the imprecise but enduring recommendations that emphasized individual responsibility and facilitated the gradual spread and acceptance of modern ideals of hygiene. This occurred via many means, from rational appeals to social learning to coercion, intimidation, and propaganda. In the end, the habits of common people, it was expected, would gradually become altered as a result of the discourses on hygiene, whether defensive, involving prohibitions and punishments; informative, involving instruction; or educational, aiming to develop, especially from the 1920s on, a certain behavior in which the values of health and hygiene intermingled with a certain ideal of beauty and modernity.

Many of these hygienic practices were eventually internalized by common people. Such internalization was due not necessarily or exclusively to the resigned acceptance of the disciplinary initiatives of the modern state but to the recognition of the evident material benefits and improvements such practices could provide. From 1870 to 1940 hygiene became not only a sort of obligation for people who wanted to feel they belonged to society, but also a new right, one which more and more social sectors demanded. Hygiene was a set of postulates that used technical language to articulate highly diverse political concerns as well as a value that, in the midterm, was celebrated by both the elite and the working classes, regardless of their political or ideological inclination. Beyond the meaning each person or social group bestowed upon it, personal and collective hygiene became "civilizing" and socializing practices.

In 1868, in inaugurating the potable water system in Buenos Aires, President Domingo Faustino Sarmiento warned that the "educated elite lavishes itself in ablutions crucial to keeping healthy; [whereas] the people, ignorant, though provided with plenty of water, will preserve their slovenliness and intemperate habits so long as their moral and intellectual state does not improve. [Potable water is] necessary and excellent; but if we do not give the people abundant and healthy education, civil war will consume the state and cholera the population."[2]

In fact, Sarmiento was one of many early enthusiasts of the virtues of education when it came to keeping common people abreast of modern methods of hygiene. Throughout the last third of the nineteenth century and into the first decades of the twentieth, new voices, some sophisticated, others less so, from a variety of ideological and political positions contributed to a discourse attentive to the improvement and strengthening of bodies and the changing of daily habits. In 1899, for instance, a pamphlet written by an anarchist and entitled *La Medicina y el Proletariado* harshly criticized the capitalist system but exalted the benefits of and need for personal hygiene.[3] In 1911 the Buenos Aires city government distributed free of charge thousands of pamphlets in seven languages that offered instructions on how to raise children in accordance with modern hygiene.[4] In the late 1920s *La Semana Médica*, a professional and academic weekly journal, stated that key factors in the struggle against tuberculosis included not only an improved standard of living, particularly in nutrition, housing, and income, but also "culture, education and teaching on hygiene for common people."[5] In 1935 both social Catholics and socialists wanted to instruct not only the poor but everyone, regardless of social status, on how to keep their homes hygienic.[6] And in 1943 a magazine financed by the owners of one of the largest textile factories in Buenos Aires included a permanent section on personal hygiene aimed at its female readership. The contents of the section were similar to those in the women's column of CGT, a labor weekly published by the Confederación General del Trabajo.[7]

These examples speak of a discourse that sought to respond to the demands brought on through urbanization and incipient industrialization. In this context, hygiene, like science and education, was presented as a universal value that went beyond social differences and could be an instrument of social change. Regardless of the disciplinary content, the language of hygiene was meant to provide a certain respectability that, it was assumed, would facilitate integration and social recognition. Consequently, hygiene was included in a group of normative and edifying endeavors in which consensus seems to have been, in the midterm, more prevalent than ideological and even political difference.

Spurred by concerns about the mortality and morbidity produced first by infectious diseases and later by so-called social ills such as tuberculosis, syphilis, and alcoholism, the culture of hygiene began to emerge in the last third of the nineteenth century. By the turn of the century it was a part and consequence of a stubborn attempt to bring together medicine, on the one hand, and the social sciences and politics, on the other. The result was called social hygiene, a corpus on which, between 1920 and 1940, public health would be based. Driven in large part by professional and political sectors strongly influenced by positivism—among them those who claimed to speak in the name of workers—social hygiene brought together a range of strategies and objectives. Two were particularly important: first, providing the elite with a safe urban environment in which epidemics were under control; second, protecting vast sectors of society from the risk of contagion in the broadest sense and, as a result, including them in the modern social world as respectable, efficient, and productive individuals. Hygienic culture was furthered by educators, doctors, politicians, and bureaucrats. Even more than education, this topic encouraged consensus; it was a terrain where the statements of liberals, socialists, radicals, Catholics, conservatives active in social reform, and even some anarchists largely coincided. This sort of lay catechism on hygiene, it was thought, would be a means to inclusion in the modern life of the city. The idea was not limited to Argentina: similar versions of this discourse, with inevitable local adjustments, accompanied the advent of modernity, as well as the struggles against tuberculosis, in many other places, from Europe to Japan, from the Americas to Egypt.

Starting at the end of the nineteenth century and through the first half of the twentieth, the ideas of collective and personal hygiene became more sophisticated. The development of modern bacteriology was decisive to their social and cultural acceptance. It also entailed new challenges for "the common man" and his efforts at understanding those novelties. At the turn of the century the catalogue of hygienic behavior demanded that one not only be free of microbes, germs, and bacteria, but also believe that these agents, no matter their inconspicuousness, were the materialization of disease. Now, in addition to the known enemy generally associated with surface dirt, there was another, invisible one. In a relatively short period the hygienic code had worked its way into an endless number of realms of social and individual life: the world of the hospital, where hygiene was supposed to be asepsis; the world of the home, where hygiene was associated with cleanliness and ventilation; the world of work, where hygiene was an issue of environmental standards at factories and workshops and, to a lesser extent, one related to overwork; the world of the street, where hygiene insinuated the risk of indiscriminate contact with other people and with any kind of trash; and also into the personal sphere, where not only hygienic daily rituals but also vaccinations were thought to be crucial to boosting immunity. Gradually, hygiene became a complex question of intersecting values. In addition to the specific task of fighting disease, hygiene was steeped in ideas of morality and respectability, as well as psychosocial phenomena that involved questions of self-approval, individual responsibility, self-discipline, narcissism, ideas about enjoying life, and the consumption of new symbolic and material goods that were thought to promote health.

For those engaged in the daily battle against tuberculosis, the persistence of certain habits and beliefs was a challenge. After decades of effort, the *Archivos Argentinos de Tisiología* suggested the need to "impose, by law, preventive rules and practices, to suppress or alter people's habits, customs, and tradition which—though they will deny it—cannot be changed without coming up against deeply ingrained concepts and modalities."[8] It was in the framework of these efforts that, in 1936, one hygienist defined the two aims of the struggle against tuberculosis: "To avoid at any cost that the disease be passed on to the healthy, and to render all organisms vigorous and resistant enough so that, even if the infecting microbe attacks them, they will not develop the disease."[9] Such talk of the struggle against contagion had already been heard as early as the 1880s, when modern bacteriology had confirmed the contagious, not hereditary, nature of tuberculosis and had begun to focus on destroying the bacillus. From then on the recurring questions were what to do with people suffering from tuberculosis, how to regulate their presence in the family unit and in society, and how to gauge the potential risks associated with their free circulation around the city. In the late nineteenth century, the isolation of the sick person, whether compulsory or voluntary, was common medical practice; tuberculars were not allowed to mingle either with healthy people or people with other infectious diseases. Later, the solutions proposed for handling the disease were modified, and phthisiology and respiratory medicine acknowledged the existence of benign, almost inevitable contagion: "It [the bacillus] is found everywhere, in streets, parks, trolleys, gathering places; there is benign contagion . . . which is hardly dangerous to those with a healthy organism." Indeed, because it is "slow, gradual, and weak," this sort of contagion "might even prevent the disease itself."[10]

Nonetheless, inevitable benign contagion did little to counteract the ethos of fear surrounding tuberculosis. Though fear was largely a constant throughout the history of the disease, there were changes in emphasis. In the last third of the nineteenth century tuberculosis was seen as just another dangerous epidemic, one of the many infectious diseases that had to be controlled through improved urban sanitary infrastructure. Over time the discourse on hygiene grew more complex. Although there were concerns with disorder, degeneration, instability, and even a certain alarmism owing to a recent history of devastating epidemics, a much more optimistic vision of the future also emerged. Based on the beneficial expansion of the drinking water and sewage systems, this discourse insisted on the need to strengthen people's bodies and to forge the "national race." There was still talk of diseases—especially of tuberculosis and syphilis, much less so of other infectious diseases that were becoming part of the past—but what was new was a focus on health, not only its preservation but also its improvement. Indeed, health became a broad metaphor that affected an array of situations, from physical education and leisure time to marital morality, from child rearing to sexuality, from nutrition to clothing, from housing to work. At the beginning of the new century, concerns with physical wellness, moral perfection, family, and social harmony were important to the agendas of all reformists, regardless of their ideology. The Primer Congreso Nacional de Medicina, held in 1916, heralded "the ideal of bestowing on all organisms, with the aid of a perfectly hygienic life, enough resistance to triumph against contagion."[11] This ideal of integral individual health, as opposed to the collective emphasis that characterized the struggle against infectious diseases, grew more and more sophisticated. In 1940 "physical robustness" was associated with "correct moral attitudes," "spiritual serenity," and "immunization against the attack of foreign germs."[12] Regardless of its real impact on people's lives, this sort of preaching was meant to prevent tuberculosis and communicate hygienic habits, as well as to bring to the poor and working classes the advances of the modern world. To some extent, then, it entailed an integrationist effort.

Between the end of the nineteenth century and the very beginning of the twentieth, antituberculosis discourse was vaguely marked by the idea of prevention. The tone of *Instrucciones contra la propagación de la tuberculosis*, dated 1894, imparted a sense of emergency, fear of contagion, and the need to disinfect almost everything.[13] But the antituberculosis advice that circulated widely in the second quarter of the twentieth century was marked by a much more educational language. Though in 1936 *La Doble Cruz* made reference to practical measures to avoid contagion, it emphasized "invigorating bodies and building resistance to microbes." This catalogue of recommendations on health, which its promoters described as "indirect tuberculosis prophylaxis," set out to develop a program based not only on a network of institutions that provided protection and care, but also on an ambitious effort to model the everyday habits of society as a whole.[14]

From very early on, starting in the mid-nineteenth century, school was seen as a strategic institution. Conveying the antituberculosis hygienic program to an audience of students demanded a great deal of specificity, but also encompassed the conviction that investing in childhood was investing in the future of the nation. However, when an effort was made to communicate this program to a wider, less clearly defined public, it was necessary to come up with a vaguer approach that made use of a battery of resources, from manuals, pamphlets, movies, and radio programs on home hygiene to newspaper articles, conferences, comics, billboards, and laws. Three topics dominated this broad message: the war on sputum and dust, the female corset, and the sexuality of those suffering from tuberculosis.

The Antituberculosis Program in Schools

From the dawn of the century, childhood was strategic to the communication of the hygienic code, which included different biomedical approaches to child rearing, new standards for child growth and development, an international movement that placed value on childhood per se, the expansion of public education, and an increasing preoccupation with and condemnation of child labor. The role of children in the plan to communicate the culture of hygiene is evident throughout the first half of the century in an array of initiatives, from children's competitions and contests to publications geared toward boys and girls. Articulated around a set of enduring basic ideas that seem untouched by political change, the discourse of child hygiene rested, on the one hand, on the values of childhood innocence and purity in a modern urban world riddled with disease, and, on the other, on an exaltation of home and family hygiene in contrast to the dangerous, dirty, and immoral world of the street. In 1900s articles profusely illustrated with photographs, *Caras y Caretas* promoted and reported on contests for the best-cared-for babies. In the 1920s the socialist newspaper *La Vanguardia* encouraged similar initiatives organized by the Club de Madres during the *Semana de Nene* in the hopes that such a "children's week" would contribute to "improving the race through the diffusion of hygienic norms." The values of hygiene and personal cleanliness as a means of avoiding contagion also appeared in *Billiken*, a magazine from the 1930s that set out to entertain while raising the moral standards of children in Buenos Aires without the mediation of parents' reading. During the first Peronist administrations, between 1943 and 1955, *Mundo Infantil* (which translates to "children's world") was another publication that sought to bring the official rhetoric of social justice to the home while reaffirming hygienic and respectable modes, habits, and customs.[15] A hygienic and healthy childhood increasingly became an objective in and of itself, as well as a key argument in advertising campaigns that found in children a very attractive and potentially lucrative market.

The tone of the communication of the hygienic program to children in schools—and, through them, the family—barely changed over time: the textbooks and brochures, the contents of the curriculum and the teaching materials evidence the enduring commitment to divulging daily hygiene habits to prevent contagion. These messages were present from an early date. An article published in the newspaper *La República* in 1871, when much emphasis was still placed on urban sanitation and general hygiene, announced an agenda that would last until the 1950s. This agenda included teaching hygiene in grade schools in order to provide "children with a physical and moral education." It underscored the need for "teachers and disciples to have at hand a booklet containing the rules of hygiene . . . [which], when taken home by the children, would contribute to eliminating the crass ignorance that reigns among the people."[16] At the turn of the century, the availability of these materials increased exponentially, and they were offered in a variety of formats. In 1899 *El Monitor de la Educación Común*, published by the Ministerio de Instrucción Pública, informed its readers, mostly teachers, of the results of a contest for the best *máximas de higiene*, or educational statements on hygiene, with which to support the teaching of this topic in grade schools. During those years and into the 1910s, the publication came with a monthly supplement entitled *La Higiene Escolar* that contained articles on educational experiences abroad as well as announcements of conferences and practical advice aimed at efficaciously conveying hygienic norms, from the importance of cleaning one's mug to concerns with children who smoke, from the supposedly noxious effects of soccer to the benefits of methodical gymnastics. In 1902 Francisco Súnico, a doctor who directed the Inspección Médica de Instrucción Pública at the beginning of the century, published a six-hundred-page book entitled *Nociones de Higiene Escolar*. In it, he examined an array of issues, including the orientation of school buildings, the size of desks, the design of bathrooms, and children's posture and oral hygiene.[17] In the early 1920s an article published in *El Monitor de la Educación Común* advocated a program that would provide "indirect tuberculosis prophylaxis by getting children used to body and environmental hygiene and [by conveying to them] notions of epidemiology"; the program was meant to "attend to and oversee" the hygiene not of "upper-class children," but rather of "the poor classes" to whom the institution of the school was obligated.[18]

Posters were among the materials geared toward grade school students. Using clear language and a writing and design style intended to capture children's attention, one of them, dated 1922, urged a child to make a "personal commitment" to meeting the "commandments of health," reading them every day "until he knew them by heart" and teaching them to his friends.

The posters stressed the recurring themes of the antituberculosis hygiene outreach campaign: from proper breathing to weekly bathing and frequent washing of hands and teeth, from the risks of spitting on the ground to the risks of drinking from a glass that had been used by others.[19] Brochures were another popular means of conveying notions of hygiene. Prepared mostly by the Asistencia Pública Municipal and the new Museo Municipal de Higiene, the brochures were distributed by the thousands. They invited people "not just to read but also to remember" antituberculosis instructions and advice, to "repeat them," to "learn to protect oneself from the disease," to "learn to live healthily . . . in the hopes that [one's child would become] a good and sound Argentine, the pride and honor of the country."[20] In grade school textbooks, personal cleanliness was mentioned time and again for decades.

High school textbooks also offered instruction on the measures to take in the war against tuberculosis contagion. The textbook written by María Arcelli, which was widely read and published in several editions during the 1930s, listed objects, goods, and daily habits that, if properly managed, would help to defeat tuberculosis and avoid contagion. The author warned readers to avoid "the dust that floated in the air in rooms and enclosed places, kisses, insects, especially flies, certain foods like nonpasteurized milk and butter, objects that have been in contact with people with tuberculosis, their saliva, sputum, sweat, and urine; drinking alcoholic beverages such as aperitifs, absinthe, wine, etc." Her list of prohibitions included "immoderate exercise"; "excesses and anything that might tend to put the body in a state of constant fatigue"; the drinking of *mate con bombilla*, a popular infusion consumed via a metal straw, especially "when the same straw is used by several people at the same time"; and "the habit of using handkerchiefs to dust soccer boots." Her readers had to beware of "constant colds" and "persistent coughs that had not been aptly treated"; long stays in "closed and damp places"; "using money, whether bills or coins, when they had touched others' mouths"; "inadequate or immoderate clothing"; and, last, "living with people with tuberculosis, especially mothers or women who are breastfeeding babies."[21]

The educational campaign was also evident in congressional bills and debates. In 1921 Congressman Leopoldo Bard, of the Unión Cívica Radical, proposed a bill to create a department for teaching social hygiene. The department would be part of the Ministerio de Justicia e Instrucción Pública, and it would emphasize tuberculosis prevention, sex education, child rearing, and the fight against quackery in schools, factories, workshops, military institutions, and large markets and warehouses.[22] In 1933, as part of a far-reaching and detailed proposal to create a Comisión Nacional de la Tuberculosis, the Catholic congressman Juan Cafferata encouraged mandatory education in tuberculosis prevention at schools. He argued that schoolchildren would communicate to "their homes the great importance of prophylaxis and set their loved ones on the way to the local clinic or doctor's office."[23] However, it was not until 1947 that these proposals were passed: Law 13039 made it mandatory to teach hygiene.

Regardless of how long it took for these initiatives to become law, schools and teachers were already imparting hygiene habits, routines, and rituals. Indeed, for quite some time both educational institutions and educators had been exposed to the issue of hygiene. Starting in 1904 these issues were discussed every three years at the International Congress of School Hygiene. Topics included school buildings, premises, and furniture, teacher training, and the curricular approach to hygiene at school and how it would differ from the approach at the military barracks. These meetings also discussed the role of the school doctor, an issue that pervaded many articles published in local professional journals. However, the distance between reality and rhetoric was great: in Buenos Aires in 1922 there was one school doctor for every fifteen thousand students, a far cry from the proportion recommended at the time, one doctor per thousand children.[24]

In the early twentieth century the official *El Monitor de la Educación Común* approached the issue of hygiene from a general perspective: it attempted to train educators in the problems of contagion and facilitated the dissemination of the *Cartilla de la higiene escolar*, a sort of brochure-form hygienic catalogue, without fully working out the curricular contents. Start-

ing in the 1920s *La Obra*, a magazine that was representative of the innovative education encouraged by those enthusiastic with the ideas of the Escuela
Nueva, promoted the replacement of hygiene as a discipline with plans organized around thematic nodes. Not until 1936 did the Ministry of Education
finally incorporate parts of this proposal, viewing personal hygiene, clothing,
and nutrition as "the needs of the children" that must be tackled from a multi-
disciplinary perspective.[25] For fifteen years the magazine contained a section
entitled "didactic practice," with articles focused on the human body from a
perspective that brought together hygienic, moral, and medical dimensions; it
recommended conduct that would prevent diseases such as tuberculosis and
prioritized hygiene, prevention, and morality over science. There were advise-
ments on how to teach children to take care of their bodies, how to live in the
modern city, which ventilation system was preferable, how to use appliances
properly, and how to inculcate the habit of and actually perform a daily bath.
In the early thirties the study of hygiene was beginning to be displaced from
its central position by the study of anatomy and the physiology of the human
body, though no mention was made of the urinary, excretory, or reproductive
systems.

In 1947 a contributor to the *Archivos Argentinos de Tisiología* used arguments similar to those found seven decades earlier in the newspaper *La República* to praise the school as a means of communicating the hygienic code:
"It is in childhood that the effort to create an antituberculosis consciousness
will be truly efficacious; there lies the soft clay, the impressionable matter
capable of receiving suggestions on new behavior and of suppressing habits,
customs, and traditions. . . . School is where the State's action must begin."[26]
Throughout the first half of the twentieth century, school was where the state
attempted to order the body; to integrate society; to combine cultural and material respectability with patriotism; and to impose an enlightened hygienism
willing to use whatever it took, starting with daily routines, to carry out the
personal cleanliness project as a defense against contagion and as a physical
manifestation of morality.

Spitting and Dust

Of the clearest signs or evidences of tuberculosis—cough, perspiration, fevers,
diarrhea, and weight loss—sputum and dust were the most feared and the
most instrumental in underlining the importance of bacteria and germs in
the fight against disease and contagion. Sputum and dust were pillars of the
prevention agenda; they were also indicative of the inevitable difficulties that

came with educational and media attempts at instructing vast sectors of modern Buenos Aires on the new ideals of health and cleanliness.

Experimental germ theory was useful in defining strategies to combat and prevent the disease. It made use of new techniques such as laboratories and microscopes, and, in the long run, it replaced "sanitary science," which explained diseases as the result of the action of miasmas and ferments that incubated in the air, the ground, and the water. Germ theory postulated that diseases were caused by living microorganisms—in the case of tuberculosis, the bacillus discovered by Robert Koch in 1882—and that the aim of bacteriology should be the elimination of these microorganisms wherever they might be, in human beings' tubercular lungs or in the objects people with tuberculosis had had contact with. In the laboratory it had been proven that microorganisms could not survive at high temperatures or in the presence of certain disinfectants. The great challenge was to control or eliminate objects that, it was thought, were infected by these germs.

Before the arrival of germ theory, disinfectants were used to purify the air in rooms; to bathe the sick and cadavers; and to clean clothing, furniture, pipes, and areas where there had been excrement.[27] Thanks to the expansion of public services in the last third of the nineteenth century and the enthusiasm of bacteriologists who were discovering new germs in the laboratory, a number of sophisticated discourses and practices were designed to reform individual daily habits. This reform project, one that condensed the private dimension of public health, demanded that a significant sector of the population become familiar with the basics of modern bacteriology.[28] People were asked to believe and accept the idea that microorganisms—those living particles, like bacilli, that could be seen only through a microscope—were the agents of contagion and that a sick person's secretions scattered them in the environment, facilitating the transmission of diseases.

Convincing people of this was not an easy task, especially considering that it was impossible to see, feel, or smell germs. Furthermore, just as the few who worked with microscopes in experimental bacteriology labs attested, these germs had a vigorous life in the human body and especially in its discharges, evacuations, and excretions. Consequently, everyday gestures like touching an object or kissing a child began to be perceived as potentially dangerous because they might aid the transmission or exposure to germs.

To confront the tuberculosis bacillus, bacteriology enlisted disinfection and the modification of the lifestyles of both the sick and the healthy. The *Instrucciones para prevenir la tuberculosis* (1894) indicated the need to control and disinfect the sputum of those with tuberculosis. It was deemed necessary to separate and meticulously clean their eating utensils and bed linens and to clean, ventilate, and air their rooms. Healthy people were advised to expose the rooms of their houses to the sun as often as possible. They were told to avoid the accumulation of dust, to boil milk, and to kill flies.[29] This arsenal of suggestions recommended not only avoiding shaking hands—something that an enthusiastic urbanite convinced of the benefits of this new custom could be expected to do—but also controlling a world of objects and monitoring an array of situations whose cleanliness could never be known for certain: clothing bought at stores or a tailor's, the handle of a neighbor's door, the water glass at a restaurant, the paper money used to pay for the daily shopping at the market. The *Instrucciones* maintained that sick people should be aware of their ability to transmit the disease and urged healthy people to live according to certain standards of hygiene in order to avoid contagion. Led by doctors, municipal and national agencies, and civic groups, the program of communicating antituberculosis behavior was directed not only at the poor, who were often connected with the disease and the unhygienic practices that propagated it, but also at the homes of the emerging middle classes and the elite, whose material well-being did not necessarily mean hygienic ways of living, at least not according to the new standards postulated by modern bacteriology.

At the beginning of the twentieth century the fervor to regulate interpersonal contact and keep objects free of infection gradually died down. The change was largely explained by an incipient understanding that contagion was somewhat more complex than mere contact, and that many of the germs were inoffensive and did not live for long. The existence of microorganisms associated with dirt and excretion could not in and of itself explain contagion. And strict compliance with hygienic standards and recommendations was illusory. Over time hygiene as an urgent response to recurrent epidemic outbreaks of infectious diseases was slowly vanishing. There was still a belief in the benefits of disinfection owing to, among other things, a lack of convincing explications of and solutions to the problem of tuberculosis contagion. However, in a context in which public medicine had proven somewhat efficacious in reducing the mortality of infectious diseases in general, staying healthy and avoiding contagion ended up being associated with the benefits of education, nutrition, individual treatment of the sick, and their separation from the world of the healthy. While around 1940 there was talk of ways to avoid tuberculosis contagion, x-rays arose and were presented as a new, efficacious alternative for early detection, one more respectful for individuals than the more traditional public health interventions—such as the "mandatory and invasive disinfections"—which were not always well received by the sick and their families.[30]

But these novelties came in the 1930s and 1940s. In the late nineteenth and early twentieth centuries, an arsenal of specific recommendations influenced by germ bacteriology dominated the scene. In both journalistic and medico-professional discourses, simple contact was confused with contagion, and life in the city was seen as riddled with the risk of infection.[31] The noxious consequences of sputum and unhealthy dust lurked everywhere: in factories, workshops, homes, restaurants, hotels, coffee shops, brothels, churches, movie theaters, military barracks, schools, streetcars, trains. Through the war on spitting and the war on dust, everyday hygienic manners were connected to a wide array of situations and objects, from clothing to new ventilation and aeration techniques, from the proper use of brooms to praise for the hygienic benefits of vacuum cleaners.[32]

"THE WAR ON SPITTING" AND INDIVIDUAL HYGIENE

Toward the end of the nineteenth century intense efforts were made to understand what made a certain individual more vulnerable to infection than another. Until the arrival of antibiotics in the late forties, controlling the bacillus became a priority of antituberculosis efforts. In that context sputum came to be seen as a source of contagion and the site where the bacillus was incubated. The sick, the potentially sick, their family members, and doctors obsessively observed spitting, coughing, and sneezing. Labored breathing along with a dry cough that produced sputum or, even worse, bloody sputum, were thought to be fairly certain signs that one had contracted the disease.

Organizing a campaign against spitting meant dealing with questions of public health and focusing on reforming everyday individual behavior. Measures aimed at the individual—the public identification and official registration of the sick, doctors' obligation to publicly declare who was sick, and the forced disinfection of patients' belongings, for example—generated an array of responses, from acceptance to rejection and even resistance. But an attempt to educate the population about the risks associated with sputum—that is, how germs might affect one's organism and facilitate contagion—necessitated a much more persuasive strategy. Unlike milk and meat, which were also associated with the transmission of the bacillus, sputum had no market value and no groups were invested in influencing the tone of what was said about the war on spitting.

On the basis of the notion that sputum was a medium in which the bacillus stayed active, the goal became to disinfect everything that might come into contact with the expectorations of people with tuberculosis. From the beginning, this crusade revolved around preventing contagion.

Three priorities were repeatedly stated in 1912 in a series of pamphlets for workers, housewives, and conscripts: "Strengthening individual resistance, limiting the spread of the germ, and preaching against spitting on the ground."[33] The potential reader of these pamphlets, which were put out by the Departamento Nacional de Higiene, received a simple and direct message: participate in the "war on spitting," whose ends, its propagators confessed, were to stop the spread of the disease and teach customs in keeping with the new gospel of hygiene: "Sputum, whether fresh or dried and reduced to dust, is the basic cause of the spread of tuberculosis. When fresh it can contaminate hands, books, everyday objects, etc. and, through the digestive tracts, be transported by flies into our organism. When pulverized and dry, these dusts can settle and reach us . . . through the air we breathe. . . . Tuberculosis spreads not because it is highly contagious but because we are careless; . . . it is an avoidable disease and the most efficacious and easiest way to avoid it is individual hygiene, taking care not to spit on the ground, whether indoors or outdoors. We must wage a war on spitting."[34]

In emphasizing spitting, bacteriology appealed to a well-established tradition that associated disease with dirtiness and the advisability of disinfecting and cleaning. Spitting was seen as a dirty, vulgar, promiscuous, and aesthetically displeasing habit; it offended and suggested ignorance, a lack of respect for social norms, and a dangerous individualism. Spitting was made out to be a transgressive habit that undermined the rules of social coexistence and that, if absolutely unavoidable, should be done in private. However, this had not always been the case. Starting at the end of the eighteenth century, for reasons that had nothing to do with medicine, many regions in Europe began to consider certain bodily smells, excretions, and fluids unpleasant. Spitting came to be seen as repugnant.[35] But between the end of the nineteenth century and the beginning of the twentieth the war on spitting articulated this repugnance through modern bacteriology, associating disease with dirt and with the need for and advisability of disinfecting and cleaning. Spitting was becoming a soiled habit, vulgar, promiscuous, aesthetically unpleasant, offensive, and disrespectful of norms.

Putting an end to the habit of public spitting and to its consequent transmission of infectious saliva entailed an array of initiatives, from the dissemination of information about its dangers to the promotion of self-control. People were advised to act in a certain way, and, starting in the early twentieth century, city ordinances against spitting on the ground were issued. Everyone, whether healthy or sick, had to adapt to these new habits that, it was thought, would break the chain of contagion. The sick must do so for obvious reasons and the healthy because they might have tuberculosis and not know it. In any case, an appeal was made to individual responsibility. In 1905 *La Semana Médica* spoke of the need to disinfect paper money and library books. It was crucial, the publication underlined, to "reeducate users" not to touch books or money "with fingers wet with saliva. Nor should they sneeze or cough over these objects."[36] Four decades later signs in streetcars in Buenos Aires read, "Anyone, even a healthy person, who spits on the ground sows microbes."[37]

The emphasis on re-education was crucial to defining the figure of a citizen who was responsible for his own health and the health of others. This entailed the notion of a subject capable of self-control because he is aware of the risks and dangers associated with sputum and saliva. This re-educational drive was formulated in messages that originated with the state, which was willing to intervene in peoples' private lives, and in civil society. The issue appeared time and again in school curricula, since schools were one of hygienists' preferred sites for shaping the hygiene habits of children and teenagers. The problem of sputum also influenced recommendations on how to manage the interpersonal relationships of adults when, for example, it was suggested to "keep a prudent distance in conversations," "cover one's mouths with a handkerchief when one has to cough," and "not spit just anywhere, and only in personal spittoons."[38] According to one hygienist in 1915, the pocket spittoon should be as common as the handkerchief: "Isn't not using a handkerchief to blow your nose seen as a sign of bad manners? Well, let's make the same thing hold true of the pocket spittoon." The personal spittoon would provide an education in mutual control, since any individual would feel he or she had "the right to point out anyone who spits nearby, protecting his health and the health of others."[39] Even the very Argentine ritual of sipping mate was addressed by antituberculosis re-education. In 1936, in a tone both imperative and persuasive, *La Doble Cruz* encouraged doing away with the "primitive and dangerous [custom] of [drinking] mate." It recommended not sharing the *bombilla*, or metal straw, "even with personal friends." *Viva Cien Años* called the bombilla a "sure vehicle of contagion."[40]

The concern with creating a hygienic citizen who exercised discipline to avoid contagion was even more intense in the case of tuberculars, for whom sputum was believed to cause reinfection and worsen their already precarious state. For those who had been admitted to hospitals or sanatoriums, the incorporation of the arsenal of small recommendations was less problematic.

These institutions not only provided rest and a healthy diet, but also served to teach prevention and foster the mindset and discipline necessary to change daily habits. Hospital staff and relatives, when treatment was given at home, were key to creating tubercular patients who were aware of their limitations and the dangers their lifestyle could imply for others. In the words of the head of a boardinghouse for people with tuberculosis in the Córdoba foothills, the sick resident must "become a cautious being, who knows how to accept what is required by the rules of commonsense and moderation, . . . who knows what he should and should not do." And the proper handling of sputum— "not swallowing it," "putting it in a pocket spittoon," and "not spitting on the ground"—was at the top of the long list of appropriate behaviors.[41]

The problem, though, lay with sick people who were not in institutions; as those who led the war on sputum well knew, this was the case of most people with tuberculosis. The great challenge was how to deal with tuberculars who still went from home to workplace, who kept going to the movies and the coffee shop, who wandered around the city coughing and spitting, not the least concerned or even aware that these acts furthered contagion. In light of this fact, the best thing to do was to undertake a broader educational effort aimed at the general public. In the process, the dangers associated with sputum were endowed with meanings that went beyond the prevention of tuberculosis and became part of an ambitious project of social and moral reform. This project assumed the need to produce a citizen who understood that the proper management of sputum was connected to obtaining a respectable and respected place in the modern world.

THE WAR ON DUST AND DOMESTIC HYGIENE

The war on spitting, addressed to men and women, adults and children, was part of an education campaign against contagion intended to "build a collective mentality" while taking into account the need to use "different messages for different publics and settings."[42] Women were the primary targets of the war on dust and the broader prevention of tuberculosis. The home, after all, was a woman's terrain, and she was the one most equipped to ensure hygiene: she could apply practical advice and impart the gospel of preventative hygiene to the members of her family.

Though women's central role in the home was nothing new, the effort to run the home in keeping with the notions of bacteriology was. Applied to very specific everyday situations, these notions formulated a sort of domestic bacteriology aimed at preventing tuberculosis and other diseases. In this way, women became part of the public and private health crusade led by men while reaffirming their decisive role in family life. The home economics manuals and antituberculosis leaflets written by doctors, as well as the instructions prepared by Asistencia Pública, exemplify the new contents of women's role in the family.[43] The information in these publications, which were published throughout this period, included the most basic concepts of home hygiene, practical advice, and fairly complex explications of how germs affected the home environment. The domestic bacteriology discussed in the manuals was presented as a practical science, capable of teaching wealthy women the benefits of using the latest appliances to improve hygiene and of providing information about the proper management of domestic help; for less wealthy women, these manuals indicated inexpensive ways, some of which were simple while others demanded great effort and organization, to keep the house clean and supposedly germ-free. Rich and poor women alike were instructed in their role of conveying basic bacteriology—that is, habits and customs that were believed to help prevent the spread of tuberculosis—to their families. However, during the 1930s and 1940s the emphasis on this role was becoming somewhat less central. This was partly because medicine had become more prevalent and advanced, partly because some of the measures recommended by domestic bacteriology had proven ineffective, and partly because public and private hygiene managed by men made substantive inroads into what had been a field controlled by women. By that time, hygiene was more connected to laboratories, x-rays, vitamins, healthy diets, vaccinations, and early education, all of which conspired to make domestic hygiene less important.

During the last third of the nineteenth century, home hygiene combined old and new concerns: what to do with excretions, stagnant water, trash, and dirt were certainly not new problems. The issues of overcrowding and the lack of natural light and ventilation were indeed new and crucial to the agendas of hygienist doctors and architects, many of whom were influenced by miasmatic theories. The advent of germ bacteriology made way for the conviction that, just like the body, a house was clean when it did not have visible signs of dirt and when it did not harbor dangerous microorganisms. It was at this point that domestic dust became a recurring concern.

Bacteriology contributed to instilling the belief that anybody could get sick by inhaling unhealthy dust. It was also decisive in making people think that any household object—furniture, dishes, curtains—could hold microorganisms that might linger for months until some circumstance like a fly or a breeze brought them into contact with healthy individuals who would consequently get sick. At the same time, bacteriology was warning that at certain temperatures and humidity levels microorganisms could survive outside the body. The sun, however, destroyed most such microorganisms quickly. Similarly, microorganisms, including the Koch bacillus, were more apt to survive in enclosed settings than in open spaces.

On these grounds the war on dust in the home was launched. In his *Gobierno, administración e higiene del hogar*, dated 1914, Angel Bassi repeated what many others, both before and after him, said about the issue: "Air can be a bearer of diseases, . . . it holds floating tuberculosis bacilli that come from dried sputum that transmits infection via the respiratory tract, spreading variolar crusts that are likely to be contagious."[44]

The war on dust was in some respects a preventive hygienic measure aimed at those who wanted to stay healthy; it was also a recognition of the fact that the majority of sick people spent most of their time at home (only a small number were hospitalized). Once again, the home economics manuals and antituberculosis leaflets and instructions show the intensity and detail with which dust was treated. Its presence as a concern was ongoing, and the way it was handled changed only slightly over the course of several decades. Among the recommendations, for example, were that damp cloths be used rather than brooms to keep dust from rising; that sweeping should be done several hours before cooking so that dust might settle; that furniture with a lot of molding should be avoided, since hard-to-clean dust gathers there; that floors should not be covered with rugs, or at least should not be nailed to the floor so they can be taken outdoors often and shaken energetically; that curtains not be used, as they collect dust and impede the passage of light and air; that dusters be avoided since, instead of removing dust, they simply move it around; and that clothing, shoes, and any other object should be brushed in open environments. In the early twentieth century, any variant of the vacuum cleaner, manual or electric, was enthusiastically recommended; it combined bacteriology and modern technology in the supreme task of sucking up household dust and outperformed traditional sweeping with brooms. Along with the problem of household dust, the need to change the air was emphasized. First there was talk of the dangers of stagnant air and the benefits of good ventilation, as well as of the best ways of letting fresh air in and pushing old air out. Later, emphasis was placed on the advisability of cross-ventilation between rooms as well as the limitation of the modern fan, which stirred up air but did not change it.

This arsenal of recommendations became even more precise when it came to dealing with rooms where sick people resided. More intense and more frequent disinfections must be performed; the sick must be put in special rooms with minimal furniture, no curtains or rugs, and abundant light and air; and disposable spittoons must be available to keep the sick from spitting on the floor. When it was impossible to provide the tubercular with a separate room, hanging disinfected sheets from the ceiling in order to improve isolation was recommended. In 1922 the physician Gregorio Aráoz Alfaro warned of the dangers of close cohabitation with those suffering from pulmonary tuberculosis and of the need to impose daily routines he considered feasible, simple, and easy. For example, the sick person should be as isolated as possible: "His bed should be at least two meters from the beds" of those with whom he shared the room; "the sick person should learn to cough as little as possible and to do so with his mouth shut." He "should only cough up into receptacles holding water or in the water closet," and he should "frequently wash his beard, hands and the area around his mouth with alcohol, soap and water." "[A person with tuberculosis should be careful] not to kiss his children or, at least, not kiss them on their faces and only do so after having disinfected." Finally, he should avoid "loud conversations within a meter and a half of an interlocutor."[45]

In 1949 a pamphlet indicated that "tuberculosis will disappear thanks to a series of apparently insignificant hygiene measures that, together, are very important."[46] How these preventive measures were received is hard to assess. The increased literacy rate in the early twentieth century made it possible to imagine the existence of a potential female reading public. There was an abundance of pamphlets written by doctors, of home economics manuals written by men and women, and of textbooks used in schools that preached tuberculosis prevention. These materials were frequently rereleased, and their print runs were considerable, indicating they were not an insignificant segment of the publishing market. In 1880 *Guía de la mujer o lecciones de economía doméstica*, by Pilar Pascual de Sanjuan, was in its sixth edition. In 1884 the *Compendio de higiene pública y privada*, by José Antonio Wilde, was printed for the fifth time. *El libro de las madres*, which Aráoz Alfaro wrote in 1899, was reissued dozens of times during the first three decades of the twentieth century. The fourth edition of *El vademécum del hogar*, by Aurora S. De Castaño, is dated 1906. The first edition of Luis Barrantes Molina's *Síntesis de economía y sociabilidad domésticas*, published in 1923, had a print run of ten thousand. And *Ciencias domésticas: Apuntes de higiene de la habitación*, by María Arcelli, was mandatory reading in all girls' high schools in the thirties.

The effect of the war on dust on tuberculosis morbidity and mortality does not seem to have been significant. Though household dust was a likely place for Koch's bacilli to grow, the infectious power of these bacilli was null, partly because they were too big to reach the lungs and begin pathological processes. But these facts came to light later, well into the twentieth century.[47] And if this revelation had an instant impact on the way the scientific community handled the question of dust, its effect on hygiene manuals was slower. Until that occurred, the lay catechism of domestic bacteriology offered fairly convincing and plausible explanations of the dangers of household dust. Legitimized in the laboratory, these explanations organized the contents of many of the tuberculosis prevention initiatives led by the state and by civil society. They also affected many of the daily routines performed by women at home, whether the lady of the house who gave instructions to her maids or women who themselves performed the task of keeping their modest homes "free of sickening dusts."

The ability to put the recommendations of the war against dust into practice was certainly affected by income levels, the willingness or lack thereof to adopt such routines, and the material conditions of the home. In any case, for both elite women and middle- and working-class women, home bacteriology reaffirmed a sort of domestic ideology that not only emphasized the importance of women in the task of disease prevention but also deemed performing this task an individual obligation to her family.

In this sense, the fight against dust, regardless of its efficacy at preventing tuberculosis, was surprisingly important. The recommendations in the manuals were not only part of a broader discourse on cleanliness; they also played a role in forging discourses on gender relations, morality, and the importance of domestic and female knowledge in the project of shaping the hygienic citizen. Written by both women and men, the manuals were geared toward a female audience, defined at times as "the true mothers, the ones that delight in the domestic chores" and at times as "all women" or "rich and poor women, housewives and students."[48] The manuals presupposed an ability to read and hoped that the practical knowledge as well as its attendant ideology would be conveyed orally, from mother to daughter, from neighbor to neighbor, from the lady of the house to her maids and cooks.

In the late nineteenth and early twentieth centuries, manuals became more specific and far-reaching, celebrating as never before the benefits of home hygiene. One of them, published in 1880, encouraged "the practice of domestic virtues" through the "irresistible power of habit."[49] The introduction to another manual, dated 1906, stated that although "school and society might polish our habits and instincts . . . the home is where intimate manners, essence, and prime material are developed" and that the manual sought to contribute to education in these customs and habits.[50] In 1914 the text used in a course on "domestic science" underlined that "organizing good homes is half the work of forming good citizens," stressing the importance of the domestic sphere in the world outside the home.[51]

Throughout the 1920s—and to a lesser extent in the 1930s and 1940s, after the advent of a public hygiene that gradually displaced the household as the key site of prevention—home economics presented itself as a form of knowledge dedicated to "conserving the well-being and wealth of the family house," to the training of "the housewife on the thousands of varied tasks that often require heterogeneous knowledge and acts, [from] knowing how to shop, cook, mend, wash, raise children, and keep track of expenses [to] decorating the house, preserving food, avoiding illness, and making her husband happy." As women shaped and fostered daily habits in the domestic world, the struggle against unhealthy dust served to articulate not only the values of hygiene but also "morality, savings, work, foresight, watching over the family and good government."[52]

Corsets, Slim Waists, Eroticism, and Sickly Breathing

From very early on women were one of the targets of the discourse against contagion. Starting in the late 1870s, essays, municipal ordinances, and the press recommended the shortening of skirts and dresses by a few centimeters so they would not be dragged on the floors of houses and on dirt roads and cobblestone streets and collect extremely dangerous dust.[53] In the early twentieth century, in keeping with changes in fashion and the presence of women in new social environments, ankles and calves were revealed for the first time; skirts and dresses gradually ceased to be considered the bearers of bacilli and eventually disappeared altogether from the educational agenda against contagion.

Concern with the noxious effects of the corset, however, lasted much longer. In medical discourses the corset was not equally recurrent as the cases of dust and spitting. But certainly it was the piece of apparel most associated with tuberculosis, the one that induced a type of breathing that tended to lower defenses and facilitate contagion. As early as 1854 the doctoral thesis of Manuel Augusto Montes de Oca originated the ambivalent terms of a discussion that, without major changes, would continue into the 1940s. On the one hand, he indicated that "the use of a corset, when poorly made or worn very tightly such that [a woman's] shape is altered, is one of the most powerful factors in causing a predisposition to tuberculosis." On the other hand, he stressed that "our beauties are determined [to believe] that its use does not cause problems." And finally, he underscored that "some doctors exaggerate its disastrous consequences for health." Indeed, Montes de Oca's position tended to value this piece of apparel in women's lives; he stated that "[since] corsets relax the abdominal walls or the curvature of the spinal column . . . , they should not only be tolerated but recommended by doctors," among other reasons because "they hold up and compress, keeping the body erect."

During the last third of the nineteenth century the debate on the corset received increasing public attention, partly because tuberculosis could no longer be ignored, and anything that might spread it had to be avoided. Some theses and essays reaffirmed without major changes most of the ambivalent reasons Montes de Oca had advanced three or four decades earlier, that is, "the custom of the corset is associated with tuberculosis and for that reason is not healthy"; "the female desire to dramatically reduce sizes is served by corset"; and "the use of a corset is acceptable only when it provides containment and adjusts moderately [but does not serve as] a prison."[54] Others articulated their opposition to the corset by indicating its negative effects on health and its tendency to promote "hysteria and nervousness." Their discourse combined physiology, gender, and morality. Arturo Balbastro's thesis from 1892 defended the right of women to engage in physical exercise and education while warning about the dreadful consequences of modern lifestyles and dress such as the use of the corset, which he considered a reprehensible erotic object.[55] But Elvira Rawson de Dellepiane, one of the first female doctors in Argentine and a militant suffragist and feminist at the turn of the century, best expressed the concern with the corset and its relationship to the undesirable consequences of modernity.

Unlike discourses from the second half of the twentieth century, Rawson de Dellepiane's criticism of the corset was not based on the notion that it was a sexist manipulation of the female body. She saw it, rather, as a consequence of the frivolity and moral laxness that had shaped how many women experienced modern life. In her "Apuntes sobre la Higiene de la Mujer," the young Rawson de Dellepiane connected issues of female physiology with an array of questions ranging from women's education to their lack of civil and social rights, from sexuality to the importance of women in the biological reproduction of the species. She spoke of women workers' living conditions, the physical and psychological changes women experience at certain moments of their lives, the rituals and practices connected to feminine hygiene and maternity, and personal ethics and morality and their relevance to marriage and home life. In this complex and public presentation of the female world, women ceased to be mere delicate spiritual figures. Rawson de Dellepiane engaged in a systematic criticism of the airs and graces of the Buenos Aires woman—that is, its affluent women—"who was far too concerned with erotic interests and courtship." The woman of Buenos Aires gave herself over to "fashions that run against her health [and encourage] the use of the corset simply to accentuate her curves and show off her body." The feminist doctor encouraged marriage, which "renders woman less frivolous and flirtatious" and "tempers and satisfies her, doing away with the excesses that slacken her morality and wear on her health, harnessing her efforts for the reproductive mission." Her criticism of the corset was in line with a view of female sexuality as being solely dependent on motherhood and family life. Sex as pleasure was either absent or criticized in this discourse. Such sexuality was called a disorder of modern lifestyles that resulted in "chlorosis, consumption, anemia, and tuberculosis."[56] Rawson de Dellepiane enunciated a two-sided criticism of the corset. On the one hand, she defended domesticity in the life of women, even while advocating new civil, political, and social rights for women; in this domestic sphere, the erotic frivolity of the corset was physiologically and morally reprehensible. On the other hand, she saw tuberculosis as a sort of punishment of modern women who had succumbed to certain fashionable trends, such as the use of the corset that were largely unhealthy and therefore irrational.

The corset in relation to medical concerns was an issue until well into the twentieth century. "The Corset's Disasters," an article published in 1914 in *Argentina Médica*, made reference to "compressed lungs whose functioning is always disturbed by the corset"; to the unheeded "advice that has been given to women as well as what experience has taught them" about the dreadful consequences of using a corset; to "the cruelty of sacrificing the future health and present well-being of a young person in order to obtain a slimmer figure"; to the paradox of "forcing our daughters to spend half of their lives within confines that hinder the normal functioning of their organs" while, at the same time, "laughing at the Chinese, who, through tight shoes, keep [girls'] feet from growing."[57] Into the 1930s doctors pointed to the continued use of the corset and bemoaned the failure of their opposition to what they called an "elusive and difficult target." They said that although fashions changed—from the "highly accentuated figure" to figures dominated by "pressing down of the hips and breasts in order to obtain a boyish look"—the "long-standing use of the corset, which hinders the functioning of the diaphragm, impedes good breathing and clears the way to tuberculosis" endured.[58] Indeed, doctors in those years, like some of their peers from the last third of the nineteenth century, stated, almost resignedly, that the argument against the corset should "be altered [since] if it goes against fashion, it will go completely unheeded."[59]

Some authors of home economics manuals published at the beginning of the twentieth century agreed with the doctors, expressing reservations or open opposition to the corset. Barrantes Molina wrote that corsets "deform women, hinder abdominal breathing, . . . weaken the muscles that hold the inner organs and cause the upper entrails to be sunken."[60] In *Gobierno, administración e higiene del hogar*, Bassi included illustrations of women's chests that he described as "monstrously deformed"; he pointed out the need for a "total reform of wardrobe" in which "a simple breast support" would replace the corset. But even though he saw this garment as an "instrument of torture or an agent of the destruction of health," Bassi conceded to pressure from the fashion industry and advocated a "rational use" of the corset that would make it possible to "shape the female torso" while avoiding "excess pressure and iron rods." In the end he recommended that corsets be made to size and not be used by "girls under fourteen."[61]

In the thirties and forties, health magazines like *Viva Cien Años* and *Vida Natural* joined the campaign against the corset. They spoke of the bad breathing habits "of civilized women . . . used to wearing tight clothes and undergarments that make it necessary to breathe from the upper chest." They claimed there was a need for "an urgent, rational revision of women's ways of dressing" and, like the domestic hygiene manuals of earlier decades, suggested adapting the classic corset to the demands of modern life so that "the form and style respect hygiene without violating aesthetics."[62]

If health manuals and magazines fought the corset while trying to accept its ongoing, if changing, place in women's fashion, in the 1920s the sports magazine *El Gráfico* openly rejected it. It called the corset "an instrument of torture that diminishes beauty . . . and natural grace, a horrible tutor that replaces admirable flexibility with rigidity." Even the new expandable corsets that were advertised as particularly useful for playing sports were not exempt from this criticism. The magazine warned that the corset was constantly changing with fashion, largely because it served "the flirtatiousness of women" who used it to "highlight their principal charms." Hence, the corset was becoming a need, especially for women who were convinced their "role in this world is to arouse the passion of men."[63] To *El Gráfico*, the problem with the corset was not so much that it epitomized a certain modern feminine flirtatiousness, an argument that had been put forth years earlier by Rawson de Dellepiane. Instead, it was seen to embody an artificiality that went against natural beauty; against comfortable, functional, light clothing; against the toning of the body through sports; and against the body's preparation for reproductive functions, all of which were key to the modern woman. And if Rawson de Dellepiane

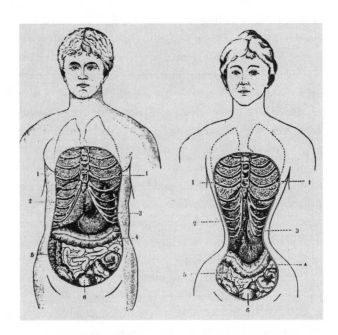

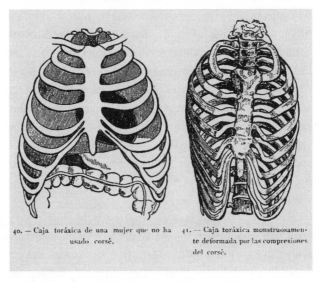

40. — Caja torácica de una mujer que no ha usado corsé. 41. — Caja torácica monstruosamente deformada por las compresiones del corsé.

The consequences of wearing corsets, as depicted by a domestic hygiene manual. (Angel Bassi, *Gobierno, administración e higiene del hogar: Curso de ciencia doméstica*, Buenos Aires: Editorial Cabautt y Cía., 1914) resoundingly connected the rejection of the corset with the early twentieth-century feminist suffragist agenda, *El Gráfico* advocated wardrobe reform and "women's moral and physical education" while putting off, for an undetermined period, women's right to vote and active participation in political life.[64]

Despite medical opposition, corsets continued to be used during the six or seven decades during which campaigns against tuberculosis contagion abounded. The unwavering popularity of the corset is evident in the advertising that, with different emphases at different times, sought to shape and reflect stereotypes of an array of women: from housewives to young modern women, from women with aristocratic pretensions to working-class women who aspired to be part of the middle classes. The messages of these ads aimed to establish a feminine canon based on flirtatiousness and charm; the eroticization of the body; and the existence of a relatively autonomous female world organized around love, sex, and certain daily rituals such as checking oneself in the mirror and adjusting—or having others adjust—the strings of a corset.

From 1870 to 1910 ads for women's corsets were very austere; they contained few lines of text and sometimes a small photograph. Newspapers at that time included a space for ads, which were placed together in a column usually entitled *avisos notables*, or noteworthy announcements. In this column, corsets were offered alongside cigarettes and cigars, watches, medicines, hats, and furniture. Without much graphic intervention, the ads informed readers of the various models and qualities of corsets. Prices were not mentioned, but a clear distinction was made between fine corsets and others, which were referred to simply as corsets. Some consumers were already buying according to brand, as the ads noted the garments' manufacturers as well as their origin—an imported corset was a guarantee of quality—and where it could be purchased, such as at large downtown stores like A la Ciudad de Londres and corset shops such as La Hermosura. By the 1890s some ads offered "perfectly shaped and hygienic" corsets in response to medical criticism and the call for a rational reform of clothing.

In early advertisements illustrations were simple; they displayed fairly static, flat, almost inert figures. In corset ads, the product appeared, but the body that bore it was hard to identify; it was suggested by the outlines of the upper torso. In the last third of the nineteenth century, such suggestiveness was truly bold, especially when compared to ads for other intimate apparel. These ads seldom contained illustrations, and when they did the product was not presented to the reader as if it were being worn on a body. The tone was one of discretion. In the case of corset ads, by contrast, there was a deliberate effort to eroticize the product. The drawing of the garment tended to accentuate the figure, especially the curves, of the female body. In illustrations in newspapers from those years there is nothing like the public presentation of the corset, which invited the reader to imagine something more than an item that could be purchased. Corset ads grew more sophisticated and suggestive in the 1890s, and the illustrations in them began to feature the entire body of a woman or her upper torso. This new modality did not replace the unseen body of the first ads or the deliberate effort to show narrow waists and prominent busts. Sometimes the postures of the bodies were downright provocative or insinuating—the hands clasped behind the neck, eyes looking straight at the reader—and sometimes the woman wearing the corset was in front of a mirror, suggesting her most intimate world as well as a certain narcissism and ideas of elegance and femininity.

These illustrations, which were presumably made by men, seem to have served masculine fantasies and desires. They allowed for a certain voyeurism that was easily concealed by the place the ads occupied in the newspaper, a place shared with other products for men. And they probably were intended to lead male readers (as most newspaper readers were in all likelihood men) to get their wives or lovers to buy the corset advertised. At the beginning of the twentieth century technological changes in the graphics industry and the impact, first, of art nouveau and, somewhat later, of art deco brought innovation in journalistic styles and in advertising design. Starting then and continuing into the 1950s corset ads were a constant in the print media; no other female undergarment was as consistently seen in ads. In general, the style of these ads is rather homogeneous. They are based on a figurine, a manual illustration, and occasionally a photograph.

During the 1910s and 1920s small-format ads were generally grouped together. Occasionally, newspapers and magazines placed bigger ads that would appear elsewhere in an attempt to take the reader by surprise. In corset ads, the stylistic innovation associated with art nouveau played a lesser role than in other areas, where image and text were much more interrelated and typography was part of a decorative scheme. Such ads were conceived as design objects, and they made use of avant-garde art tendencies. In any case, by the end of the 1910s some corset ads took up more than a fourth of a newspaper page and a full page in magazines; these ads were much more elaborate and modern. Smaller, less costly ads were still published, and they continued to use the stylistic resources of the last third of the nineteenth century. But even in those ads a certain degree of innovation was visible, the illustrations featuring a looser line, a flatter perspective, and a marked stylization of the face and body.

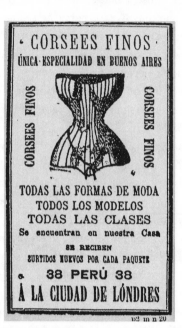

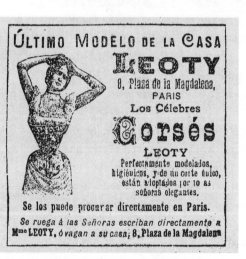

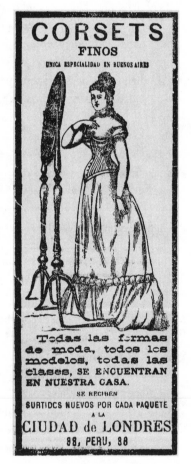

Late nineteenth-century advertisements for corsets. They stress not only variety and quality but also "hygienic condition." (*La Nación*, December 2, 1880; *La Patria Argentina*, June 8, 1885; *La Nación*, March 20, 1895)

In the ads from the first three decades of the twentieth century, the curves of the female body are less accentuated than in ads from the late nineteenth century. In these later ads, the corset appears to be dressing the natural figure of a woman's body. Corsets no longer pressed the body but gave back "to today's woman her natural figure, which the old corsets had destroyed."[65] The corsets that highlighted the bust and buttocks to form an S-shape had lost ground to the more modern straight corsets that, it was thought, did not cut into the waist. All of this was possible in part because of the use of new materials like latex, which provided elastic fabrics; cotton and poplin, which provided a lighter, more porous product; and rayon, which looked like silk or satin but was much cheaper and served to further democratize and expand the female corset market. There were now advertisements for corsets for young women that did not hinder dancing or playing sports, corsets that came in an array of qualities and price ranges, revealing a market that was varied in terms of material resources and expanded the ability of female consumers to choose. These ads appealed to elegance and slenderness, hygiene, fashion, and the ability to move: "strong, flexible, hygienic, elegant, and comfortable corsets that keep the body in place while beautifying the slenderness of the bust"; "perfected and unique corsets that combine hygiene and aesthetics and provide the true figure of today's fashion"; "corsets that are absolutely necessary for *la vie au grand'aire*, tennis, polo and all other country sports"; corsets that were not "overly tight," making it possible "to cultivate the hygiene of elegance"; corsets that "do not have bones and give back to the body an ability to perform its habitual movements"; and corsets, girdles, and corselets made from lighter, more porous fabrics that were, as a result, less rigid and could be used in great comfort.[66] And even the ads that continued to praise the traditional corsets that accentuated curves and used rigid materials were influenced by the modern cult of movement: "a very elegant and cleverly boned model that makes movements highly flexible."[67] Some ads spoke of the hygienic virtues of the corset, pointing out the approval of the French National Hygiene Board and the Hygiene Society. These ads articulated a sort of recent history of the corset as a product that could be improved on to accommodate the recommendations of medical science: "Men of science [and] their medical associations, which always anathematized the old corset, have examined these new hygienic corsets and changed their opinions."[68]

Starting in the mid-1930s, advertising began to make use of graphic resources developed in North America. The image became central; the text lost importance and became a secondary resource that served only to reinforce the image. Ads spoke of innovations in style, price, and materials used. The fact

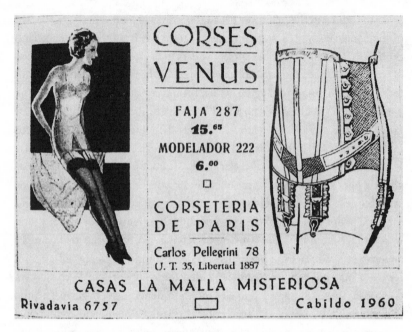

In spite of the recurrent medical critique of corsets as a close-fitting undergarment that predisposed one to tuberculosis, corsets were still advertised for sale during the first half of the twentieth century—revealing their continuing presence in women's intimate wear—but later ads stressed new designs and new materials. (*Para Tí*, March 10, 1925; *La Razón*, August 8, 1945; *La Razón*, March 8, 1950)

that these were hygienic corsets was mentioned only sporadically in order to highlight that they did not cause "early deformation of the body." There was greater freedom of line in rendering light, quick figures, and any decorative pretense was left behind. The ads featured stylized bodies and the art deco tendency to elongate the female figure. They accentuated the breasts more subtly than before. The waist was also stressed, though not excessively, revealing that the flapper style of the 1920s—that is, flattened breasts, loose clothing, and no corsets—had been just a passing fad partly because it could only be adopted by young, extremely thin women.

During the 1940s these tendencies grew more pronounced. In corset ads, which also promoted corselets, girdles, and trusses, the figure of the woman with wide hips, a small waist, and a generous bosom reappeared. The ads emphasize that these corsets do not restrict. The drawn images they contain were generally less rigid than the ones from the turn of the century; they did not make use of art deco design or geometrism. In keeping with the tenets and styles of North American graphic illustration, the image was placed at the center of the ad, and the text was clearly secondary. Some ads were influenced by caricatures the illustrator Divito developed in a series of popular magazines, some of which were humoristic, like *Rico Tipo*; others, like *Chicas*, were directed at an emerging young female audience.[69] Divito's girls, with their long hair, statuesque bodies, slim waists, childlike (if heavily made up) faces, and super high heels, were always hyperbolic representations of the feminine, models for emancipated women and manifestations of the dreams of many men. They combined humor, based on the emphasis on imposing sexual features, and indirect eroticism. One ad in *Chicas* announced a corset "as stretchy as the body required . . . ; it performs the miracle of the thinnest waist and the loveliest hips you ever dreamed of. It is cool and allows for absolute freedom of movement."[70]

Corsets began to disappear from ads in the 1940s, displaced by elasticized girdles, but they had proven capable of adapting to changes in fashion and retained a loyal group of consumers. The medical discourse against corsets was largely ineffective and irrelevant to the efforts to decrease tuberculosis morbidity and mortality by means of re-education in daily habits. From the 1850s on, people concerned with the negative effects of corsets were aware of the limited impact of their discourse. In 1854 Montes de Oca stated that "beautiful women's stubborn use of corsets, despite the opposition of doctors, must be based on something other than fancy."[71] Somewhat later, Wilde wrote that there are many women who "despite everything . . . and even at the cost of getting sick or dying . . . have chosen to be slim and elegant."[72] In 1914 Bassi pointed out the problems caused by the "blind and passionate abuse of the corset in pursuit of elegance and a certain figure [despite the risk of] harming health."[73] And in the 1920s, in a tone of resignation, Barrantes Molina blamed "women's impulse and instinct toward flirtatiousness" for the fact that they "subject themselves to the tortures of the corset in order to reduce their figures, wherever and whenever fashion demands it."[74]

Para Tí, a widely read women's magazine that circulated from the 1920s on, offered a different view. It criticized the rigid corset, which for nearly "two thousand years . . . shaped women to suit its fancy," but it celebrated the advent of the new "delicate and flexible" corsets that "provided support without taking away freedom." This type of corset, "made by worthy manufacturers whose staffs include not only experts in fashion but also doctors," made "the Greek ideal of the slender woman" possible, an ideal that was affronted by the sedentary nature of "modern life in large cities." *Para Tí* postulated that the modern woman "has discovered that if she wants to keep her beautiful figure and charms she has to ask art to help nature." In this way, she will be able to make intelligent use of her freedom and avoid what happens to women from the tropics who, "without corsets or any support whatsoever are lovely at sixteen and old and deformed at twenty-five."[75]

The popularity of the corset was based on what it could do for the body. The corset outlined the body, kept flesh firm, hid any visible stomach movement, made breasts rise and fall suggestively while supporting them, and anchored the torso so that it looked elegant. The corset made it possible to feign a slim waist and ample breasts, two highly celebrated attributes that would certainly have tempted women who lacked them. And for working-class women the corset offered a way to cultivate the elegant figures of wealthier women, making it one of the many resources at the disposal of women seeking to climb the social ladder, on the upper rungs of which appearance mattered a great deal. For this reason, not surprisingly, lower-class girls and working women consumed corsets. The low price and quality of some corsets made them accessible to a wide range of budgets.

For many elite and nonelite women alike, the corset was an instrument of seduction as well as an indirect way of rejecting, at least to some degree, the domestic and passive space patriarchal society had assigned them. Both the rigid and the elastic corset eroticized women. Such eroticization—the "irresistible flirtatiousness" condemned by doctors and celebrated by *Para Ti* as an exercise in freedom—was steeped in ambiguities. On the one hand, corsets entailed a sexist manipulation of the female body, a sort of confinement. On the other, they were a resource to be used in constructing a sexuality both appealing and restricted, demure and rebellious, refined and bold. This ambiguity is evident in ads in which women wearing corsets pose, play, and look at themselves, in either relaxed or intense stances, in a mirror. In the intimate setting of the bathroom or the bedroom, they seem to be speaking of themselves, revealing something of their private worlds, staging their femininity or desires. But since these ads circulated in a patriarchal society, their ambiguous message was fetishized and, in this sense, served the sexual or even quasi-pornographic expectations of men.

This ambiguous eroticization of the corset helped shape not only medical and moral discourses but also a feminine sensibility that was more directly associated with disease. The symptomatology of this sensibility was linked to tuberculosis, chlorosis, neurasthenia, hysteria, depression, multiple anxieties, pains in the head, the chest, and the back, uterine disorders, repeated vomiting, and fainting.[76] In the case of tuberculosis—in addition to warnings about the corset and its dreadful physical and physiological consequences—doctors, suffragists, and clothing reformers emphasized the passionate side of the garment. They maintained that the corset expressed or even enhanced the unbridled eroticism and uncontrollable desires that were believed to characterize women with tuberculosis. In addition, as they constricted the ribs and the diaphragm, corsets were seen as contributing to the production of "tubercular matter" and the triggering of coughing fits "accompanied by bloody sputum." The corset was seen as a double evil: an expression of excessive sexuality and a goad to contagion.[77]

Some women seem to have found in the corset a means of expressing an ambiguous sensibility that involved, on the one hand, the sensitive, refined spirit associated with gentleness, sadness, and weakness and, on the other, an intense sexual ardor and open eroticism. This image rested on a notion of tuberculosis as a romantic disease of the soul and the passions, a notion that was certainly present in the last third of the nineteenth century and, to a lesser extent, into the twentieth century. Putting the corset to implicit uses, women with tuberculosis as well as healthy women could seduce. They could display gestures, postures, and traits that at times suggested a physical weakness that bespoke an elegant, aristocratic moral refinement, and at other times an exceptional eroticism. In the end, the pale, languid faces, the respiratory difficulties that soon became sighs, the inexplicable fainting, the unbridled sexuality—all of which were associated with women who used corsets—embodied not only a medical and moral discourse that considered tuberculosis a disease of the passions but also a feminine way to exercise seduction.

Infectious Kisses, Tubercular Sexuality, and Eugenic Records

In 1946 the tuberculosis lung expert Antonio Cetrángolo recalled how widespread the fear of catching tuberculosis was among doctors during the first decades of the twentieth century and how these fears were reproduced among the general public.[78] It was in this context that the dramatic image of the so-called infectious kiss emerged. This image rested on the idea that contagion was possible not only through the respiratory system but also through the digestive and even reproductive systems. Saliva was pivotal to this fear of contagion and countless everyday situations—some more or less predictable, others totally arbitrary—were thought to cause tuberculosis.[79] Anticlericals, for instance, used the opportunity to stress that the "parishioner not kiss habits, chains, and holy symbols."[80]

But it was in interpersonal relationships that kissing was considered most dangerous and, as a result, became the target of an arsenal of recommendations which, if put into practice, were believed to reduce the risk of contagion.

These recommendations were aimed at both the general population—which, for a long time, had kissed as a common form of greeting—and at those who lived with people with tuberculosis. "Adults should not kiss children and children must be taught, from the time they are very small, not to let themselves be kissed," indicated an antituberculosis pamphlet in the early forties.[81] Much earlier, in 1906, a report issued by school doctors proposed banning kissing—"an almost certain means of transmitting germs"—between children and teachers.[82] Those who lived with tuberculars were encouraged to teach them "habits that avoided the spread of their illness," such as "standing no less than two meters" away from healthy people.[83] "Misunderstood mother love," said one doctor, "leads [mothers] to give kisses to children without understanding that these displays of affection result in the transmission of the disease."[84] Consequently, one must "forget about kisses, avoid any close contact, and not permit caresses."[85] This was the dramatic scenario experienced by Luisa, a woman with tuberculosis in the play Los derechos de la salud by Florencio Sánchez, when, in a desperate condition, she discovers a sort of "family conspiracy" to prevent her from having any physical contact with her children.[86] Such precautions were consistent with the recommendation, common as of 1875, that mothers with tuberculosis not breast-feed because the fatigue resulting from lactation might worsen her condition and the disease might be transmitted through her "dangerous milk."[87] In 1915 the hygienist Nicolás Lozano took this reasoning further, suggesting that "single women with tuberculosis should not marry or have children," but if they did, they "must not breastfeed them."[88]

Until the early 1940s it was common to advise avoiding kissing. Some doctors warned of the danger of "prolonged, intimate kisses on the mouth," and others recommended that everyone, healthy or sick, do without "kisses on the lips."[89] Indeed, the discourse on contagion hovered around married life, bodily contact, and sex in general, not only in the case of the sick but also of the healthy. As a result, some connected a moralizing discourse with medical knowledge, using a battery of professional and ideological traditions—among them even anarchism and feminism—to condemn "certain sexual perversions, especially oral-genital relations." Others targeted "prostitutes' kisses [which are] sure transmitters of tuberculosis."[90]

The image of the infectious kiss epitomized the fears that accompanied a marriage between a person with tuberculosis and a healthy person. When one of the partners had active tuberculosis, doctors strongly discouraged marriage. If one partner had been cured of the disease, marriage was not ruled out, but it was necessary to know if "[the couple was] in proper shape to enter into matrimony."[91] Some doctors considered raising this issue as a matter of their professional duty and obligation. Others did not hide the difficulty of harmonizing medical reasoning and the feelings of the interested parties.[92] In any case, everyone agreed that if one of the members had tuberculosis the couple had to be closely watched over: "There is the risk of contamination from a sick member of the couple to a healthy one. In fact, kisses and shared daily life are almost sure causes of contagion because the practices that can if not eliminate then at least diminish the risk of contagion are not sufficiently known." To a man with tuberculosis only "very occasional sexual relations" were recommended. Before sex, his mouth had to be "impeccably clean, and his beard and moustache carefully tended." Single people with tuberculosis, both men and women, were advised to get married only after they had been fully cured and had "sufficient resources not to have to work too hard."[93]

As part of the effort to control contagion, there were initiatives geared toward regulating marriage and pregnancy. Attention was focused on the risk to offspring of sexual unions in which one or both of the parties were sick. In the early 1940s Carlos Bernaldo de Quirós stated this perspective: "Public social morality as well as home and institutional order make it necessary to hinder, avoid, and make it impossible for foul genetic elements, which are a public menace, to work unconsciously or criminally toward the breeding and transmission of their degenerative defects to their offspring."[94] This sentiment was not in keeping with the dominant eugenic approach in Argentina during that time, an approach which, generally speaking, aimed at the improvement of individual and collective health through the prescription of behaviors and education. This positive eugenics was shared virtually across the whole ideological political spectrum, from liberals to Catholic conservatives and from socialists to libertarians and radicals. Nonetheless, throughout the period there was no lack of voices, even within diverse ideological groups, eager to include in population policy recommendations a series of measures that promoted segregation as a means to prevent and impede the reproduction of those considered unfit. Bernaldo de Quirós's statement asserted an urgent demand for drastic intervention aimed not so much at gradual genetic improvement as, in his words, at "hindering, avoiding, making impossible" marriages that were perceived as degenerative. It was in this context that Argentine eugenics, which was mostly positive, contemplated notions and projects for drastic and cruel intervention in terms of selection and sterilization. Others who came before de Quirós, in the late nineteenth century, had expressed similar concerns. But these were not the dominant voices, and they did not set the tone of the debate.

In 1880 Eugenio Ramirez's doctoral thesis argued that "it would be a true service to people with tuberculosis to legally prohibit them from getting married." Matrimony, he said, unleashed passions that "increase the causes that have led to their illness, hence hastening death."[95] Three decades later the Argentine antituberculosis conferences of 1917 and 1919 discussed the issue, and *La Semana Médica* celebrated vasectomies, which were being performed in the United States. The journal stated that such drastic measures should be considered "after having assessed the inefficacy of prohibiting marriage to degenerates and criminals as well as to those with syphilis and tuberculosis."[96] Somewhat later, in popular pamphlets and professional forums, the Uruguayan Paulina Luisi, a major figure in Buenos Aires socialist circles, enthusiastically advocated what were then called the "negative procedures such as sterilization, abortion, anticonceptive practices" as well as prenuptial physical examinations. Her arguments connected birth control, women, and children's rights; a great confidence in medical science's ability to regulate human reproduction; and the long-standing discourse of national efficiency: "Birth control should be . . . geared toward . . . [producing] . . . the desired excellence; . . . all beings that are temporarily or permanently inferior and, hence, likely to give rise to poor quality offspring should abstain from procreating. First by selection and then by breastfeeding, man will devise a way to obtain resistant, strong, and vigorous offspring." In this context, she understood that abortion was not only "a right but an obligation . . . in particular when it came to expunging the unhealthy fruit of someone with tuberculosis, someone insane, someone with syphilis, an alcoholic." She was convinced that though "the tuberculosis germ" could not be inherited, a terrain fertile to tuberculosis could be: "The child has inherited an organism with poor resistance which renders it vulnerable to infection; even if he is not born with tuberculosis or syphilis, he is born full of tuberculosis toxins, . . . [and is] predisposed to all infections."[97]

Faced with these risks, Luisi proposed sterilization, a procedure that was "wholly inoffensive to men" though somewhat more "delicate" when performed on women. However, in the socialist paper *La Vanguardia* she adamantly expressed her confidence in science and medicine, and wrote that the procedure would become simpler with "the advances of modern surgery."[98] Some doctors spoke of therapeutic abortions, claiming that tuberculosis progressed more quickly during pregnancy, and since for poor pregnant women both hospitals and good nutrition were not guaranteed, "it was advisable to interrupt the pregnancy."[99]

In the 1920s and 1930s many advocated contraception as a eugenic resource. *Viva Cien Años*, which supported a modern discourse on marriage in which social, biological, and moral obligations were combined with the psychology of love and desire, stressed that "no one has the right to generate beings defective in their physical capacity or diminished in terms of their human value."[100] Some tuberculosis experts encouraged temporary sterilization of married women with tuberculosis, putting forth arguments that focused on the negative effects of pregnancy on the health of sick women.[101] In those years, Juan Lazarte, a doctor active in anarchist and libertarian circles, recognized not only the need for sterilization, which should "be considered a right, not a punishment," but also the advisability of "making understandable to the people the norms of negative eugenics, [while] avoiding bad press and unwanted attention."[102] His approach echoed the early twentieth-century anarchist language on birth control, free love, and the need to make available "noncompulsive, mechanical, and chemical means of avoiding pregnancy."[103] The issue served to articulate an array of anarchist concerns such as individual rights, revolutionary spirit, and social transformation. While the carpenters' newspaper *El Obrero Ebanista* postulated that "numerous and poor offspring enlightened the workers' consciousness," most anarchist publications, like *Brazo y Cerebro*, pointed out that "the limitation of the family" made it possible to raise better revolutionary children.[104]

In those decades and into the 1940s there was an effort to define the circumstances in which sterilization and abortion might be acceptable. Some professional publications spoke of "sterilization when there is a state of need." Sterilization could not be questioned when the mother was suffering from "a serious illness and pregnancy or delivery put her life at risk" or when "the future mother or father or both had an infectious, degenerative disease that would be transmitted to the offspring." For women with chronic tuberculosis, sterilization was advocated by stressing the harm caused by "successive abortions" and "unsafe methods of contraception."[105] Some discouraged sterilization in cases of nonvirulent and cured tuberculosis, recommending contraception in order to limit pregnancies to one every two or three years. Others suggested temporary sterilization as a means to deal with "evolutionary tuberculosis" before pregnancy or what were believed to be cases of tuberculosis reactivated by pregnancy. Others prescribed surgical sterilization of mothers with several children who were approaching menopause or unable to undergo antituberculosis treatment for economic or religio-cultural reasons.[106]

The issue of sterilizing tubercular women also appeared in books with large print runs like *Fertilidad e infertilidad en el matrimonio*, the second volume of the trilogy *El matrimonio perfecto* by the Dutchman T. H. Van der Velde. Reprinted more than twenty times by the mid-twentieth century—and sometimes as often as twice in a single year—this book, like many inexpensive manuals and scientific pamphlets sold at newspaper stands, was aimed at fairly educated readers who were interested in self-instruction on topics usually discussed only in academic circles.[107] The tone in which *Fertilidad e infertilidad en el matrimonio* suggested definitive sterilization in women with tuberculosis was more persuasive than prescriptive: "Pregnancy could expose women to great dangers and even death." Thus, more than eugenics, the rational, self-interested choice for sick women was sterilization.[108]

If, in the emerging sexology proposed by Van der Velde, the issue of procreation took on new meanings which combined eugenics with questions like desire, individual impulse, and erotic love, most medical voices spoke of sexuality in terms of the long-standing and vague discourse on the "strength and health of the race." The emphatic declarations in support of abortions, sterilizations, and contraception, that is, of the need to keep people with tuberculosis from procreating, had highly active opponents. The Catholic doctor Ricardo Schwarcz, for instance, added a statistical quantitative dimension to the debate. His study revealed that from 1925 to 1935 the number of pregnant women with tuberculosis in the maternity ward of the Hospital Tornú, where he was a doctor, had increased steadily. In 1935 a new administration at the hospital prohibited abortion, but this did not increase the mortality rate among birthing women with tuberculosis. In his conclusions he added that more than 70 percent of children born to mothers with tuberculosis—all of whom participated in a program that separated mothers from their children after birth in order to prevent contagion—were perfectly healthy. In view of this, Schwarcz did not believe abortion offered any benefit to pregnant women with tuberculosis, though it did serve to "destroy the life of many children."[109]

Also based on hospital cases, though lacking statistical support, Juan Munzinger's thesis, dated 1920, did not conceal his concern about tubercular women with several children—the condition of some of whom improved after birth, while others' worsened.[110] In keeping with an agenda common in the twenties and thirties that sought to increase the birthrate, many people saw the "negative procedures" as "brutal zootechnics" or "irresponsible approaches in countries in need of population."[111] Catholics also opposed these practices, claiming that any effort to regulate reproduction in marriage was unnatural. Nonetheless, some said that the Catholic Church "never officially defined its stance" on the issue of "special cases." Furthermore, the issue of sterilization was "very complex given that it has not been satisfactorily proven that [mothers with certain diseases] may affect or threaten the well-being of the nation."[112]

Throughout this period some advocated limiting the reproduction of people with tuberculosis, while others believed people with tuberculosis did not in and of themselves constitute a danger to the "national race." The pro-abortion position gained ground in the new political context brought on, in part, by the military coup of 1930. At that time conservative sectors began to discredit biologist transformism and to look toward the modern genetics programs and practices of Nazi and fascist regimes in Europe as well as some U.S. states. Nonetheless, while the Asociación Argentina de Biotipología, Eugenesia y Medicina Social—among whose members were doctors who enthusiastically supported negative eugenics—others continued to favor policies to increase the birthrate and to oppose any regulation of reproduction.

These diverse discourses and, to a lesser extent, medical practices occurred in a period when the decreasing birthrate was a growing concern, and ideas about procreation and marriage were becoming more complex and ambiguous. Thus, while women had fewer children, evidencing a growing use of contraception, procreation in marriage became not only a religious, moral, biological, or eugenic mandate associated with the forging of the national race, but also an outgrowth of impulses and desire increasingly accepted as part of the human experience. It was in this context that the degenerative nature of people with tuberculosis was discussed. The talk of negative eugenics by those who saw tuberculars' sex lives, marriages, and offspring as a risk to the national race was not in keeping with dominant notions of progress promoted for more than half a century by positive eugenics. Moreover, this negative eugenics was to a great extent merely a rhetorical exercise, given the fact that its application seems to have been marginal.

The prenuptial certificate, contemplated since the 1870s, was another resource meant to regulate reproduction. Article 175 of the Civil Code outlines premarriage procedures, stipulating that both parties must have a certificate of health. In his *Curso de Higiene Pública*, first published in 1878, the doctor Eduardo Wilde, who would later have a distinguished career as a hygienist and politician, wrote, "Today, men of science deem it essential that families see their doctors to determine a person's physical fitness for marriage. Parents must think of the problems that tuberculosis and scrofula bring to spouses and offspring."[113] Thus began the debate on the best way to determine a bride's and groom's aptness for marriage: which infectious diseases could lead to population deterioration and therefore should be deemed cause to prohibit marriage? In the early twentieth century, in keeping with the discourse on national efficiency, the hygienist Emilio Coni argued that if "livestock is controlled to improve its quality" there was no reason not to mandate the "certification of the health of a bride and groom."[114] Others said that if one had to take a physical exam to join the army, "the same should hold true for those interested in marrying." Consequently, by "legal means or less compulsory . . . medical advice," the marriage of people with tuberculosis when the disease is still in a virulent phase should be discouraged.[115] By the 1930s the question of prenuptial medical examinations was an important part of the eugenic agenda and, in 1940, four years after the law to prevent venereal disease was passed and the prenuptial certificate was required of men, some hygienists insisted on the need for a "mandatory, categorical, individualized and official prenuptial medical certificate for both sexes that would impede marriage due to chronic, contagious, or hereditary disease."[116]

But tuberculosis was never specified as a legal cause to prohibit marriage; instead, its regulation was voluntary, combining personal desires, family and social pressures, and doctors' opinions. In the case of people with active tuberculosis, marriage was openly discouraged. The controversy arose in terms of those who had been cured or were recovering. A pamphlet from the 1930s recognized that in these cases there was an evident "clash between the feelings and the interests of the person with tuberculosis," a tension whose risks "varied according to sex." In the case of cured tubercular men, family life, "as an ordering factor, was beneficial"; in the case of women, by contrast, "household responsibilities, pregnancy and childbirth [were] dangerous."[117] In the 1940s Bernaldo de Quirós demanded a more precise legal framework, urging the legislature to look to foreign examples in which tuberculosis was cause to prohibit marriage. He called Law 12331, which regulated the prenuptial medical examination, "preventive and prophylactic but not eugenic." As a result, he demanded that "all diseases with consequences for offspring . . . such as tuberculosis, essential epilepsy, dementia, and other nervous and mental diseases" be included in the law in order to render it "a veritable law of eugenic marriage."[118]

Starting in the late nineteenth century, ideas about marriage were an integral part of a discourse that, in the more general framework of positive eugenics, emphasized a sort of rational hygiene of reproduction. In different ways and with different nuances almost everyone participated in this climate of ideas, from hygienists and social Catholics to socialists and the more radical eugenicists. By the 1930s a prenuptial medical exam was largely deemed necessary. *Viva Cien Años* encouraged "overcoming resistance arising from modesty, denial, and family complications" since "the eugenic attitude consists of fully accepting that no one has the right to generate physically defective beings or beings whose human value is diminished." And to achieve the goal of eugenic marriage it was necessary "to carry out a prenuptial physical examination as a way of taking stock of health."[119]

These discourses on aptness for marriage, risks of pregnancy, and the nature of the sex lives of those suffering from tuberculosis were no more than that, regulating discourses. They, like many of the recommendations in the antituberculosis hygienic code, constituted a project whose social acceptance and effectiveness were by no means assured. One initiative that was expected to help spread these behaviors was the eugenic card. The surveillance of those predisposed to tuberculosis entailed early diagnosis, medical examinations, and very detailed follow-ups. Starting at the beginning of the century, and in part as a result of the increasing acceptance and legitimacy of statistics, there had been talk of ways of recording individual biological histories. Some emphasized the importance of material living conditions, pointing out correlations between certain lifestyles and certain diseases, especially tuberculosis.[120] Others promoted a "sanitary card for the tubercular [that] would record in detail the course of the person's pathology."[121] The most ambitious and sophisticated of these registering and monitoring proposals was the "biotypological card." Starting in the 1930s such records aimed not only at monitoring the physical and psychological evolution of individual cases but also at classifying the population. The Asociación Argentina de Biotipología, Eugenesia y Medicina Social proposed the card, one of its many initiatives, along with training programs in "biological eugenics and puericulture" and in "legal and social eugenics."[122] In some of these initiatives, especially the biotypological card, the influence of Italian biotypology led by Nicola Pende and its earlier local impact on the psycho-physiological laboratories in factories proposed by the socialist Alfredo Palacios were apparent.[123]

Biotypology recognized that certain characteristics were hereditary while acknowledging the importance of environmental factors in determining an individual and his or her biotypological type. It defined six types according to racial and constitutional features. And even though certain features were considered hereditary, in the Mendelian sense of the word, the inherited capital of each individual, it was said, could be influenced by the environment. The regulating and modeling of biotypes was part of an agenda that sought to improve the biological structure of the nation. And given that certain biotypes implied different abilities, anthropometric characteristics, and susceptibility to disease, the careful recording of biotypes would make an important contribution to forging a nation of apt citizens. Children, women, and workers were the focus of the eugenic effort. The "student hygienic card" contained a range of information that went from "the child's health and hereditary and personal background to the sort of prenatal care and delivery he had undergone, . . . his nutritional and neuro-psychic development, his prophylactic vaccinations, his preventive health care visits . . . and all the traits decisive to his personality."[124] The "eugenic fertility assessment card" given to women echoed ideas on maternal and reproductive functions that had been present as early as the 1870s. The card also contained the sort of information found in health records in public hospitals starting in the early twentieth century; it was reminiscent of experiences abroad in a wide range of political and ideological contexts, from liberal democracies to Nazi Germany.[125] Information about race, phenotypic characteristics, and religion was recorded; fertility was monitored in order to avoid miscarriages; and education on maternal obligations was provided.[126] In order to register information about workers, so-called psychophysiological laboratories were started in factories. There, "workers would be examined periodically, recording their individual aptitudes in order to direct them to proper posts as well as to diagnose their constitutional predisposition to morbidity and weakness." In this way, it was said, "thousands of workers could be saved from tuberculosis [by being] examined and warned of the terrible calamity within them while it was still in a latent form."[127]

Biotypology certainly provided a frame of reference for Law 12341, dated 1936, which mandated the keeping of health records for mothers and children. During the first Peronist administration, biotypology influenced many of the Secretaría de Salud Pública's preventive health recording instruments for school age and teenage populations: the *ficha sanitaria*, which was supposed to keep track of the results of periodical medical examinations and vaccinations, including the antituberculosis vaccine; the *libreta sanitaria*, which was a private document for personal use; and the *certificado de salud*, a public document that evidenced having received certain tests and inoculations. In 1946, at the height of the parliamentary debate on health cards, a congressman eager to make public the outcome of an examination of thirteen thousand schoolchildren announced that "fourteen [were] carriers of serious tuberculosis, ten had somewhat serious tubercular lesions, and 726 children with cured tubercular pathologies" had been detected.[128]

Like so many other preventative projects, the ambitious biotypology plan did not result in a mass recording of the population; it did, however, exercise a more general influence on an array of preventive medical initiatives aimed at shaping daily habits and avoiding tuberculosis contagion.

Reacting to Tuberculosis Phobia

During the decades in which the fight against tuberculosis was conducted, the intense, almost militant communication of everyday hygiene practices believed to prevent contagion managed to affect, to a certain extent, the lives of people and their ideas about not only what was healthy but also what was respectable. Regardless of their influence in preventing the disease, the influence of these discourses was felt throughout the second half of the twentieth century via widely accepted habits and behaviors.

Starting in the late nineteenth century and well into the 1940s, the arsenal of hygienic recommendations was boosted by fruitless efforts to control tuberculosis mortality and morbidity. From private doctors' offices to public hospitals and from widely circulated newspapers to radio conferences, advice was given on how to combat the bacillus and its possible breeding grounds. Soon, these efforts, which were celebrated by the medical establishment and increasingly accepted by a society that was frightened of contagion, were the object of criticism. In 1921 Cetrángolo wrote that "everyone has become a propagandist dispensing advice on tuberculosis, and newspapers spread these recommendations with a dedication that frightens even the bravest." He also stated that "in more than thirty years, this preaching has led only to failures [and generated] . . . endless fears and a vicious hate of the bacillus."[129] During the first half of the twentieth century some doctors and social critics coined the term *tuberculosis phobia* to refer to the obsession with contagion and the discourse that sought to spread the antituberculosis code at any cost. They used the term to refer to actions that, they said, "start off making war on the bacillus and end up making war on the person with tuberculosis."[130] This distrust of the vehement desire to spread the hygienic code articulated two concerns: on the one hand, a concern with tuberculosis as a product of the injustices of the prevailing social system that clearly went beyond issues of hygiene; on the other, a critique of the exaggerated efforts to normalize daily habits in general, that is, the habits of the healthy and the sick, adults and children, men and women.

These two perspectives, or combinations of them, were in the making as early as the last third of the nineteenth century, before tuberculosis phobia had fully taken hold. In 1870 Eduardo Wilde wrote, "When there is poverty, hygiene is impossible [and even] the wealthiest man necessarily commits a hundred thousand hygiene sins per day. There is insufficient time and resources to verify the demands of hygiene, [and anyone who sets out to follow all hygienic advice will become] a tormented and miserable victim of its exacting cares.

[Hence], and due to its impossibility, hygiene has been expressly put together in order not to be obeyed on the whole."[131] Years later, in 1905, an article published in PBT, a magazine with a huge circulation that bitingly recorded the advent of modernity in Buenos Aires, wondered if "the respected hygienists believe in the positive usefulness and undeniable efficacy of their advice. Do they want us to duly heed their high knowledge? Well, start by giving each one of us an income of 10,000 patacones [the Argentine currency], and then we will see if we have to follow your so healthy and redemptive teachings. If this is not possible, let's see if you can come up with some advice that can be used by rich and poor alike. Anything else is just a waste of time."[132]

In the early 1920s and into the 1930s a few doctors spoke of a "mental plague of contagion." They were speaking ironically when they referred to "forty years of Homeric battles around the world, efforts against the life and reproduction of the bacillus." They criticized the "absurd contagionist aberrations that have led some to adopt precautions so excessive that they seem victims of blind panic." These doctors characterized the "war on spitting" and its emphasis on the regulation of daily habits as "practices inspired by doctors who dream of quarantines, making use of old systems of terror."[133] They listed individual and group reactions that could be explained only as the result of "atavisms," "mad fears," "false medical legends," and "groundless beliefs." They scorned behavior resulting from tuberculosis phobia, like the habit of "covering one's nose and mouth with a handkerchief to keep from inhaling the contagious air" in areas where people with tuberculosis circulated. They criticized the residents of a neighborhood who did everything they could to prevent the establishment of antituberculosis dispensaries and summer camps for pretubercular children in their neighborhoods out of a fear that such institutions would increase the risk of contagion.[134]

Somewhat embarrassed, Luisa G., who grew up in a tenement in the 1930s, recalls how she felt in the presence of a person with tuberculosis: "I went into a panic. For many years, I did everything I could not to take the bus that went by the Hospital Tornú. The truth is, when I heard the word tuberculosis I was terrified." Newspaper obituaries reported deaths from tuberculosis in a language that mixed pain, respect, and feigned concealment when, in fact, they concealed nothing and exacerbated fear. The deaths of Carolina Muzzili and Francisco Cúneo, two members of the socialist leadership, were covered in two long articles in La Vanguardia; not once did the word tuberculosis appear in the articles. Reference was made to Muzzili's stay in the Córdoba foothills and to "her ardent temperament and delicate physique"; Cúneo's obituary spoke of "the terrible disease that produces so much ruin among the proletariat." Curiously, such self-contained language was also a main concern of a socialist legislator who, in a congressional debate, said that tuberculosis has become "the phantom of the entire world, the working-class bogeyman," "a fear of evil that easily becomes the evil of fear."[135]

Newspapers and magazines contributed to tuberculosis phobia in both long articles and brief notes that included a wide range of messages and tones. They satisfied the reading public's thirst for stories with unhappy endings, while exposing social injustice and praising science as a source of solutions to human problems. At the same time, critical perspectives were often represented in the printed media. In 1906 *PBT* contained a page-length comic strip entitled "The model street" that made fun of the "war on spitting" and "the war on dust."[136] The strip cited spittoons, like "works of art" that were designed to help passersby "not spit on the sidewalk." Hygienic places were provided for used "paper handkerchiefs," and there were "antiseptic deposits every thirty paces where the city's inhabitants could exterminate the microbes that infested their hands and, hence, offer their hand to others without fear of contagion." The comic strip depicted "monetary disinfectants" that cleaned the money in circulation as well as macadam pavements and sidewalks that combated the "homicidal dust." One scene in the comic strip depicted "globes of oxygen" that renewed the air when many people converged on sidewalks. The main characters in the strip are by no means impoverished; they are respectably dressed men and women who probably have already internalized the anticontagion message, though they still need the watchful eye of a policeman in charge of making them comply with the hygienic habits that make this street a "model street."

Somewhat later, during the 1920s, in a popular science column in the newspaper *La Razón*, an article signed by a certain Doctor B. A. Cterio (as Doctor B. A. Cterium) made fun of the signs that were already part of the Buenos Aires landscape. These signs read, for example "No spitting on the sidewalk" or "Please do not spit on the ground for reasons of hygiene." In a tone quite similar to the one used a decade earlier by the magazine *PBT*, the article dealt with supposedly "hygienic conduct" as well as the sensible use of science in daily life. In it, Doctor B. A. Cterio wrote that "passersby [should be encouraged] to spit anywhere at all because spit left on the street is the least dangerous [since] the bacillus cannot survive in direct sunlight." He questioned the aspiration to "live under a crystal ball that was always being sterilized" and stated, earnestly it would seem, that all individuals should attempt to increase their defenses, producing enough "antibodies, the true barriers that the organism uses to oppose the invasion of bacillus."[137] B. A. Cterio criticized the signs against public spitting because they were based not on a concern with hygiene but on the idea that certain habits should be eradicated because they were seen as immoral or impolite.

Opposition to tuberculosis phobia was grounded in science and common sense. Along with these doctors and journalists, there were also anarchist and libertarian opponents of the hygienic excess. Tuberculosis phobia opened a space where it was possible to articulate an ideological criticism of customs and capitalist society. On a certain level, anarchist positions ruled out any dialogue with the dominant antituberculosis efforts, stating that "the capitalist system is responsible for the advancement of tuberculosis" or that "it is impossible to improve the existence of the poor who die of tuberculosis without the advent of a new society."[138] This brand of fatalism denied any possible cure or prevention. For some anarchists, tuberculosis was seen not only as the denial of the natural right to health and happiness, but also as a sort of betrayal of the natural harmony of things and life in society. In 1900, *Ciencia Social* said, "What we see everyday in the newspapers is a brand of sarcasm. The Galenic sirs are either dumb or they act dumb. To combat disease they call on hygiene. But under a regime of lies, social injustice, and exploitation, hygiene is like cutting off the branches of a tree that is infected at its roots and leaving the trunk, which will later reproduce even sicker branches."[139] The same tone was used in the 1920s and 1930s. *El Obrero en Madera* questioned the right of a few supposedly enlightened people to "hygienize" the life of the workers: "First, they take away [the workers'] bread and then, in the name of hygiene, they want to teach them how they can and must live."[140] *Acción Obrera* criticized those who "consider themselves protectors of the poor" and pretend to explain the lack of hygiene as a consequence of people's ignorance. Instead, the workers' newspaper claimed human beings were hygienic by nature, but the difficulties of the material environment in which they lived prevented them from practicing what they already knew.[141] *Ideas* called "the gentlemen in favor of antituberculosis prophylaxis very evil or very stupid," especially when they attempted "to ignore that workers cannot follow their prescription for vaccinations, trips to the country, moderate work, and good nutrition."[142]

Nonetheless, when it came to dealing with the more concrete and daily aspects of contagion — that is, when the discourse was removed from the patently ideological — anarchists became somewhat less countercultural. Though they criticized the "hygienic impositions" of the powerful sectors, they did not cease to recognize hygiene as a resource that, if well implemented, could promote some of the social harmony promised in the new libertarian age. This was the context of the debate on how to support the war on spitting, the use of spittoons, and "the spread of habits which, in the name of hygiene, would prevent contagion."[143] *El Obrero en Dulce* newspaper deemed "hygiene a means to emancipation since, without it, there could be neither progress nor health. Hygiene is born of the same consciousness as man, so it cannot be regulated. Everything that has been done, ordinances and laws, has failed in the face of the workers' unconsciousness." The blame for this regrettable situation lay not with the men whose natural rights, like the right to health, were being curtailed, but with the degraded social environment in which "a poverty of spirit and . . . antihygienic ways of living" prevailed. The state was powerless, and the solution was in the hands of "workers' societies, [in charge of] sowing this love of hygiene, morality, and education."[144]

Acción Obrera supported educational campaigns geared toward avoiding contagion, but it emphasized that "antituberculosis measures should be kept within practical and rational limits." Such measures would be "complements to the true prophylaxis, which consists of improving the human environment to make it resistant to evil."[145] *Ideas* recognized the importance of "material and spiritual poverty" in the life of workers; it acknowledged their "vulgarity, moral filth, and physical carelessness" and saw that social innovation might be possible if "hygienic, rational, and delicate ways were put into practice."[146] Not surprisingly, the anarchist press published handbooks on child hygiene and disease prevention, promoted books like *Guía de las buenas madres* — a guide on how to be a "good mother" that was also recommended in the media with no connection to anarchism — and passionately helped disseminate parts of the antituberculosis code, recommending that "healthy and sick alike should only kiss on the forehead and the cheek, never on the lips."[147]

Francisco Súnico, a doctor sympathetic to socialism, characterized tuberculosis as "a process of collective malnourishment, mainly economic in nature, which undermines the animal resistance of the human species." He relativized its contagiousness, stating, "Where there is no breeding ground, whether innate or acquired, there is no contagion; the disease will vanish or become inoffensive when the social causes that make man prone to it disappear." His view was quite different from the prophylactic approach advanced by social hygiene, and he declared that "the fight against tuberculosis is not a fight against microbes, it is a fight against regimes, persons, media, and environments." As a result, the primary means to defend against and remedy the expansion of tuberculosis lay in "the transmutation of the economic values of our society. . . . Changing and reconstructing our organic, political, and social institutions will automatically eliminate the calamity. . . . The definitive prophylaxis for social tuberculosis is the equality of social classes."[148] Nonetheless, in numerous articles and books Súnico offered practical advice on hygiene in general and the fight against tuberculosis in particular.

The criticism of tuberculosis phobia became more important in the 1930s and 1940s. By then, many doubted the extreme contagiousness of the disease. They emphasized the need for x-rays and institutionalized health care and doubted the importance of disinfection, the war on spitting, unhealthy dusts, and the exaggerated risk of tuberculosis in marriage.[149] In 1936 *Viva Cien Años* warned of "excessive fear and even terror that make many see every person with tuberculosis as an enemy." In *La Doble Cruz* Aráoz Alfaro wrote about the need to communicate that agents of contagion "are, in fact, found everywhere, in streets, parks, trolleys, gathering places . . . they are benign, slight, attenuated, and hardly dangerous to those with a healthy organism." Indeed, because of its attenuated nature, this sort of contagion "might even prevent the disease" by boosting immunity. According to Aráoz Alfaro, "[the contagious agents] released by those who are seriously ill and cough a great deal are dangerous and terrible." That is the contagion "one must avoid, and especially protect children from." Preventive measures must be combined with "care to the sick" and "promoting overall well-being, economic, hygienic, and social improvement for all classes, good nutrition, a healthy bedroom, comfort, rest, and even happiness."[150] In 1947 the Secretaría de Salud Pública added its voice to the voices of doctors concerned with tuberculosis phobia. It warned of the need to "combat the fear of contagion," not only among people in factories and in the army, but also among doctors, teachers, and authorities who were resistant to setting up tuberculosis wards in general hospitals.[151] The warning reveals that even when tuberculosis mortality was clearly declining, tuberculosis phobia continued to grip vast sectors of society.

······················· ✤ ·······················

CHAPTER SIX

A Disease of Excesses

At the Second Pan-American Scientific Congress, which took place in 1917 in Washington, D.C., the hygienist Nicolás Lozano stated that, along with the "biological cause" of tuberculosis, that is, the Koch bacillus, some "sociomedical factors predisposed to the disease." These factors included "alcoholism, unhealthy housing, poor or inadequate nutrition, and excesses of all sorts."[1] This way of explaining the disease began to take shape in the second half of the nineteenth century. By then, it was no longer considered an "inflammatory disease" but a "disease of exhaustion." The human body was seen as having limited capacity for resistance and, in certain conditions, this resistance could break down, paving the way for various pathologies. An endless number of human actions and behaviors could, if carried out to excess, overstimulate certain organs and dramatically reduce vitality. Some of these excesses were strongly emphasized at certain times, while others were more fleeting; all of them, however, reveal not only uncertainty and powerlessness in the face of tuberculosis, but also the strange, often arbitrary narratives of why certain people caught it. There were biomedical explanations of weakened immunity, some of which centered on the individual or on the environment. Others focused on lifestyles or morality, always discussed in general, imprecise, and quite often derogatory terms.

In this framework, a catalogue of excessive behaviors that could facilitate the onset of tuberculosis gradually emerged. In 1886 the newspaper *La Educación* cited "the muscular cerebral fatigue" resulting from "excessive school duties [and] physical inactivity" as causes of tuberculosis in children.[2] Several decades later, in the 1920s and 1930s, the "restless and feverish life of cities" transformed the urban experience into a "tuberculosis factory."[3] At other times, certain excessive lifestyles were associated with dangerous frivolity that, it was said, weakened the organism and reduced physical and spiritual resistance. An article by Augusto Bunge in 1900 that focused on "the social causes of phthisis" warned of the effects of the diets of "wealthy women who are always anxious to achieve the graceful aesthetic." Bunge's view is certainly in keeping with the nineteenth-century European image of the languid, sophisticated woman with tuberculosis, mostly intense aristocratic women who aspired to be artists or elegant prostitutes.[4] Along the same lines, three decades later an article on tuberculosis prevention stated, "Unbalanced diets affect the organism, produce a sudden nutritional imbalance, lower defenses, and favor the spread of the bacillus." Diets were criticized as a type of excess that came from "female fashion which, both yesterday and today, subject[s] women eager to improve or keep their figure to regimes of starvation of what is called our aristocracy." Similar terms were used to speak of the benefits of outdoor life and sports. Their virtues, "disinfection and the strengthening of organic defenses," were never doubted, and time and again they were presented as decisive to disease prevention. Yet, starting in the mid-1920s, when sports, outings to the beach, parks, and vacations became commonplace, there were warnings about "a trend that has led to reprehensible excesses."[5] In the case of actual and aspiring professional athletes, the combination of "a not very ordered life," "overly developed muscles," and "the fatigue resulting from excessive physical demands" tended to "weaken the organism's proper balance." Such concerns were voiced also about common people "who exercise too much" and "seek success at all cost."[6] Excessive exercise was another piece of a complex puzzle: in addition to "physical excesses [that], far from strengthening, depress defenses," the "lack of sleep, excessive mundane pleasures, and alcoholic beverages . . . paved the way for tuberculosis."[7]

But excesses of diet and exercise were not at the core of the worry over tuberculosis. Excesses linked to sexuality, drink, and work were more persistently present in the ways doctors, essayists, and journalists discussed the disease. With a lack of restraint that often resembles a sort of free association of ideas, these views of tuberculosis joined hypothetical social etiologies of the disease; biomedical, moral, and psychological explanations; and sociopolitical agendas as well as economic interests and the interests of bureaucratic and administrative groups. The disease was used to organize and legitimize a series of discourses that attempted to forge a consensus about lifestyles governed by notions of individual responsibility and moderation.

The Hypersexuality of Tuberculars

Though sexuality was hardly studied at the Universidad de Buenos Aires Medical School between 1870 and 1940, many doctors expressed their opinions on the matter. To a large extent, they based their views on the increasing medicalization of culture that took place starting in the last third of the nineteenth century. Medical doctors articulated very odd, often capricious notions, some of which dealt with the physiology of sexual organs and their connections with hormonal metabolism and certain reproductive problems.

In the late nineteenth century and early twentieth, medical, especially psychiatric, discourses on sex were part of a climate in which old taboos were being challenged. At the beginning of the century, José Ingenieros's was one of the few voices that dared to tell individual passionate stories that contravened the dominant morality. By the 1920s much more was being said about the subject of sex and sexuality. The *Biblioteca científica*, a collection of books by foreign authors with a surprising range of viewpoints, manifested this change. On the one hand, the *Guía sexual*, by J. L. Curtis, defended "the holy sacrament of marriage" as the only state within which sex should occur. On the other, G. Mac Hardy championed free love and defended "the abuse of love [due to] the anguish of modern celibacy." Between those two extremes, the *Enciclopedia del conocimiento sexual* by the physicians A. Costler and A. Willy set out to present a "modern ideal of love" in which there was room for both physical and spiritual attraction.[8] This range of viewpoints was considerably less evident in texts and commentaries by Buenos Aires hygienists and doctors, who approached sexuality in terms of sex education and the prevention of venereal diseases. They stressed the physiological side of sex and did not say anything about eroticism. Only a few, many of them anarchists, went beyond that kind of discussion, encouraging debate and reflection that connected sexuality to love, sensuality, family, and long-term relationships.[9]

In this context so-called sexual excesses were seen not only as a cause or consequence of tuberculosis, but also as a means to prescribe a certain morality.[10] Discourses that combined physiology with new developments in the fields of psychology and psychoanalysis prescribed the frequency and type of sexual activity. People wrote on "endocrine arousal disorders that came from the toxins of the Koch bacillus and were often accompanied by strong psychic anguish" and on "a libido that was produced not only by the sexual organs but by all the body's organs." There was confidence that this new interdisciplinary approach would be able to "explain perfectly all the psychic-sexual phenomena of the person with tuberculosis."[11]

During the late nineteenth and early twentieth centuries matrimony for someone with tuberculosis was seen as dangerous. In the 1880s one thesis said, "Owing to the passions [marriage] brought on, [it] could accelerate the death of a person with tuberculosis." Another recommended that "tubercular patients who have not been cured should not marry."[12] Even in the 1930s some doctors upheld the idea of "nuptial tuberculosis." This was a "consequence of the weakening of organic defenses due to sexual exhaustion, [a situation that] led to greater predisposition to contagion or caused a latent case to become active."[13] Given the impetuous nature of sexuality, usually associated with men, doctors recommended moderation and periodic abstinence as a preventive strategy.

Frequent masturbation, whether by the healthy or the sick, by women or men, by adults or children, was also seen as a cause of tuberculosis. In his "Opúsculo sobre la Tisis Pulmonar," dated 1843, Eugenio Pérez indicated that "masturbation and an excess of venereal pleasures" created a predisposition to tuberculosis. In 1878 a doctoral thesis emphasized that "the deplorable habit of onanism" could trigger the disease in the young. In the early twentieth century "the evil effects of masturbation" were discussed in a newspaper geared toward the Spanish community of Buenos Aires; it discussed the promiscuity and moral decay of the tenement room, where "parents have sexual relations regardless of the attentive ears of their children," a goad to "masturbatory practices in boys and girls," practices that "diminish their already poor defenses, exposing them to tuberculosis and other ills that lurk in poor homes." In the 1920s an anarchist newspaper that was not the least bit prudish when it came to discussing free love and bourgeois prejudices indicated that, along with the known "tuberculosis-inducing factors in schools like overcrowding and fatigue, one must consider onanism, possible because of an almost absolute lack of supervision" by teachers. Some hygienists related the supposed noxious effects of masturbation and ardent sexuality to the discourse on social inequalities. Bunge postulated that "puberty and the dawn of sex" did not have the same effects on "the weak organisms of the poor," who, unlike those with a more comfortable background, at the onset of sexuality were subject to "polarizing energies [which invite] a fatal outbreak of tuberculosis." Francisco Súnico, a doctor who often underlined the social dimensions of tuberculosis in the poor, linked the disease to a sort of antimodern criticism; he believed the rich could be victims because "the errors and social vices of the bourgeoisie are so deep [that they drive] girls, especially fragile virgins who have just come to the sweet dawn of youth, to blindly give themselves over to the dangers and excesses of modern life [which is] a terrible collection of virulent factors in the etiology of what has been called social 'tuberculosis.'"[14]

Especially after the 1920s this critical tone was much more nuanced in the books of the *Biblioteca científica*. Curtis, the author of *Guía sexual*; Gregorio Marañón, a Catholic doctor from Spain; and the Argentine Luciano del Carril, a frequent contributor to the magazine *Viva Cien Años*, all condemned masturbation with arguments based on the physical and moral risks it entailed. Del Carril's stance encouraged sexual abstinence for youth as a way to stay healthy for marriage. On the other hand, the *Enciclopedia del conocimiento sexual* strongly disapproved of the demonizing campaigns against masturbation, while recognizing and celebrating the various forms of erotic life of individuals and couples. Supporters of this line, which recognized and accepted masturbation as a part of life, included Ingenieros at the beginning of the century. And in the 1920s Roberto Arlt, whose well-known story *El juguete rabioso* had among its characters a masturbator, a homosexual, and a prostitute, stressed the inevitable, as opposed to the pathological, disorder of the world of sex and love.[15]

Masturbation was also an issue in relation to inpatients with tuberculosis at sanatoriums. One doctor spoke of "guys who lived in a permanent state of hormonal arousal owing to the accumulation of semen" and gave themselves over to "the imperative mandate of their young natures, to aberration and onanism." He also referred to "women with tuberculosis, with intact hymens and excitable temperament, who struggled against a voluptuous desire that betrayed their morality and indulged in onanistic satisfactions."[16] The magazine *Reflexiones*, published by inpatients at the Sanatorio Santa María in the Córdoba foothills, went on at length about this topic in frequent articles; attempts at education—such as "genital fatigue is frightful for people with tuberculosis; it causes fever and hemoptysis, diminishes strength, and removes minerals from the organism"—were published in the magazine, revealing that at least some tuberculars were convinced of the harmful effects certain behaviors might have on their efforts to overcome the disease.[17]

The ardent sexuality of people with consumption and tuberculosis had been an inevitable topic of French medical essays since the end of the eighteenth century.[18] These essays were often cited by Argentine doctors in their doctoral theses. In 1880 Eugenio Ramirez wrote, "The person with tuberculosis is a more ardent individual, one inclined to sexual pleasures, the satisfaction of which quickly brings on death."[19] At the beginning of the century an article published in *Archivos de Psiquiatría, Criminología y Ciencias Afines* spoke of the "heightened sexual appetite of people with tuberculosis," citing cases of women for whom tuberculosis meant overcoming "years of sexual numbness" and men whose "genital arousal" coincided with "periods of their

tuberculinization."[20] In the 1930s there was talk of "the hungry lips of tubercular lovers" and in the 1940s of the advisability of avoiding their "sexual excesses."[21]

The supposedly heightened sexuality of people with tuberculosis seems to
have given free rein to all types of explanations. One hypothesis, for example,
indicated that "people with tuberculosis, skeptical and with no hope of being
cured, are determined to enjoy, in the few days they have left, what they would
have enjoyed if they had lived for many years." Another suggested that "the
bacillus that sickens the lungs sends toxins that arouse the individual, [hence]
the idea that a man might come down with tuberculosis due to excesses mis-
takes the cause for the effect. In fact, the man engages in sexual excesses because he has tuberculosis." Others maintained that heightened sexuality was
the result of a "simple coincidence between infection and hysteria and senti-
mentalism"; that "the rest treatment makes way for a genital sexual appetite
that is heightened by arousing medication and fevers"; that "tuberculosis ex-
aggerates preexisting sexual tendencies"; that "analogies between spermidine
and tuberculin explain the sexual precociousness and heightened libido of
men with tuberculosis."[22]

Parallel to this figure of heightened sexuality was the image of the fragile
sick person, for whom doctors recommended "sexual rest" or "total abstinence."[23] It was suggested that single people with nonacute tuberculosis avoid
"emotional excesses, including flirting," whereas the supposed order, moderation, and self-control that married life entailed were celebrated.[24] Supposed
fragility was evidenced in a novel published in 1943 in which Federico, a sanatorium inpatient, warned another patient of the inadvisability of the affair he
was having with a tubercular woman: "It won't do anyone, neither you nor her,
any good to get so excited."[25]

Warnings about the sex life of people with tuberculosis were connected to
the phantasm of syphilis. It was said that the weakened defenses of persons
with syphilis made them more vulnerable to tuberculosis, and that persons
with both tuberculosis and syphilis were less likely to recover from either.[26] To
a large extent, this message was meant to dissuade illegitimate relations that
usually took place in the "bacillus-ridden nightclub environment."[27] This association, based on mainly moralist assumptions, was also found in the anarchist
press, which in the late 1920s warned of the dangers of prostitutes' kisses, "certain carriers of both the ill of syphilis and of tuberculosis."[28] In the 1930s belief
in the possibility of tuberculosis contagion through the genitals made it possible to speak of "the role of sexual perversions in the transmission of the disease," specifically "the contagion through saliva during oral–genital contact."[29]

In the case of women, sexual risk was associated with contagion in marriage—something that supposedly affected men as well—and potential pregnancy. Women with tuberculosis were advised to avoid sexual activity until they were cured, and doctors insisted on viewing "pregnancy and breast-feeding as facilitators of tuberculosis in women."[30] In this climate of ideas a councilman did not hesitate to state, "There should be no mothers with tuberculosis given that they commit a social crime."[31] In the late 1920s the nature of the association between tuberculosis and the dangers of motherhood began to change. Some doctors maintained that in cases of cured or inactive tuberculosis it was not essential to interrupt pregnancy. This approach was in part a result of the questioning of the hereditary interpretations of tuberculosis and in part a consequence of the accepted strategy of placing newborns whose mother had tuberculosis—the so-called *bebés tuberculizables*—in the hands of a healthy wet nurse in a "hygienic home or a children's health center."[32] Though medical views linked the sexuality of married women exclusively to reproduction, in terms of single women with tuberculosis, especially "women whose hymens are intact," the dangers of motherhood were replaced by concerns with an impetuous sexuality or eroticism. This led some to advocate for marriage between tubercular women and castrated tubercular men as a way to avoid hindering the "depuration of the races" on the one hand, and an advisable mode of channeling their "instincts," on the other.[33]

A few people questioned the association between tuberculosis and hypersexuality. At the beginning of the century some anarchist newspapers offered the exact opposite account. *La Voz de la Mujer* (The voice of women) defended "the noble and elevated practice of masturbation" without invoking the troubling specter of tuberculosis, and *El Rebelde* stated that "it is rare that a woman who has reached twenty without knowing sexual sensations is not threatened by tuberculosis."[34] Similarly, a dialogue between the protagonists of *El balcón hacia la muerte*, a novel that takes place in the Córdoba foothills sanatoriums in the late 1930s and early 1940s, refutes the supposed insatiable sexuality of people with tuberculosis: "You must have realized that here chastity is not impossible. There is no bigger lie than the one that says that we, people with tuberculosis, are madly sexual."[35] There were also some doctors who refused to accept these assumptions. One of them explained, "The increase of sexual desire often seen in sanatoriums and similar places is attributable to very common things. [First,] the [fact that] people with tuberculosis are, by and large, young, the increase in their metabolism, fever, the protein-based diet they tend to have, material and moral rest, the lack of everyday concerns, the reading of sentimental and erotic literature, sexual continence, all of these suffice to explain the phenomenon."[36] Another perceptive doctor pointed out that "the sexual energy of which certain authors speak seems more like a projection of a fantasy onto these sick people than a characteristic observed in reality."[37]

The enduring idea of the heightened sexuality of people with tuberculosis was evident enough for Manuel Puig to repeat it in his *Boquitas pintadas*, published in the 1960s. The novel, which takes place in the 1930s, depicts Juan Carlos, a patient with a fairly incipient case of tuberculosis, receiving advice from his doctor: "Hey, kid, you are in a delicate state. Don't go too far with the chicks because then you've had it. Try to cut back; if not, as your family doctor, I will tell your mom."[38]

Alcohol and Tuberculosis

Regardless of their ideological alignments, all discourses on degeneration associated alcoholism and tuberculosis. In an article in the *Archivos de Psiquiatría, Criminología y Ciencias Afines* published in 1907, a drinker's organism was described as "a paradise for tuberculosis" in that "the disease settled [in the alcoholic's lungs] as if in a ruined and defenseless house. Alcohol [seems to] call to tuberculosis, and tuberculosis helps it in its dark task of bringing the drinker to his end as soon as possible. Or tuberculosis pushes him to his grave and alcohol speeds up his fatal decline."[39] Others, like Súnico, found in alcohol "a sign of decay," "a virulent factor in tuberculosis [that furthers] dissolution and the moral and physical inability and degradation of peoples and races [that culminate] in the loss of will." According to Súnico, tuberculosis and alcohol lead to a "lack of discipline and of the desire to get ahead," "the absence of dignity," and "withdrawal of good feelings."[40] A few years later, *El Obrero Panadero*, the newspaper of the bakers' union, pointed out that "alcohol stultifies, degenerates the senses, and denigrates; it produces squabbles, dissension, crime, wretchedness, disease, insanity, and it prepares the body for consumption and tuberculosis."[41]

Heavily influenced by the new perceptions of drinking that had been championed in French academic circles since the mid-nineteenth century—perspectives that not only considered drinking perilous and degrading but also distinguished between fermented and distilled beverages—several doctoral theses in the 1870s and 1880s discussed the question of alcoholism in social and moral as well as medical and pathological terms.[42] In all of these theses, alcoholism was associated with issues like vagrancy, public disorder, and criminality that had been discussed since the early nineteenth century.

There were also newer concerns related to life in the modern city: unemployment, indolence, extreme sensuality, prostitution, labor absenteeism, leisure, public unrest, family crisis, moral decline, degeneration, and threats to the forging of the "Argentine race."[43]

One thesis, dated 1896, stated that "using the term disease to explain the tendency to drink is recent in the history of medical science." The figure of the alcoholic, who was almost always poor and often associated with the dissolute or the insane, began to be seen as an "individual whose spirit had a pathological inclination"; the alcoholic was not necessarily "a degenerate," but one who suffered from a disease that could not "be cured by fines and punishments."[44] During the first decades of the twentieth century the medicalization of alcohol consumption became more widespread, and the figure of the drinker, no longer necessarily poor, was increasingly associated with the sick. No wonder that by 1945 the headline of an article in *Viva Cien Años* read, "If he is a drinker, call the doctor, not the police."[45]

The association between alcoholism and tuberculosis was already present in the 1870s.[46] In 1900 an article published in *La Semana Médica* indicated that "the steady increase in [the rate of] tuberculosis coincides with an increase in alcoholism" and that in alcohol lay the cause "of the vital impoverishment produced by tuberculosis, the greatest of all misfortunes."[47] Throughout the early twentieth century, alcoholism was omnipresent in speculations about hereditary predisposition to tuberculosis. In 1918 a doctoral thesis stated that "the tightness of the thorax of those born to alcoholics favors the disease."[48] And if in 1907 it was said that "60 percent of men with tuberculosis have alcoholic backgrounds," in 1939 a well-known doctor affirmed, equally oversimplified, that "the only major medical antecedent of many people with pulmonary tuberculosis is chronic alcoholism."[49]

From 1870 to 1940 moderate consumption of fermented beverages and abstinence were the two main recommendations offered to tuberculars in terms of alcohol. Although both sought legitimacy in science, the absence of a convincing medical assessment of the nutritional qualities of fermented beverages made it impossible to close the debate.[50] In this context of uncertainties, the consumption of a certain drink was associated with certain dangers or certain benefits; there was speculation about how much alcohol one could drink without losing one's respectability and becoming stigmatized as degenerate or sick. Hence, two discourses emerged: one viewed alcoholism as a disease, an unnatural habit, and evidence of abnormality, disorder, and dangerousness; the other saw the consumption of fermented beverages as a natural, healthy, normal habit that increased one's ability to work. Not unexpectedly, the latter judgment was encouraged by numerous and diverse interests, among them large wine and beer producers, small taverns, politicians from wine-producing provinces, and fiscal-oriented policymakers in the federal government.

There were many positions between these two extremes. Some hygienists and doctors who had become politicians emphasized the nutritional value of certain drinks yet recommended abstinence, since it was "very difficult to know the amount of alcohol that each individual can consume safely, keeping in mind variations in weight and diet."[51] There were those who supported prohibition on principle yet were aware of how difficult it was to put into practice.[52] There were others who saw alcohol as a food, but "the worst of all foods," and others still who regarded beer and wine as not only "millenarian drinks" but also "sources of national wealth," and, particularly in the case of wine, "a potion that does not pervert but rather civilizes."[53]

FORTIFYING WINES

Not everyone accepted the association of tuberculosis and alcoholism, which was usually based on generalizations, impressions, tautologies, or a dubious use of statistics.[54] Various theses from the 1870s considered wine a resource to treat pulmonary tuberculosis. Avelino Sandoval postulated that the moderate consumption of nondistilled alcohol was beneficial in that such drinks were "nourishing nervine [that is, soothing] beverages"; furthermore, a portion of what is consumed "is expelled without undergoing any alteration whatsoever," and the rest "remains in the tissue to eventually become energy or be burned off." Consumption of fermented beverages should not be thought of as a practice of "the lazy or inactive" but as a resource for "the man who works hard and eats little; like coffee, *mate*, or coca leaves, it is a means of defense that offsets the hard work and poverty that deteriorate the human machine."[55]

In Buenos Aires, doctors and essayists alike considered fermented beverages part of a varied, healthful diet. Moderate consumption of such beverages was an old Mediterranean tradition which, since 1860, had been praised in numerous manuals and health-oriented books published in France, Spain, and Italy. Beer was seen as a "lactogenic beverage" advisable for pregnant and breastfeeding women and as a harmless, nutritious drink for adult men.[56] Beer-producing interests emphasized these qualities when they pressured the government to establish unrestricted sale on Sundays, pointing out that, like almond-milk *horchata*, beer was a "soft drink, a tonic with very little alcohol that helps to ward off the consumption of harmful alcohol."[57] Wine was also considered a nutritious drink. At the beginning of the century it was praised not only for helping to sterilize water and prevent infection but also for reinforcing the body's resistance.[58] Turn-of-the-century doctoral theses as well as travel guides with information about rest treatments against tuberculosis also recommended moderate consumption of wine.[59] In 1917 an instruction booklet on how to care for soldiers with tuberculosis recommended that they drink moderate amounts of "reddened water, that is, very watered down wine, or light beer." The booklets ruled out "alcohol and liquor in general, as they impeded recovery."[60] In 1940 a medical journal emphasized the nutritional value of wine: "Its chemical composition renders it a foodstuff, an energetic drink. A good table wine consumed in a moderate dose (250 cc.) cannot harm anyone with tuberculosis."[61] The same qualities were attributed to the so-called medicinal wines, for decades specifically prescribed for "tuberculosis, neurasthenia, neurosis, anemia, and chlorosis" and also persistently marketed as potions used to "nourish people with tuberculosis and convalescents."[62]

DISTILLED DRINKS THAT WEAKEN

In 1936 an essay published by the Departamento Nacional de Higiene stated that "the concurrent and indirect influence of chronic alcoholism on tuberculosis contagion cannot be categorically denied." Indeed, even when no direct toxic action can be attributed to alcohol, "it is certain that alcohol intoxication is an agent of physical decline, moral decay, and poverty, which, together, undeniably diminish individual resistance to the disease."[63]

In this context, it was not easy to define the figure of the alcoholic, the moment when someone who drank became an alcoholic, or even how to interpret the symptoms. In any case, as in most wine-producing countries, in Argentina the wine drinker was not considered sick or a social menace. The drinker of distilled beverages, however, was considered both. Many doctors saw such drinkers as being "physically and spiritually wretched" and as a sure target of tuberculosis. Yet throughout this period, drinkers of distilled beverages were caught in a crossfire. On the one hand, they were assailed by those who, supported by newspapers ads and also by some short stories published in the labor press, believed in the invigorating, healing, and energizing qualities of absinthe, cognac, grappa, liqueurs, and aperitifs. On the other, they were attacked by medical discourses, the moral criticism of social reformers, and the salvos of wine-producing sectors and some labor publications that questioned the common belief among workers that the hardest jobs required the strongest drinks in the largest quantities.[64]

The supposed rapid increase in the consumption of distilled beverages was an idea deployed by critics of those beverages.[65] The increase, however, was in fact minimal; distilled beverages never challenged the preeminence of fermented drinks or significantly altered the average annual alcohol intake per person.[66] The militant opposition to distilled drinks on the part of doctors, social reformers, and union leaders seems to have resulted from at least two questions. First, the conviction, now disproved, that the concentration of alcohol in distilled beverages had a faster, more pronounced, and thus more toxic impact on the circulatory system and on a drinker's health.[67] Second, the anxiety produced by the rapid acceptance of distilled drinks in Buenos Aires, where fermented drinks were traditionally more common. The range of distilled drinks on the market ended up being perceived as dangerous. It was associated not only with decline, suicide, crime, madness, and tuberculosis, but also with the presence of distilled drinks that competed with fermented ones in the marketplace. At the same time, the act of drinking became more visible. The increase in the number of taverns and clandestine distilleries, which occurred alongside an increased consumption of liquors, reaffirmed militant prohibitionists' beliefs about the dreadful effects distilled beverages had on health and morality.[68]

In this context, a mass of evidence—from the number of drunks reported to the police to the alcoholic pasts of the inpatients at hospices or those receiving care at tuberculosis neighborhood dispensaries—was produced to demonstrate the dangers of distilled beverages. On the basis of impression and arbitrary statistical speculation, a sort of agenda emerged that attempted to model the ways common people drank. This agenda linked watchfulness, punishment, and a series of initiatives aimed at the individual improvement of the urban masses and an ordered society engaged in the process of perfecting itself. Geared toward "making drunks into workers" and "inculcating the idea that true physical and moral comfort lies in the home and not in the tavern," this vision suggested a clear idea of the decent, hygienic, and tireless worker.[69]

If for liberal and Catholic social reformers this idea privileged moderation, predictable conduct, self-control, hard work, family, and the strengthening of the national race, for socialists and anarchists it also included a strong work ethic and the conviction that greater sobriety entailed greater awareness of and inclination toward social change. Among socialists the alcohol issue was part of an ambitious effort to transform workers into an influential and respectable political force capable of making good use of political and social rights. Some socialists called for abstinence, but more seem to have understood the advisability of "facilitating the production of hygienic and inexpensive drinks, given that the total suppression [of drinking] would be impossible." This thinking found in "wine a popular and universal drink" that, "if unadulterated and consumed in moderation, does not do any harm." Nonetheless, socialists indicated that "it is good to remember that a loaf of bread is worth more than a glass of wine, and thus wine must come after basic and even certain superfluous needs are satisfied."[70] For certain anarchists the question was "to free oneself from both the bourgeois and the alcoholic yokes [since] the worker drunk on hard liquor can hardly be drawn to ideas of emancipation." Other anarchists demonstrated a curious flexibility: they spoke out against alcoholism and supported "vegetarian and antialcoholic restaurants" while— probably out of an acute need for funds, included advertisements in their publications for gins and beers, labeled "the workers' choice."[71]

As potential drinkers and as antialcohol preachers, men were at the center of all discussions on the consequences of drinking for people's health. Women were only marginally present, and they were always associated with the noble task of keeping drink out of the home.[72] In the debate around tuberculosis and alcoholism, the ideas of alcohol as poison and as nourishment coexisted, as did the notions of moderate consumption and total abstinence and the different impacts of fermented and distilled drinks. Indeed, perceptions of the alcohol issue seemed to speak more to the agenda of those who sought to control tuberculosis morbidity and mortality than to people's actual experiences with drinking and its effects on health. Even though Buenos Aires was hardly a city of drinkers, any narrative on tuberculosis seemed to use alcoholism, especially in association with distilled liquors, as a means of explaining and fighting the disease.

Work Fatigue

In October of 1900 the newspaper *El Rebelde* reported the death of an anarchist activist: "The consumptive existence tolerated by those who are exploited by the monstrous capitalist machinery cruelly wounded comrade Carlos Valpedre, who died after enduring a long illness caused by an excess of work."[73] By no means an exclusively anarchist notion, the association between excessive work and tuberculosis had been taking shape since the late nineteenth century.

Unlike excesses of sex and drink, excessive work was not a choice but an imposition and consequently difficult to attribute to a lack of individual self-control. Its association with tuberculosis articulated at least two problems, both particularly relevant in the relationship between this disease and the factory, domiciliary work, the extension of the workday, night shifts, piecework, industrial hygiene, and the pace of production. The first of these problems had to do with medical controversies and judiciary cases that argued whether tuberculosis was a professional disease. The second referred to tuberculosis as a disease in which excessive work was just one of the many factors that paved the way for contagion.

Starting in the late nineteenth century, in the context of debates on the social question, there were vague commentaries about "workers' diseases." Later, in the 1910s, the concept of workplace diseases began to take shape and, with it, a discourse of specialists that offered litigation services and promised material compensations. Within this framework there was discussion of whether tuberculosis was a work-related disease. In 1909 one study concluded that such a categorization was problematic, partly because tuberculosis was very common among workers and partly because it "entailed numerous contributing causes that might determine or aggravate it."[74] The issue was also current in 1915, when Law 9688, which dealt with workplace accidents and work-related diseases, was passed, although tuberculosis was not included in the legislation. Nor was it included in executive branch initiatives that, starting in 1916 and continuing into the 1920s, set out to regulate, modify, or broaden that law.

In the 1930s and 1940s, on the basis of the mass use of x-rays, many studies emphasized the high rate of the disease in certain occupational groups and work processes.[75] During the same period workplace illness became a solid medical category that consisted of pathologies that were "indirectly acquired at work" and could not be considered a consequence "of the sort of work carried out by the victim."[76] It was in this context that jurisprudence began to discuss tuberculosis in quite different terms than in the past. In 1936 an executive branch decree expanded the list of professional diseases to include tuberculosis whenever a causal relationship between a job or working environment and the beginning of the disease could be proven. With these very general guidelines, the idea of "indemnifying any disease or harm where work could be shown as a cause" was put forward.[77] In 1941 a congressional bill cited the advisability of including tuberculosis in the work-related diseases specified by Law 9688, arguing that jurisprudence which "at the beginning vacillated now clearly leans toward" considering "tuberculosis a disease worthy of indemnity."[78] In the late 1940s this tendency became more evident, especially when it could be demonstrated that tuberculosis was the "consequence of a specific, sudden, and violent event" that might worsen a preexisting condition or "when tuberculosis has been encouraged by a pernicious environment."[79]

The idea that tuberculosis was a disease caused by excessive work had been expressed in the workers' press since the late nineteenth century, and it continued to be voiced into the 1940s. In 1894 *El Obrero Panadero* bore the headline "Night work is the seed of tuberculosis"; in 1912 *El Obrero Textil* declared that "the cause of tuberculosis lies in the factory, which is an evil stepmother, a prison that steals everything: strength, health, youth, joy"; in 1928 *Acción Obrera* described workshops as "breeding grounds for tuberculosis," and in 1941 the textile union's newspaper claimed that "cotton spinning mills engendered tuberculosis."[80] Some years later, in a poem probably influenced both by the early twentieth-century social poetry of the eclectic Pedro Bonifacio Palacios Almafuerte and also by 1930s tango lyrics, the association between tuberculosis and excessive work allowed Peronist labor leader María Roldán to make sense of the death of one of her coworkers at a meat-processing plant: "Bloodied daughter of the people, cannon fodder for the shop floor / Tell them that yesterday a comrade died, / poor and exploited, defeated by evil. / Tell them that not long ago you entered the factory, beautiful / and yesterday you lay dying, consumptive, / in the last bed of a miserable hospital."[81]

Work fatigue was a concern of intellectuals, doctors, and politicians active in reform and social change. In 1899 Ingenieros warned of the "excess of work established by the present form of industrial exploitation [that] contributes to weakening the resistance of the organism [of the] worker who toils beyond the physiological limits of fatigue." Ingenieros blamed not the worker for his condition, but the way industrial work was organized. Excessive work thus became a central point in a regeneration program aimed at viable improvement of working conditions as well as an issue in the advocacy of what Ingenieros called a "new right where social interests outweigh individual interests."[82] In 1906, in a congressional debate on whether the federal government should buy a sanatorium in the Córdoba foothills, a legislator categorized tuberculosis as "a disease [tied to] excessive work and poor living conditions."[83] Somewhat later, in a report of 1910 requested by the federal government, Bunge spoke of the harm done by "intense work, long workdays, . . . a lack of fresh air, [time spent in] crowded places, dust, the lack of ventilation, and sunlight." In addition to the muscular fatigue that might lead to general anemia, he mentioned a form of "workers' neurasthenia" attributable more to the "increasing intensity of work" than to "intense and excessive mental activity." Tuberculosis was a "disease of muscular or nervous burdens," and fatigue an "aggravating factor" or a factor that "predisposed to the disease."[84]

By the 1920s, the issue of work fatigue was frequently mentioned by social critics. Súnico said that "devitalizing work" ended up "provoking tuberculosis."[85] The socialist politician and intellectual Alfredo Palacios was the major local figure in an international network of experts dedicated to studying, with a strong empirical basis and quite sophisticated quantitative methods, the connections between work processes and the worker's body. The concern was part of a socialist and liberal tradition that saw science and moral appeals based on science as a means to overcome social conflicts and to make work a legitimate source of wealth and property. The metaphor of the human engine and scientific regulation of the body's movements was in conversation with this concern. And, although the topic was soon politicized in debates on the length of the workday, as well as on workplace and military service accidents, the way experts dealt with the issue of labor fatigue indicates that they wanted to offer an objective, nonpartisan response to what was increasingly perceived as a serious problem. They saw the worker's body, not social relations in the workplace, as the realm in which to resolve conflicts. The language of the rational use of energy was employed worldwide by many ideological, political, and professional groups, from liberals, socialists, and fascists to Taylorists and Stajanovists. If with different nuances, all of them focused not only on the idea of a worker in full control of his physical capabilities and accordingly resistant to fatigue, but also on a "productivist calculation" as a means of balancing material well-being and social justice.

Fatigue, weakening, and exhaustion were described in modern terms: decline and a loss of power, of energy, and of the will to live. The question of fatigue appeared in Europe in the last quarter of the nineteenth century and gained ground at the beginning of the twentieth, when it began to be defined as an inability to perform mental and physical tasks resulting from labor excesses. This is certainly different from premodern fatigue, which was an agreeable sensation, a sort of recognition of achievement, a resource that could even permit the recovery of health. By contrast, the discussion of modern fatigue was dominated by a sort of transcendentalist materialism. It understood the body as a system of economies with a finite amount of energy and medicine as a key instrument in the effort to rationally use that energy and to control the reproduction of the labor force.

In 1923 Palacios published *La fatiga y sus proyecciones sociales*, an investigation that analyzed "in the factory" physiological and psychic phenomena related to "the exhaustion of workers' energies." The goal was "to prove, as if in an algebra problem, that the man who works a given number of hours under certain conditions suffers from certain alterations in his physical state, and that after a determined period of work total exhaustion strikes."[86] According to Palacios, fatigue produced "pathological phenomena, organic degeneration, general ruin of the organism, a psychic and physical inferiority that determines a predisposition to tuberculosis, favored by other concurrent causes like the factory environment and poor diet." In addition to work-

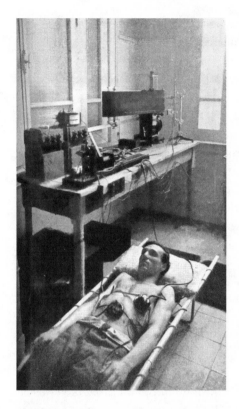

Measuring fatigue in the workplace. (Alfredo Palacios, *La fatiga y sus proyecciones sociales: Investigaciones de laboratorio en los talleres del estado*, Buenos Aires: La Vanguardia, 1935)

related fatigue, Palacios spoke of a "premature fatigue" among poor children or children who worked, and a "fatigue in women" that grew out of the combination of working in the workshop and housework, the demands of breast-feeding, and deficient diet.[87] Written in the period between the wars, *La fatiga y sus proyecciones sociales* was unsparing in its criticism of Taylorism, which it described as a system solely interested in productivity and incapable of contemplating exhaustion because it was so focused on performance. Palacios' book stated that it was not possible to study the workers' question "without using an experimental method offered by physiology and psychology." It saw tuberculosis as evidence of the negative impact social and economic inequalities could have on the physical and moral health of the working classes and on the efforts to consolidate nationality.

Along with the concept of work fatigue, the image of tuberculosis as a disease of exploitation took shape. It circulated widely among anarchists, who stated that the "blame for tuberculosis lies in the capitalist system" and that "it is impossible to improve the existence of the poor who die of tuberculosis" in a capitalist society.[88] Such fatalism, which ruled out any hope for cure or prevention, was much more commonplace at the beginning of the twentieth century than in the twenties and thirties.

In the two decades after the publication of *La fatiga y sus proyecciones sociales*, the issue of work excesses was still on the experts' agenda. At the Primer Congreso Argentino de Sociología y Medicina del Trabajo, in 1939, it became clear that workplace or industrial medicine was gaining ground, and with it several studies addressed the correlation between tuberculosis and fatigue, certain occupations, and work processes. In 1948 another study whose focus was on work fatigue cited significant improvements in the labor conditions of many workers in the industrial sector, while pointing out the ongoing need to deal with issues like psychological questions, the commute from home to work, the excessive physical demands still common in workshops, unskilled piecework, and the long workday of those who worked at home. It mentioned "nonapparent or lesser fatigues" that common clinical exams could not identify but that "laboratory methods" could demonstrate. The study also referred to occupations in which work processes tended to favor "the development of pulmonary tuberculosis in the worker."[89]

Jobs that Weaken

In 1948 an article published in *El Médico Práctico* criticized professionals who thought of tuberculosis as a "disease related to environment but not to work."[90] The prevalence of the environmentalist approach was evident in the statistics, and there was no lack of supporting proof for that view at the beginning of the twentieth century and in the 1940s. In 1927, for example, a report from the Departamento Nacional de Higiene warned of the limitations of any attempt to relate occupations with tuberculosis mortality: "Suffice it to say that out of 9,434 men over the age of 15 who died of tuberculosis, 4,191 did not have a specific occupation. Indeed, in the case of women, out of 6,616 almost all of them — 6,503 — did not report any specific profession."[91]

In a certain way, these statistics were the result of the dominance of the environmentalist approach to tuberculosis in medical and hygienist circles, which were more inclined to scrutinize the connections between disease, individuals, and housing.[92] In any case, starting in the late nineteenth century, work and occupation came to be seen as "factors that [might] cause tuberculosis," though it is true they were not formulated as decisive to the discussion of the social etiology of the disease. In addition to the meagerness of the statistics, there were specific problems resulting from the characteristics of the Buenos Aires labor market, which was marked by a high presence of unskilled workers, the importance of seasonal labor, and the simple fact that working people tended to change jobs quite often. In addition to housework, women did paid work in workshops, factories, and the service sector, but usually only for a certain period of their working lives. All these issues were relevant when it came to establishing a causal relationship between the loss of physical resistance and its attendant predisposition to tuberculosis and a certain occupation.

The only study available from the first half of the twentieth century that explored the relationship between occupation and tuberculosis was published in 1918. It concluded that average tuberculosis mortality from 1912 to 1916 constituted 18.3 percent of all deaths of people over the age of ten, and that in the printing industries these figures reached 35.5 percent, in the leather industries 30.8 percent, and in the clothing industry 29.0 percent. Among public employees the figure was 21.6 percent, among metallurgical workers 22.1 percent, among transport workers 21.2 percent, woodworkers 19.6 percent, food industry workers 19.2 percent, and construction workers 18.8 percent.[93] Many years later, in 1957, the issue was still being discussed, and there was still insistence on the need to "systematize the study of the causal relationships between work and tuberculosis." It was considered advisable to focus on "jobs that [diminish] organic defenses, jobs that [produce] other diseases associated with tuberculosis and jobs carried out in dangerous settings."[94] In any case, beyond the fairly unsuccessful efforts at systematization, the fear of contagion; the demands of specific sectors; and the willingness, for whatever reasons, to statistically examine mortality and morbidity in a certain occupation produced a mass of knowledge that served neither to consistently identify the occupational groups most affected by the disease nor to convincingly explain its causes.[95]

WORKING WOMEN: DOMICILIARY WORKERS, DOMESTIC SERVANTS, AND SEAMSTRESSES

From 1870 to 1940 the relative presence of women in the workforce diminished. According to the census, during the first decades of that period the decline was marked: women's presence in the active workforce dropped from 58.8 percent to 27.4 percent. Between 1914 and 1947, the rate leveled out at around 20–25 percent. Even in periods like the late 1930s, when the economy became more diverse and complex, women's presence in the labor market was concentrated in a half-dozen largely traditional occupations. Almost three-quarters of the women doing nonhousehold work tended to perform domestic service or domiciliary work. A distant second, with significant variations according to the industry and period in question, was the group working at large textile, food, tobacco, and match factories. Next came teachers, saleswomen in shops, nurses, and other occupations in the service sector. Last were the women holding what were called modern jobs, like telephone operators and secretaries.[96]

In 1918 a university thesis maintained that the primary characteristic of women's work was, in financial terms, its complementary relationship to the work of men. This idea had already been put forth by an inspector for the Departamento Nacional del Trabajo, Celia Lapalma de Emery, in 1911, when she reported that paid work performed by women was simply a "prudent supplement, used to help out with the expenses of modest families."[97]

Starting in the late nineteenth century, tuberculosis mortality among domiciliary workers—seamstresses, dressmakers, women who took in ironing and washing, milliners, all of whom worked in their homes or at someone else's, for themselves or for others, but not at a factory—was associated with the burden of long workdays, daily household responsibilities, the high cost of housing, and, when performed in a seamstress's home, low hygiene standards because rest, work, leisure, and meals often took place in a single physical space. It was also associated with poor pay, mostly because of the large number of women performing such work as well as those working in clothing factories and in the workshops of charitable organizations. Because it was largely piecework, which was usually erratic and involved intense labor and tight deadlines, the seamstresses' domiciliary work was, in the opinion of hygienists, unhealthily sedentary. Seated and leaning over for hours, seamstresses placed excessive demands on their bodies in a work routine marked by repeated movements and a posture that hindered respiration and made way for tuberculosis. However, contrary to the common belief that lack of ventilation in the rooms of overpopulated *conventillos*, or tenements, was the cause of seamstresses' predisposition to tuberculosis, a study from 1915 emphasized that their salaries and their seasonal workloads—not the lack of ventilation— were largely to blame for their predisposition to tuberculosis; indeed, most seamstresses worked in a courtyard or next to a door or window.[98]

The garment industry also employed many women in factories. It was one of the manufacturing sectors able to substitute imports with relative success and speed. In the 1870s and 1880s the garment industry was not very economically concentrated, and there were sewing workshops and tailors' shops scattered throughout the city. Many were using sewing machines, and production was mainly geared toward meeting the needs of the nonluxury local market. Quite flexible, the garment industry had effected an increasing division of labor that demanded more and more of dressmakers, tailors, and embroiderers. After the economic crisis of 1890, and largely as a result of the exchange rate and tax policy that quickly ensued, some foreign companies that used to export to Argentina set up factories in Buenos Aires in order to satisfy the local demand for massive nonluxury items, while continuing to import more expensive items. Now concentrated in a group of large and medium-sized companies, the garment industry's domiciliary workforce constituted about half of its workers, maybe more, considering that the seamstresses who worked at workshops often took home extra work.[99] At the beginning of the century a hygienist reported that "for every ten garment workers who work in a workshop, there are one hundred who work at home, and this proportion sometimes increases when demand calls for it."[100] Somewhat later, the newspaper *La Nación* reported that the workshops that supplied the army and navy provided home labor for more than ten thousand women and that in terms of the garment workshops belonging to the large stores, more than five or six times as many people worked at home as in the production plants.[101] In 1912 the tuberculosis mortality rate for women working in the garment industry, whether in factories or in their homes, was 32.7 percent (40.9 percent if all diseases of the respiratory system are taken into account). This was almost twice as high as the average rate of tuberculosis mortality.[102]

The industrial dust from spinning mills, textile plants, burlap sacks, and hemp sandals were "predisposing factors" that "facilitated the spread of the bacillus."[103] In 1902 Gabriela L. de Coni claimed these work settings fostered "coughs, abundant sputum, and respiratory fatigue," which, over time, caused "anemia and consumption."[104] A few years later a survey of working conditions in garment factories, some of which employed up to seven hundred people, included the words of a girl who worked in one of them: "I am very strong. I have worked here for a year and I have not yet gotten sick, but there are others who cannot go on. They say they caught tuberculosis."[105]

Tuberculosis was also found among those who performed what were then called modern jobs. Among typists it was said to result from "the obligation to keep up an appearance" beyond the possibilities of "their lean salaries"; these women spent money on presentable clothing while sacrificing good nutrition, and "their health inevitably weakened." This "paved the way for the disease."[106] Among telephone operators, tuberculosis was considered a consequence of fatigue rather than the result of trying to look like a member of the emerging middle-class, white-collar employee: "For several hours, with a ten-minute break, telephone operators must wear a heavy apparatus on their heads. Hence, their nervous systems necessarily suffer, and so they are a legion of people with anemia and tuberculosis."[107]

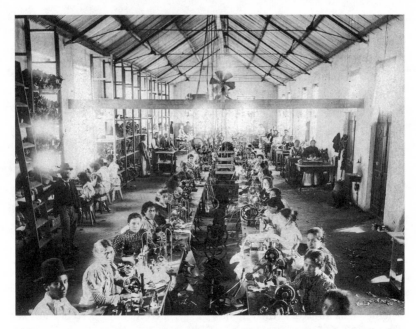

Female garment industry workers. Garment industry jobs were
consistently associated with high female tuberculosis mortality rates.
(Archivo General de la Nación, 1912 and 1920)

At the beginning of the century domestic workers constituted 39.8 percent
of the female workforce, and by the end of the forties, 30.5 percent. According to hospital statistics from throughout this period, a striking number of
women with tuberculosis specified having a profession, "particularly cooks,
maids, and servants."[108] In the case of cooks, the disease was associated with
"sudden changes in temperature," while in that of the "domestic servants," the
result of work performed "in closed spaces and poor lodging conditions."[109]

WORKING MEN: BAKERS, SHOEMAKERS, AND DOCKWORKERS

In 1924 *La Vanguardia*, the socialist newspaper, stated that the workers most
affected by tuberculosis were bakers, painters, cart drivers, carpenters, shoemakers, and tailors.[110] The list was far from exhaustive. Unlike working women
who had died of tuberculosis and were largely concentrated in a small group
of occupations, men with tuberculosis worked in a wide range of fields. In
1909 a hygienist spoke of this fact, contradicting what was then considered a
proven truth in saying that tuberculosis affected people who worked in closed
settings as much as those who worked outdoors.[111] Later, in 1947, catching the
disease was related to "fatigue, inhaling dust, vapors and gases, poor posture

or repeated movements and the work environment." Those holding unskilled jobs that entailed "difficult tasks and long workdays" had a tuberculosis mortality rate "two and a half times higher than the general population."[112] But while some emphasized the strains of manual labor, the statistics from tuberculosis hospitals revealed that in both 1918 and 1933 the vague category of employees constituted the majority of patients.[113] Indeed, in the specific case of grocery store employees the mortality rate was said to be a good deal higher than the overall rate.[114]

As with teachers, domestic employees, and prostitutes, the place of waiters and postal workers in the contagion chain led to studies of their tuberculosis rates. In 1910 it was thought waiters grew sick owing to the "poorly ventilated setting" in which they worked. Three and four decades later, explanations included the pace of work, inadequate and irregular breaks, and alcohol and tobacco abuse.[115] In the case of postal workers, the list of factors that predisposed them to the disease included the closed office setting, overcrowding, and the absence of natural light. The physical demands of the job were not "what affected the health of these workers." It was, rather, the fact that they spent all their time "receiving and handling mail sacks that had not been disinfected" and items "that after going through eight or ten sets of hands were a sure source of contagion."[116] In addition to these reasons, which had been cited since the early twentieth century, an equally vague new explanation referred to "the personality of the postal worker," who "religiously performed his responsibilities and had a spirit of obedience and resignation. Over time, this leads to a state of moral depression. . . . When a character of this nature coincides with a . . . weak physical constitution, tuberculosis finds the best terrain to spread."[117]

Starting at the end of the nineteenth century there was much talk of the "tuberculosis-causing factors" that characterized the work of bakers.[118] A report published in the *Anales del Departamento Nacional de Higiene* mentioned "small, filthy, shops with poor ventilation and worse lighting," and *El Obrero Panadero* spoke of night shifts that "diminish the workers' vitality, deny them natural light and fresh air that might oxygenate their lungs," and forces them "to make extremely intense muscular efforts."[119] In addition to these factors, the workers' press spoke of "irregular diets," "long workdays," and "the lack of muscle tone and physical endurance which drives bakers to drink, where they believe they will find stimulation and reward."[120] Night shifts often forced many bakers to participate in a world of single men that went from the bakery to the tavern to the brothel. A study from 1904 concluded that, considering the combination of poor diet, precarious and insufficient rest, and moral degradation, "it is surprising that not all bakers succumb to tuberculosis."[121] In 1928 *El Obrero Panadero* admitted that "most people believe that every baker is inevitably a future resident of the Hospital Muñiz and Hospital Tornú."[122]

Bakers' perception of themselves coincided with the opinion of many doctors, who affirmed that "the number of bakery workers with tuberculosis has risen to 70 percent."[123] These impressions, which were shared by both doctors and the labor press, contradicted hospital records. In 1912, at least, of a total of 250 bakers seen and later released from hospital, only 15 were diagnosed with tuberculosis; the total for all respiratory diseases was 27. In any case, a study in 1913 demonstrated that 20 percent of bakers died of tuberculosis; the number rises to 30 percent if one includes those with other respiratory diseases. Both numbers are significantly higher than the tuberculosis mortality rate in the food industry and the overall rate among the employed population.[124]

Hospital workers, in addition to experiencing a poor diet, long workdays, and overcrowding, had "direct contact with people with tuberculosis."[125] In 1922 the newspaper *Idea Hospitalaria* reported that "the apocalyptic monster of tuberculosis turns nurses into patients."[126] Later, in the early 1950s, an exhaustive study that compared workers at tuberculosis and general hospitals showed that there was no "specific risk" of contagion at tuberculosis hospitals. Indeed, contrary to the extreme contagionist approach, this study concluded that in tuberculosis hospitals the disease was more common among "poorer [workers] such as laborers or kitchen workers" than among those "who worked in contaminated environments or in close contact with patients," such as the nursing staff, which, starting in the 1910s, was mostly female.[127]

According to studies from the beginning of the century, polishers and metal sharpeners who used sandpaper and emery, those who worked with sand in the glass industry, potters, stonemasons, and bricklayers seemed to suffer from inhaling inert dust that "did not actually constitute the disease but did cause slight alterations in the respiratory apparatus that are the gateway to infections and diseases like pulmonary tuberculosis." The conclusions of studies from 1950s were similar, although at that time the debate centered on whether "silica or silica-ferruginous dust paved the way to tuberculosis . . . or if tuberculosis is followed by silicosis."[128]

Tuberculosis in people who worked with paint, whether making it or using it in construction, was often associated with lead poisoning. At the beginning of the century, some refuted this correlation, but later studies verified it.[129] Apparently, frequent contact with white lead, metallic salts, and other chemicals was the main cause of work-related health problems in painters and of their predisposition to contracting tuberculosis.[130] In 1912, 22 percent of painters died of tuberculosis, a number that rises to 32.8 percent if all respiratory diseases are taken into account.[131] Workers in the printing trade who were affected by the turn-of-the-century expansion of the publishing industry and of journalism also suffered the effects of the lead dust created by typesetting machines.[132] Some added piecework to the list of tuberculosis-causing occupational hazards, warning that "in one hour a worker may do more work and earn a little more, but his chance of catching tuberculosis also increases by 80 percent, since, in his eagerness to finish off a given number of galleys, he becomes a machine, constantly moving his arms and causing his lungs to work nonstop while breathing in the dust of a box impregnated with antimony."[133] In the early 1920s, 25 percent of deaths of workers in the printing trade—46 percent if those with general respiratory diseases are included—were caused by tuberculosis.[134]

In 1912 tuberculosis mortality among shoemakers reached 19.2 percent, just above the average of 15.9 percent and is notably higher, 28.4 percent, if all respiratory diseases are taken into account. Some of the causes mentioned were "the partial and excessive muscular effort that leads to underdevelopment of the thorax," "long workdays," "poor living conditions," "sedentary tasks that require little effort," which, it was said, attracted "men already with tuberculosis but still able to work."[135] Piecework was often added to these causes. It played a major role in the shoe industry starting in the 1880s, especially in the common, nonluxury segment of the market. Though the industry grew considerably, its level of mechanization did not, and for a long time the work of the shoemaker—whether in large factories, small workshops, or at home—was manual.[136] In all of these settings, piecework was fundamental. It tended to lower production costs in a labor market where there was often great pressure to increase productivity.

Among dockworkers, death from tuberculosis in 1912 was around 43.8 percent and almost 50 percent if those caused by other respiratory diseases were included.[137] This elevated rate was associated with "a very physically demanding job, poverty, and alcoholism."[138] The labor of dockworkers, mainly that of shoveling grain, was considered "particularly dangerous and tuberculosis-causing," as these workers were constantly straining "to keep up with the enormous pipes that tossed grains endlessly, [where] there is a lack of oxygen and [the workers] are constantly breathing in fine dust . . . and, soon enough and to a heartbreaking degree, they fall victim to tuberculosis."[139]

In spite of all these very speculative associations—a sort of epidemiology based on some statistics and plenty of impressionistic suppositions—between 1870 and 1950 work was not considered a decisive cause of predisposition to tuberculosis. Though the explanatory power of work was noted in the late nineteenth century, it was largely unheeded until at least the 1940s. Such neglect resulted from the difficulties posed by a social disease; the limitations of statistics; and the tendency, for unclear reasons, to pay attention to certain occupations and overlook others. As was evident in the attempts to forge the association of alcohol and tuberculosis, for example, that of tuberculosis and work was also complex, multifaceted, very speculative, and at times even arbitrary.

Housing that Weakens

During the last third of the nineteenth century and the first half of the twentieth, tuberculosis was interpreted as an inevitable consequence of social relations in the urban environment, in particular the overcrowding and promiscuity that predominated in housing of the urban poor. This environmentalist explanation informed almost all efforts to identify the social factors that caused the disease; it largely overshadowed the importance given other factors, like excessive work or an unhealthy diet.

In 1866 the *Revista Médico Quirúrgica* indicated that "the atmosphere [in Buenos Aires] was once richer in oxygen than it is today, and that explains why, previously, someone with tuberculosis could be cured [while living] downtown or [at least] survive for several years."[140] Twenty years later the municipal census warned that in Buenos Aires "tuberculosis lurks in old walls and brick pavements."[141] The emphasis on the environment was important when it came to trying to understand "tuberculosis in the comfortable classes," which, according to hygienists, was related to "the fashion of having papered walls, dark rooms with too much furniture." But this environmentalist approach was even more important when it came to discussing housing for the urban working class, especially the *conventillo*, which for over six decades was called "an unhealthy nucleus," "a damned house," "an unwholesome residence," "an unhealthy islet," and "an unhealthy and overcrowded room."[142] Its material precariousness and quaintness roused social and moral critics, reform politicians, public officials, and naturalist or realist writers.

The filthy water tanks, clogged drains, and unventilated rooms found in tenements were seen as breeding grounds for tuberculosis as well as other diseases that marked the demographic history of the late nineteenth century. "Let's keep in mind," one hygienist said, "that in the poor person's home germs reproduce by the thousands; that, unseen, poisoned air . . . comes in houses, even those that are well equipped and well located."[143] The urgent concern with housing was understandable in a city which, from 1870 to 1900, housed thousands of newly arrived immigrants in a variety of ways. It was in this context that tuberculosis became bound to the inadequacy of the sanitation networks, which were growing, but not fast enough, and to the housing of the poor. More in keeping with the miasmatic theories of Max Joseph Pettenkoffer than with Edward Koch's bacteriology, in the 1890s the physician and politician Guillermo Rawson wrote that tuberculosis "can be explained only by the increase in the dampness of the city's subsoil, along with the common causes of unhealthiness," including the "mephitis produced by accumulation, the imperfect circulation of air, the lack of light and the gases let off by decaying organic matter, which spread and threaten everyone."[144] For some, this notion of menace epitomized the essence of the urban world, where the risks of contagion could easily ignore social differences. It was not in vain that, in 1883, Eduardo Wilde wrote that as soon as "an individual becomes sick in a city, he harms not only himself and his family but also the distant and immediate population." In the following decades this argument was taken up by others, who were also concerned with this issue when they warned that "tuberculosis radiates out over the city" from "the basic and unwholesome settings" of the tenements; they warned that the "unseen germs and poisoned air that incubate in the houses of the poor can get into homes in even the best neighborhoods."[145]

During the last third of the nineteenth century there was an unambiguous conviction that the material environment of housing for the poor was not only a passport to disease but also a nucleus for pernicious influences "on the physical and moral well-being of the community."[146] Housing for the poor brought together a hodgepodge of social, moral, political, and biological concerns. In 1883 a university professor was appalled to see in every tenement room not only "a pandemonium where four, five, or more people breathed the same air, despite hygienic recommendations and the demands of the body itself," but also an affront to "the laws of common sense and good taste."[147] A few years before the Memoria Municipal—a periodic, sometimes yearly account of city governmental affairs presented by the mayor—stated that the "insalubrious and noisy" tenement is "a moral and physical risk that impedes a tightening of family bonds; it presents obstacles to sociability, and it is a risk to the health not only of those who live there but to the general population."[148]

These preoccupations latched onto the specter of degeneration, of decaying bodies and souls which Rawson, once again, articulated clearly: "Once reduced to the physical and moral decay of the tenement, a vigorous and healthy family, with honest and hardworking parents, undergoes a physical and moral depression that renders the strong unfit for work and the children [deprived of] the health necessary to grow up naturally."[149] This persistent association between rundown, overcrowded housing, on the one hand, and tuberculosis and moral decline, on the other, was a cornerstone of the discourses of almost everyone who discussed the issue. In 1900 the hygienist Samuel Gache described the Buenos Aires tenements as "residences where all sentiments are corrupted, all affection lost; . . . they are a risk to public health since all diseases incubate there; . . . they are also a risk to morality, because these residences are the stage for shameful scenes of licentiousness and brothels."[150] In 1907 President José Figueroa Alcorta referred to tenements and boardinghouses as "environments devoid of light and air [and that, hence, foment] libertine misconduct, . . . which extends its pernicious influence on the future and hinders the fight for good and social progress."[151] In 1918 *La Vanguardia* reported that life in the tenement was marked by a "promiscuity that brings violent, forced intimacy and harms cordial relations between neighbors."[152] In 1920 a Catholic politician involved in the housing question stated that "overcrowding in tenements affects hygiene and morality; the germs that live in the body bear the vices that kill the soul. Promiscuity paves the way for prostitution, and poverty leads to tuberculosis." One year later, in 1912, the anarchist magazine *Ideas* referred to the tenement as "a hovel, a site of tuberculosis and moral decline."[153] And in 1942, when Europe was in the throes of the Second World War, the *Anuario Socialista* stated that "morality is a problem of square meters. The tenement is neither moral nor immoral: it is simply amoral, and as such a threat to health and productivity; . . . it is the urban concentration camp of nations in times of peace."[154]

This long-lasting association between tuberculosis and the overcrowded, precarious tenement room reinforced the common, if erroneous, perception that these collective residences were the most common form of housing for the Buenos Aires working class. This gave rise to an interconnected set of beliefs: one got tuberculosis by living in a tenement, poor people lived in tenements, poor people had tuberculosis. But the censuses revealed that neither before nor after the emergence of new neighborhoods in Buenos Aires did tenements house more than one-quarter of the population of the city. Individual housing, whether a modest house made of durable construction materials or a simple shack, was the most popular form of housing and the most decisive contributor to the city's rapid urban growth. It's not surprising that of all deaths from infectious diseases, including tuberculosis, recorded in 1892, only 14 percent were people whose declared residence was a tenement. Furthermore, the rate never reached 50 percent, even when unspecified hospital deaths of people whose declared residence was a tenement were added to that total. At least half of all deaths from tuberculosis occurred in homes and, though tenements (5 percent of the city's housing) did in fact see a relatively high proportion of these deaths, they were in no way crucial in terms of the overall rate.[155]

In the last decade of the nineteenth century Gache called tenements "a Pandora's box that holds the secret to the spread of tuberculosis among the poor and malnourished." He pointed out that "there is less tuberculosis in Catedral North and South, Buenos Aires neighborhoods where wealthy people live" than in Balvanera and San Cristóbal, where "tenements abound, the population is denser and poorer, [and where] workers, craftsmen, and everyone whose hygiene leaves a great deal to be desired live."[156] A study by the demographer Gabriel Carrasco distinguished tuberculosis mortality by neighborhoods for the years 1897–99. He concluded that in San Cristóbal and Balvanera Sur, which had numerous tenements, tuberculosis mortality rates were 380 to 400 per 100,000 inhabitants, whereas in the San Nicolás and Vélez Sarfield neighborhoods, where there were few tenements, the rates were 64 to 52 per 100,000 inhabitants.[157] The study seemed to reaffirm the direct association between poor housing and tuberculosis, despite the problematic case of the San Juan Evangelista neighborhood, where the tuberculosis rate was about 51 per 100,000 inhabitants and tenements housed 26.6 percent of the population, as opposed to an average of 14.5 percent for the city at large.[158]

Carrasco's study quickly circulated in local medical and hygienist circles. Bunge cited it in an ambitious work on the social etiology of tuberculosis, and the socialist physician Nicolás Repetto mentioned it time and again at his tuberculosis conferences, which were geared toward educating and politically engaging the residents of La Boca, as the San Juan Evangelista neighborhood was called. Both Bunge and Repetto explained the paradox of low tuberculosis mortality in an area with so many tenements by pointing out that while the housing was precarious, the ventilation was good. They also pointed out that the population, which was not terribly overcrowded, mostly worked outdoors, on the docks. They were also largely of Italian descent, a group with a relatively low rate of tuberculosis.[159]

Emilio Coni was the first to criticize Carrasco's conclusions. He noted that the design of the statistics inevitably exaggerated tuberculosis mortality in neighborhoods with hospitals. Using a different model, he correlated hospital mortality and the origin of the person who had died, and his conclusions gave another picture of the geography of tuberculosis in Buenos Aires. In his study the tuberculosis mortality rate of La Boca doubled, San Cristóbal's rate declined dramatically to well below the average, and three neighborhoods with

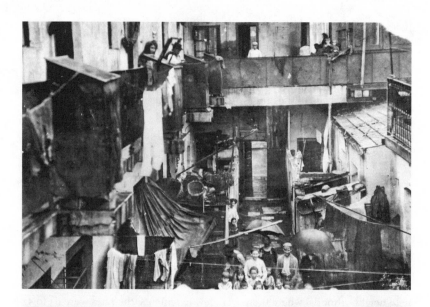

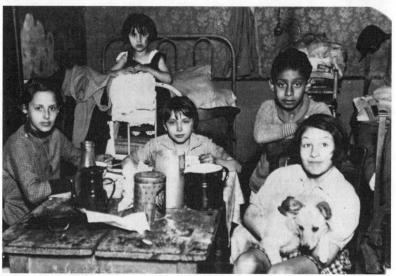

(*above and opposite*)
Poor housing and overcrowding in tenements were two recurrent
and long-lasting topics associated with tuberculosis contagion.
(Archivo General de la Nación, ca. 1900–1915)

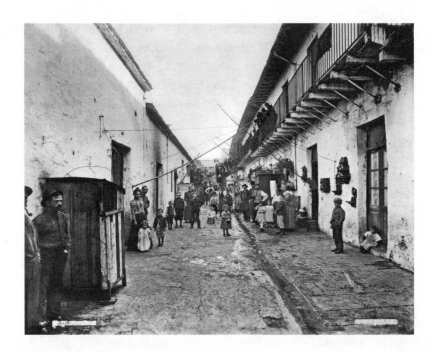

modest health infrastructure and, for him, inhabited by a socially heterogeneous population — Catedral South, Pilar, and Catedral North — had high rates
of tuberculosis mortality. Coni stated that "it is not clear there is a relationship
between tuberculosis mortality and population density" and that "the topo-
graphical distribution of tuberculosis mortality includes tenements and other
unhealthy mud dwellings with dirt floors, where the rate of deaths from tuberculosis is much higher than in tenements." His study warned not only of the
presence of other, equally unhealthy, dwellings but also the multiplicity of "still
unknown" causes that might explain the "true foci of tuberculosis."[160] Years
later, in 1918, an article published in *La Semana Médica* reaffirmed this complex
social etiology, concluding that from 1908 to 1917 the neighborhoods most affected by the disease were San José de Flores, Belgrano, San Benito de Palermo,
Las Heras, and San Carlos South. These were all relatively new areas with a high
proportion of single-family homes and average population density.[161]

In addition to the problem of tenements, in the 1920s and 1930s there was
concern with "modern apartment buildings, which are antisocial and have no
soul." In apartments, social reformers thought, the old problems of poor lighting, small quarters, and poor ventilation reemerged. In the end, their position revealed that the debate about the tuberculosis-causing effects of different
sorts of dwellings was becoming more complex; the old tenement, the modern

"antihygienic apartment," the "dark, low-ceilinged, overpopulated, and damp" houses in poor neighborhoods and suburbs, the shacks, the "modest dwellings located next to industrial centers and docks," all reinforced an environmentalist explanation of tuberculosis.[162] *La Vanguardia* stated that "tuberculosis mortality could easily be prevented" if "modern buildings" allowed "sunlight into the apartments."[163] By that time, it was becoming clear that population density, overcrowding, and lack of hygiene could not in themselves explain the variations in tuberculosis mortality. In this context of acknowledged biomedical uncertainties, a study was released by the Departamento Nacional de Higiene in 1936. It emphasized that "the supposed causal relation between poor housing and tuberculosis is too absolute; there have been many cases of unhygienic dwellings in abandoned areas that have been inhabited by the same families for many years and where there has not been a single case of tuberculosis."[164] In the mid-1940s, a complex, multicausal etiology was recognized, and it was possible for the many medical studies to affirm that "organic and environmental factors are tightly bound under the common denominator of social position, expressed as questions of housing and overcrowding, nutrition, and economic situation that can not be separated but are intrinsically correlated. Consequently, economic situation is not only the most important of the environmental factors in tuberculosis epidemiology; it is also the immediate and basic cause of these factors."[165]

In Buenos Aires, as in so many large cities, the vision of tuberculosis as an essentially urban disease related to housing, overcrowding, and promiscuity informed the specific knowledge constructed around it. This approach, which was present to a greater or lesser extent in all discussions of the social dimensions of the disease, led to an enduring notion of tuberculosis as either a cause or an effect of a poor, degraded environment. This approach brought together the social dimension of tuberculosis, the impact of Koch's discoveries, and a notable expansion in health statistics. Tuberculosis came to be seen as the result of faulty relations between society and its environment. The social etiology and epidemiological knowledge developed around this relation deeply influenced the thinking of doctors, academics, technicians, professionals, and politicians. Not until the beginning of the 1940s was this approach able to significantly diminish the emphasis on housing and allow for greater recognition of the multicausality that marked the presence of tuberculosis for over seven decades in the history of Buenos Aires.

CHAPTER SEVEN

Immigration, Race, and Tuberculosis

In the mid-1930s and particularly in the 1940s several medical essays discussed points previously made in European and North American scientific circles, namely, that "race seems to play no part in the resistance or the predisposition toward tuberculosis" and that "everything leads to the conclusion that given equal living conditions, tuberculosis affects all human races in similar ways."[1] This conviction was relatively new. Since at least the end of the nineteenth century and especially during the first decades of the twentieth, racial predisposition was considered a major factor of tuberculosis.

In the first half of the nineteenth century, the disease was considered the result of a body's imbalance. This etiological explanation was based on a very simple mechanistic logic. It spoke of an alteration in the flow of bodily fluids owing to an external matter; at some point, the alteration would give rise to physical deterioration. The matter was a sort of poison that consumed lung tissue. After a while, small nodules, the tubercles, were produced. In them, the residue of the affected tissues was deposited, evidencing the degenerative taking place in the sick body. This explanation was advanced in a book by D. J. Pérez published in 1854 and in many doctoral theses written around the mid-nineteenth century at the University of Buenos Aires. The work of European doctors was cited to support this explanation, though the experts in Buenos Aires acknowledged a lack of medical certainty about the disease, primarily because the source of contagion was still not clear. Domingo Salvarezza's thesis, dated 1866, indicated the existence of a greater susceptibility among individuals of "poor, meager and weak constitution," who have "pale skin and a narrow chest," and live in "humid and poorly ventilated" urban environments; these individuals were undernourished, suffered from moral passions, practiced venereal excesses, sunbathed infrequently, and led sedentary lives. Those whose work fatigued the breathing organs and those exposed to noxious substances were also potential victims of the disease. Heredity issues were another concern: it was deemed likely, if not infallible, that a "father or mother sick with pulmonary tuberculosis engendered tubercular children." Contrary to the thinking of the past, this hereditary influence was now understood to mean that "children inherited a [corporeal] organization similar to that of their parents," and "an aptitude or predisposition to suffer from the same diseases."[2]

By the last third of the nineteenth century, other interpretations appeared. Based on studies with new empiricist and scientific pretensions, these works explored the problem of contagion. After the discovery of the tuberculosis bacillus in 1882, the idea that tuberculosis was not a hereditary but an infectious disease caused by a microorganism became increasingly accepted. Yet Koch's findings were not immediately or automatically assumed, and there were many contradictory interpretations during much of the nineteenth century and even the first decades of the twentieth. This multiplicity of views was due, in part, to the still-mysterious unequal distribution of tuberculosis mortality in the population. The doctoral theses of the time reflect this moment in medical knowledge, evidencing that the new scientific information provided by bacteriology was still far from widespread. A thesis written by Abel Domingues in 1895 spoke of tuberculosis entering the body as the result of inherited contagion and inherited predisposition. A year later Marcelo Viñas entitled his thesis "The heredity of tuberculosis." In 1918 Leticia Acosta affirmed that tuberculosis was not inherited, though there was a predisposition in the children of tubercular parents. In 1919 Leónidas Silva thoroughly questioned Koch's conclusions and the theories of contagion, and even as late as the early twenties two theses on tuberculosis and pregnancy insisted on the hereditary nature of the disease.[3]

By the beginning of the twentieth century it was widely known that a certain segment of the population had the disease but not manifest symptoms. Exactly who got sick was still a mystery; medical explanations largely focused on heredity and constitution as well as on the idea of individual, family, and group predisposition. Those who accepted the existence of the bacillus and the infectious as well as the social dimensions of the disease also wondered about hereditary factors and predisposition. No matter which theory was accepted, the fact that one individual became sick while others didn't tended to be explained by their relative susceptibility. The contracting of tuberculosis could be the confirmation of a natural predisposition. And even if the disease was inactive, that didn't necessarily mean there was no predisposition. In 1945 Antonio Cetrángolo, one of the most renowned lung specialists in Buenos Aires, summarized in a semiautobiographical book how biomedical explanations of the time were confronting the problem of individuals' relative susceptibility and the transformation of tubercular infection into disease. These explanations blamed bad living conditions, underscoring that "when facing the germ, only the strong prevail" and that "some phenotypes and races are more predisposed to the disease than others."[4]

In Buenos Aires the association between race and tuberculosis was articulated around two issues: first, a broad approach that discussed ethnic and racial mixing, the forging of the "Argentine race," and the construction of nationality in the context of an immigrant society; and second, a more specific approach that dealt with racial, ethnic, and national groups that were somehow viewed as more or less predisposed to the disease.

The Nation, Immigration, and Ethnic Mixing

Imagining a wholly uncertain future and trying to escape from the past—either colonial times or the turbulent years following independence—nineteenth-century Argentine intellectuals heralded a belief in social and political order and faith in the progress of the young Argentine nation. They engaged in a scientific culture strongly influenced by French, English, and German ideas and attempted to conceive of and shape a specific, distinctive national identity. Their insights, mainly influenced by positivism but also by decadentism, vitalism, and modernist spiritualism, in the end, were used to support criminologist, anthropological, cosmological, biological, and psychological visions of the nation.[5] While discussing how to influence the development of the human species, scientists, politicians, essayists, and journalists reflected on race as a highly relevant and at the same time highly imprecise concept.

In nineteenth-century Western thought, racial groups were classified on a scale that considered the organic and the spiritual, and skin pigmentation and phenotypic traits, as well as language, tradition, morality, and psychology. Physico-anthropological interpretations and historico-cultural visions competed and coexisted, often producing hybrid results. Thus, there were many and varied definitions of race, including decidedly racist perspectives that stigmatized as inferior particular groups and racialist views, that is, doctrines on races and populations that didn't necessarily stem from racist and supremacist beliefs.[6]

In Argentina, from the mid-nineteenth century to the 1940s, racial thinking developed as part of the broader and crucial question of populating the
country with immigrants. It displayed a remarkable continuity over time, quite
often erasing ideological differences that would have been insuperable when
other issues were under debate. In the second half of the nineteenth century
it dominated the goal of attracting immigrants from northern Europe.[7] The
policy was epitomized by the phrase "To rule is to populate." Later, in response
to the massive and conflictive presence of immigrants who demonstrated that
the foreigners who were settling in Argentina were not "the right ones or the
sought-out ones," this agenda mutated into, "To rule is to sanitize."[8] In the
1920s and even into the 1930s and 1940s the same concern was present, expressed in the phrase "To rule is not merely to populate, but to populate well,"
emphasizing the need for selection.[9]

To a large extent the racial question in Argentina was actually the immigration question. And if during those decades that question was dominated by
the possibilities and pitfalls of imagining and constructing a modern nation
with immigrants, in Buenos Aires those discussions were shaped not only by
ideas about the best immigrants but also by the recognition of immigrants'
massive presence in the demographic and cultural realities of the city. The key
issue revolved around accepting or rejecting certain immigrant groups. Some
saw the massive arrival of foreigners as a harmonious process of integration,
an investment in the future. Others had nativist reactions and advanced an
unsettling discourse that associated massive immigration with degeneration.
Though xenophobic outbursts did take place from time to time, they were
determined more by political, social, and religious problems than by racial
concerns. All in all, the integrationist discourse, which viewed immigration
as central to making a modern Argentina, more accurately reflected the way
most people thought at that time.

Indeed, between 1870 and 1940 very few resisted the temptation to use
racialized language when talking about population issues. Some justified the
notion of inferior and superior races by combining notions taken from biology, history, culture, and geography. Liberal reformists, Catholics, socialists,
and anarchists thought they were using scientific concepts to reflect on the
present and to conceive the future. Accordingly, *race* could signify the human
race, the country's population, the national race, or the people. Other issues
associated with this vague concept of race emerged: ideas of social justice, national interests, the responsibilities of particular individuals and of the state,
political concern for the nation's demographic future, and others.

This welter of ideas motivated both nuanced and vulgar discussions about how to forge the population best suited to guarantee Argentina's future. Though there were variations, the prevailing tone did not appeal to a search for racial purity or the notion that hereditary traits were immutable or the violent segregation of the unwanted. It appealed, rather, to the ability of the environment to transform the organic, mental, and moral constitution of individuals as well as of ethnic and racial groups. Indeed, the racial question in Argentina was by and large how to mix people with diverse backgrounds. In the mixing of natives with foreigners, and of foreigners with other foreigners, lay both the risks and the possibilities of a new "national race." Native, black, and Asian peoples were decidedly marginal to this discussion, even though certain voices, in the last third of the nineteenth century and in the Congreso Nacional de Población in 1940, considered the surviving native population as little more than a set of races supposedly doomed to extinction.[10] With transatlantic immigration at its core, racial mixing and how to fully take advantage of it were discussed as crucial elements in the nation-building project.

In Argentina, these discussions were richly nuanced and went from a biological conception of race—that is, race as blood—to a more culturally rooted concept of race as a nation in the making. Especially at the beginning of the century it is easy to find in a single author—indeed, in a single work—the influences of both positivism and spiritualism. But despite the broad range of visions, few invoked the idea of racial purity; most based their thinking, instead, on the idea of racial and ethnic mixing in which the Argentine environment and the European immigrant would be decisive. This common and enduring emphasis arose from the addition of ideas connected with very specific conjunctures rather than from doctrinaire agendas or more or less planned exercises of social engineering.

Considered a device for advancing progress and civilization, the composition, proportions, and prevailing characteristics of such racial and ethnic mixtures were recurrent topics among political and intellectual Argentine elites. The second half of the nineteenth century was marked by the fruitless attempt to attract Anglo-Saxon races to Argentina. At that time European immigration was encouraged, while an open-door policy for every immigrant group was established in the Constitution of 1853. In 1910, when Argentina had been receiving immigrants for fifty years, the demographer Juan Alsina spoke of the advisability of keeping the Argentine population connected with the "Christian nations of Europe." He suggested the need "to distinguish between desired, neutral, and undesired immigrants," stating that Latin groups were particularly compatible with Argentina. In the name of order and social defense, Alsina demanded that new legislation be created to further specify the contents of Article No. 32 of the Immigration Law of 1876, especially in regard to the physical and moral traits of the most desirable immigrants.[11] This idea was present throughout the 1930s, emphasizing time and again the advantages of Latin races and arguing that "the mixture of culturally or racially distant groups ought to be avoided."[12]

The turn of the century saw myriad diagnoses and formulations of the future of the Argentine race. In 1894 the university professor and writer Calixto Oyuela was convinced that the "Argentine type" lay in the "Spanish race" and that newly arrived races would serve to fertilize the traditional Argentine spirit, which would be able to absorb these races in the best way possible.[13] And if the tone of the writings of the former governor, senator, and professor Joaquín V. Gonzalez and the academic and politician Estanislao Zeballos was similar, in the writings of Juan B. Justo, the physician, essayist, and founder of the Socialist party, European immigrants are seen as the model that the native *criollo* population should aim for. According to Justo, criollos were "incapable of heading to the superior social type on their own."[14] The painter and essayist Eduardo Schiaffino was convinced that immigrant groups became part of the "boiling melting pot" in which "the [Argentine] race is forged, modeled, transformed, and transfigured," a process whose final outcome was unknowable.[15] The physician and politician José Ramos Mejía maintained that the local environment—mainly its pleasant climate, diet, and civilized life—would regenerate the weak immigrant masses, which had shown limited ability to bring progress, despite the predictions of Juan Bautista Alberdi and other members of the elite who launched the ambitious project of populating Argentina with immigrants. According to Ramos Mejía, it was in future generations, the Argentine offspring of the ethnic mixture, that the "forging of the [immigrants'] noble metal" was going to yield its best products.[16] In some of his writings the essayist Carlos Octavio Bunge maintained that the crossbreeding of very different races was actually counterproductive and that in order to build a biologically sound society it was necessary to get rid of the inferior groups. But in others he articulated a concept of a nationality capable of embracing all ethnic groups in a veritable celebration of a social blend that would give rise to a "single Argentine type."[17] The physician, writer, and professor José Ingenieros announced that the new Argentine race would grow out of the Argentine environment's effects on European races.[18] And even the journalist and writer Ricardo Rojas, who unsuccessfully tried to revalorize Native American cultures in Argentina, was optimistic about what a "patriotic education" could produce out of mixing the immigrant and the criollo.[19]

The literature of the period offers numerous examples of a shared sense of the possibilities and risks of racial mixing. In the naturalistic novel of the 1880s the immigrant's ubiquitous presence led to antagonism and fed intolerance and prejudice. This was the case in Julián Martel's *La bolsa*, which gave rise to a wave of anti-Semitism. Similarly, the novels *En la sangre* by Eugenio Cambaceres and *Inocentes y culpables* by Antonio Argerich unleashed anti-Italian feelings. But there was also an abundance of literature that expressed and created the opposite reaction. *Irresponsable* by Manuel Podestá and *Libro extraño* by Francisco Sicardi emphasized the regenerative power of European immigration. Enrique Larreta and Manuel Gálvez celebrated Spanish immigration, and in *La gringa*, Florencio Sánchez spoke of the blend of criollos, or natives, and gringos, or foreigners, that would give rise to the "strong race of the future."

In 1919 Emilio Frers, a former president of the Sociedad Rural Argentina and politician with a liberal background who worked for years in conservative administrations, suggested that all ethnic and cultural particularities should be forgotten in order to "create a national type of our own . . . through the fusion of all the races." He considered this the best strategy for assimilating and nationalizing immigrants.[20] In the twenties and thirties, imagining and modeling the Argentine race was increasingly the task of specialists, most of them influenced by the eugenic movement. The debate stressed the advisability of the Latin races, a point of view clearly influenced by the biotypology of the Italian doctor Nicola Pende.[21] Some, like Lucas Ayarragaray—an essayist with an extreme, sometimes openly racist voice—went even further and proclaimed the need to filter immigration with a "selective and restrictive sieve," stating that white Europeans would purify the inferior Indian and mixed-race populations, hence "consolidating a noble, expansive, and strong civilization."[22] But most of the participants in the 1940 Congreso Nacional de Población were more moderate and advocated mixture, stressing not only the advisability of encouraging Latin immigration—though not to the exclusion of others—but also the need to select immigrants according to their physical, occupational, intellectual, and moral aptitudes.[23]

The idea of ethnic mixing as a resource that could ensure the improvement of the national race was greatly influenced by eugenic theories and Lamarckian transformism. According to this vision—also present in other parts of Latin America—the changes to living beings brought about by external forces could be passed on to future generations.[24] It saw evolution as a slow, intentional process of adaptation to environmental changes. Its tone was fundamentally optimistic. This vision trusted in environmental improvements, assuming they would modify and benefit the population's genetic capital. The problem of nature was thus limited, whereas nurture—that is, upbringing, social context, education—was decisive to producing more fit individuals. In a tradition closer to the Enlightenment spirit than to the more systematic Darwinism, human will and environment were seen as strategic resources to be used in the effort to improve ethnical and racial types. In this context, the multiple forms and strategies associated with constructive hybridization took shape in Argentina and the rest of Latin America. These strategies considered certain aspects of the construction of national identities as "racial dilemmas," in which allegedly inferior races would be absorbed by superior ones. The new national races would arise from these mixtures. By the end of the 1930s and especially in the 1940s this eugenic thinking and its dominant positive tone began to decline. On one hand, the growing recognition of Mendelian genetics gave rise to a revision of Lamarckian transformism and its ambiguities, particularly in terms of the problems of heredity. On the other, social thinking was retreating from posivitism and organicism, while other perspectives, born of psychoanalysis and irrationalism, took hold.

In this intellectual climate in which the topic of the best racial and ethnic mix had a relevant role, the discussion revolved around how to get rid of elements that caused the inherited capital and health of the population to deteriorate. Tuberculosis was quickly identified as a degenerative threat, and hence it was important to know if it was a hereditary disease, if the entry of tubercular foreigners should be impeded, and if it was appropriate to discourage the immigration of groups with a high rate of tuberculosis mortality. It was crucial to know if varying degrees of predisposition to the disease were determined by heredity (that is, by national or ethnic group) or by environment (that is, the life they lived in Buenos Aires). Between 1870 and 1950 these questions, though endlessly debated, had not been answered, and indeed they weren't convincingly answered in the second half of the twentieth century either. In a widely used book on internal medicine published in Buenos Aires in 1966, Rodolfo Pasqualini indicated that predisposition factors, individual immunity, and race are as important as the bacillus to the development of tuberculosis.[25] Similarly, an essay written in the 1980s stressed how difficult it is for biomedicine to determine relative susceptibilities as a result not only of genetic and environmental factors but also of the duration and intensity of exposure to the pathogenic agent.[26]

The long-lasting uncertainty about a convincing understanding of tuberculosis and how to control it made the disease into a way to speak about many things. In a city where, during certain periods, foreigners constituted more than half the population, tuberculosis was a means of articulating or justifying the supposed advisability and necessity of selecting who would be granted the opportunity to try their luck in the Argentine capital.

Selection of Immigrants

The concern over which immigrants were desirable was present in Argentina starting in the 1860s. Immigration legislation issued in 1876 encouraged an open-door policy that, at the same time, aspired to become much more selective in terms of the quality of the immigrant: without distinguishing between nationalities, it prohibited the immigration of all foreigners with a contagious or infectious illness that rendered him or her unable to work.

The selection of immigrants, a relatively soft eugenic resource in the late nineteenth century and early twentieth, always entailed the exclusion of people with tuberculosis. During these years discourses and practices surrounding emigration and immigration hygiene were widespread not only in Argentina but also in most places involved in the transatlantic crossing. By the end of the nineteenth century and the beginning of the twentieth, there were debates about enacting more restrictive measures. Most of them revolved around health concerns, though the Laws of Residence (1902) and Social Defense (1910), which dealt with exclusion on the basis of ideology and culture, were also debated. Further regulations included a municipal edict of 1893 authorizing health inspectors to monitor arriving ships and examine immigrants staying at the recently created Hotel de Inmigrantes. There were also doctoral theses, like Alsina's, on this issue, as well as instructions for ship captains to report the cases of passengers with contagious diseases.[27] The sheer number of immigrants arriving before the First World War gave rise to attempts to avoid the undesired effects of massive, unregulated immigration, which was said to be attracting political agitators and exotic groups such as the Russian Jewish and the Syrian-Lebanese. In 1904 an international treaty to stop the spread of foreign diseases was signed. The agreement, enacted by Argentina and its neighboring countries, aimed to place South American doctors on European ships bearing immigrants; in 1913 an unprecedentedly detailed decree stated that diseases were grounds for impeding entry into the country. The idea of selecting immigrants continued into the twentieth century and gained strength thanks to a peculiarly Latin American tendency to connect European immigration, eugenics, and the forging of better "national populations." In that context, other issues, together with those focused on health and sanitary matters already well defined by the immigration law of 1876, were shaping ideas and policies on the best and most needed foreigners Argentina should seek. One of them was how to keep unskilled urban workers out and attract immigrants willing to settle in rural areas. Questions of ideology and culture were also discussed, often articulating vaguely defined concerns with racial affinity, habits, and lifestyle that were assumed to facilitate assimilation into the Argentine social fabric. Some never lost their faith in northern Europeans as the best resource for bettering the national race, although by then it was impossible to ignore the prevailing presence of immigrants who originated in southern and Mediterranean Europe. Others did not hesitate to stigmatize certain foreign groups as retarded and dangerous or useless. Others deemed those critical qualifications of immigrants—and more generally the lexicon of social defense used to justify immigrant selection or to expel so-called politically dangerous immigrants—as unsuitable strategies for confronting the social challenges posed by modern Argentine politics.[28]

In 1923 an ambitious bill on immigration was sent to Congress. It maintained the open-door policy, but this time offered more specifics with respect to sanitary and criminal controls as well as to immigrants' age, which had to be under fifty-five. A policy of discouraging single mothers with young children and excluding political activists, prostitutes, beggars, and alcoholics was also made explicit. The bill largely sought to systematize common practice but generated heated debates and controversies in the Congress. Taking note of that, the government decided to implement administrative regulations that were in the spirit of the law of 1876.[29] These regulations, which were full of ambiguities, gave immigration authorities the power to keep undesirable immigrants from getting off the boats. Moreover, the selection process was to begin at the immigrants' birthplaces: presenting a certificate of good health, economic viability, and a clean criminal record to the Argentine consulate before departing was to become mandatory.

Although there are no statistics on the total number of immigrants rejected, immigration reports from those years reveal that very few people failed to get into the country. None of the politico-administrative initiatives seemed capable of accomplishing their goals, largely because they were very difficult to put into practice. Several reasons might explain this outcome. One was the unsatisfied labor demand—remarkable in certain years, less so in others—as a result of the growth of the Argentine economy during the European wars; another, the increasingly restrictive U.S. immigration policies that led many to try their luck in Argentina. And finally, a lack of enthusiasm or the outright difficulties in enforcing the approved regulations—because economic prosperity made them easily forgettable, or because the shipping companies did everything they could to avoid transporting rejected immigrants to their home countries gratis, or because local ethnic associations or national consuls supported the immigrants' desire to stay. There was another quite obvious explanation for the failure to enforce these policies: mainly, the limited number of health inspectors available. There were no more than a dozen, a fact that reveals, yet again, the distance between a certain policy, its discursive and symbolic relevance, the difficulty of putting it into practice, and the more than modest results.

The efforts to select immigrants at the Buenos Aires port didn't significantly affect the mass arrival of Italians and Spaniards, nor were these efforts particularly effective when it came to selecting central and eastern European immigrants or people from the Middle East. Flexibility prevailed most of the time, and very few were rejected. The inspectors were strictest in dealing with those with evident handicaps, young women traveling alone who were assumed to be prostitutes, and those who couldn't hide their disease. The sanitary control was relatively clear: it specified that every staff member who failed to inform on the presence of a sick person was breaking the law as well as his obligation to indicate the reasons and justification for rejecting that individual. However, identifying a tubercular person wasn't easy, as clinical and bacteriological analyses were still far from conclusive. A medical examination performed by a doctor, whether at the immigrant's birthplace or at the Buenos Aires port, was far from conclusive. The laboratory analysis of saliva was not simple because it demanded not only specific equipment and time, but also a good sample, which could be obtained only if the sick person was willing to collaborate, and that was by no means certain. Furthermore, the saliva analysis was reliable only in very advanced cases, when the presence of the bacillus in the saliva itself was a clear indication of the destruction of the lung tissue. Outside the laboratory, the process of identifying a person with the disease took place under the inspector's gaze. It was difficult, if not impossible, to identify symptoms or physical signs that could establish if a person had tuberculosis. Doctors were aware of these limitations, and this explains why the number of immigrants rejected because they had tuberculosis was relatively small. Indeed, determining that a newly arrived person had tuberculosis was as hard and arbitrary as affirming that he or she would become a criminal or a radical political activist, two other grounds for banning entry.

Though the achievements of immigration policy on immigrant selection were really modest, evidence of the effective social integration of immigrant children and discourses about the "racial qualities" of each immigrant group suggest how complex, nuanced, and even contradictory experiences and ideas about immigration were in the making of modern Argentina. In terms of social integration, significant participation in the public education system, mandatory military service, rituals associated with national holiday festivities, involvement in politics, homeownership, and social and employment mobility reveal the existence in Buenos Aires of a relatively open, mixed, and quite inclusive society.

In Argentina, as in other immigrant countries between the 1900s and 1940s, discourses about the racial qualities of each ethnic or national group largely consisted of subtle or clumsy distinctions articulated by many ideological groups, from left to right, and were based on prejudices and stereotypes. Southern Italians never enjoyed the warm welcome reserved for their northern compatriots; Russians and so-called Turks, peoples coming from areas under control of the former Ottoman empire, were deemed exotic and Chinese and Latin Americans undesirable. Europeans from the north were consistently sought out, whereas those from eastern and central Europe were rejected. Unfitness for agricultural work, inherited mercantile tendencies, "linguistic distance" from Spanish, religion, and skin color were the most frequent reasons to build a stereotype or articulate a prejudice. Naturally, a supposedly inherited predisposition to tuberculosis of a certain ethnic or national group was instrumental in discourses aimed at organizing the elusive reasons for rejection, despite very sketchy associations between race or ethnicity and disease.

In the end, the five or six decades in which racialized and ethnicized discourses of tuberculosis sought to define the best immigrant group and to establish who should be excluded were just that: discourses. Tuberculosis was always among the justifications for these selective and exclusionary policies. However, despite those highly imaginative and oftentimes arbitrary discourses, only rarely was tuberculosis the reason an immigrant was not allowed into the country.

Spaniards and Tuberculosis

It was common to speak of the perceived numerous tuberculars who entered the country undetected, as well as of foreigners who had been in Argentina only briefly before coming down with pulmonary tuberculosis.[30] The concept of imported tuberculosis quickly became connected with immigrants from the Iberian Peninsula, the European immigrant group most affected by the disease and suffering a tuberculosis mortality rate twice that of Italians. There were two main perspectives on the so-called Spanish tuberculosis question.[31] On the one hand was the hereditary explanation, which claimed there was a predisposition in the Spanish race, grounding this view not only on the rate of tuberculosis mortality in Spain—one of the highest in Europe—but also on the growing numbers of first-generation Argentines of Spanish descent to catch the disease.[32] For example, in 1920 Ayarragaray stated that even among hardworking immigrant groups and "superior types," such as Italians and Spaniards, there were the "lowly leftovers of old European populations . . . bearing the stigmas of alcohol, syphilis, tuberculosis, epilepsy, and every form of mental and physical degeneration."[33]

By the late 1920s a different point of view questioned this alleged hereditary predisposition. Gregorio Aráoz Alfaro, a doctor very close to the Spanish community and also very active in the antituberculosis movement in Buenos Aires as well as state public health institutions, said that the explanation for this elevated tuberculosis mortality rate did not lie in "a lack of organic resistance," or constitutional weakness. The explanation, rather, was the type of jobs the Spanish immigrants had, mainly "doormen, servants, grocers, hotel workers and waiters." Such workers were "locked up in poorly ventilated places"; their jobs were excessively sedentary, "requiring very little exercise."[34] But before and after Aráoz Alfaro's perceptive analysis, other voices did not hesitate to cite cultural reasons in order to racialize the Spanish predisposition to the disease. By the end of the nineteenth century, in a much more bigoted impressionistic account, a doctor working for the city government underlined what he understood as "very Spanish traits" that could lead to tuberculosis: "the workings of greed" that permitted some Spaniards "to make solid fortunes" in Argentina meant that other Spanish immigrants, who had come with delusions of grandeur, "lived in a voluntary beggary, subjected to tuberculosis, . . . haunted by nostalgia and febrile dreams of quick, certain prosperity."[35]

These interpretations of the high tubercular mortality rate among Spanish immigrants in Buenos Aires partially resonated with the theories advanced by Galician intellectuals and doctors since the beginning of the century. Miguel Gil y Casares, a specialist in lung diseases who was very influential in Galicia, the northern region in which most of the Spaniards emigrating to Buenos Aires originated, wrote a number of essays on the hereditary nature of the disease. In these essays, published between 1912 and the mid-1920s, he questioned the relevance of contagion and warned against the "unexplainable belief" that insisted that the infection was always acquired after birth.[36] Less empathically, E. Hervada García pointed out in 1923 that although contagion existed, among Galicians tuberculosis was "undeniably due to hereditary factors."[37] These explanations dominated the Galician academic milieu until at least the early 1930s, when, after Gil y Casares's death, they were dismissed by explanations of contagion.[38] Nonetheless, as was true of most explanations elsewhere, these statements were not solidly grounded in epidemiology. Often they were linked to environmental factors and the reigning metaphor of the "propitious territory for the growth of the tubercular seed." Facing the problem of the quick spread of the disease, the experts in those years connected hereditary factors to circumstances that, in their opinion, heightened the congenital predisposition to the disease. Expatriation, multiple pregnancies, and alcoholism were the most frequently mentioned factors. A term used to mean the act of emigrating and then returning, *expatriation* became a very particular issue in the social and cultural construction of tuberculosis in Galicia, where, as in Argentina, the massive migrations of people had many meanings and were a way to speak about many things.

Although significant throughout the nineteenth century, Galician emigration became massive at the beginning of the twentieth century owing to a complex combination of factors: the stagnation of the possibility for economic growth and modernization of poorly diversified small farms; demographic pressure; increasing circulation of information by several means but especially personal letters about the possibilities offered by emigration; and cheaper transatlantic tickets, which were often purchased with money sent over by relatives in America or with funds obtained by mortgaging a small rural property. The impact of the successful emigrants who returned served to reinforce the image of overseas immigration as a sure ticket to social mobility. All these factors contributed to an emigration process with very limited social selectivity in comparison with what was happening in the rest of Spain, except the Basque country. More than 50 percent of Spanish emigration to Argentina was from Galicia, and it was centered in Buenos Aires. The Argentine capital soon became the most desirable destination for those leaving both the coast and highlands of Galicia and thus the city with the world's largest population of Galicians—around 150,000 in 1914, two and a half times the number of Galicians living in La Coruña, the largest city in Galicia.

According to Gil Casares, the "greatest reason for the rise of tuberculosis" in Galicia was the return of emigrants who had caught "acute tuberculosis" and had "reduced organic energies because of the suffering and work they have endured in America."[39] In 1930 A. Gutiérrez Moyano, the director of the medical journal *Galicia Clínica*, didn't hesitate to say, "In Galicia, tuberculosis has been imported from overseas." In his view, the reports of the doctors caring for the rural population indicated that the geographical distribution of tuberculosis mortality and morbidity was directly proportional to the presence of emigrants who had returned home.[40] In this finding, Galician specialists saw further proof of the disease's hereditary nature. They said that the sick emigrants who returned to their birthplaces facilitated the spread of the disease not so much by direct contagion, but by transmitting the disease to their offspring. Statistics, however, offer a less clear picture. Doctors who supported Gil Casares's theory were inclined to point out that 20 percent of the tuberculosis patients examined in hospitals had been emigrants and that their relatives made up another 20 percent of the cases. Official reports indicated that in 1925, 60 to 80 percent of the 31,000 returnees arriving in La Coruña had tuberculosis. Meanwhile, somewhat contradicting the association between returned emigrants and tuberculosis, the Inspección General de Emigración placed at just 175 the total number of tuberculars who reentered all Spanish ports in 1931 and 143 in 1932, hardly enough to account for the Spanish tuberculosis morbidity and mortality.[41]

Not medical but equally based on intuitions and inconsistent statistics, the explanations provided by certain Galician intellectuals, like Alfonso Daniel Rodriguez Castelao, were similarly limited. A celebrated sketcher, painter, writer, and politician who died in exile in Argentina in 1950, Castelao connected emigration and tuberculosis to voice a blistering, patently negative vision of Galician emigration. In 1931, at the Cortes Constituyentes of the Spanish republic, he accused emigration of siphoning off thousands of young people dazzled by the American myth; such emigration separated families, impeded the search for collective solutions to the problem of poverty, and drained away the leadership and commitment needed to regenerate and transform Galicia. He stated that "the wealth of a few 'Indianos' [Galicians who had come back from America] with more or less philanthropic inclinations cannot make up for what the returned tubercular emigrants have brought to us."[42]

Time and again, Castelao's political speeches referred to a sort of archetypal character, that of the Galician who returns to his home village, defeated and sick. Nonetheless, it was in his drawings, which were generally accompanied by succinct, incisive phrases, that his criticism of emigration and the figure of the defeated emigrant who returns were most poignantly expressed. The drawings are deliberately simple and synthetic, and, rather than exaggerating features, they select and leave out what is not essential. By using plain strokes to capture a gesture or a physiognomy, the focus is on individuals, not landscapes. His characters are like abbreviations, and they grow more and more precise as he repeats the same motif in different versions.

All of Castelao's drawings, but especially the ones published between 1914 and 1920, alluded to village politics and local political bosses, *caciques*; social injustice; and emigration in a style that employs Expressionism and hyperrealism. His work was published on both sides of the Atlantic: in *El Sol* of Madrid and in *Galicia*, *El Noroeste*, and *Faro de Vigo*, all of which circulated in Galicia, as well as in newspapers and magazines printed in Buenos Aires, such as *La Voz de Galicia*, and *La Semana Universal*.[43] One of Castelao's drawings that refers to the experience of the sick, defeated emigrant is especially suggestive. Published for the first time in Buenos Aires in 1915, it tells the story of a Galician who returns to his village sick with tuberculosis and beaten down. There's no text in the piece, just the image of the dying Galician man lying naked, hopeless, and weak on a bed. His mother is taking care of him. The label on the trunk in the room reveals the poor man's port of departure: "Buenos Aires." The drawing was republished in Galician newspapers with a few changes and additional text. In one of these versions, the dying man says to his mother in Galician, "I didn't want to die there, you know, mom?" In another drawing Castelao chose laconic titles like "The repatriated ones. The doctor says: I'm late to save them."

This was not the archetypical image of the Indianos or Americanos. As returning emigrants, they strived to make their emigration experiences seem triumphant. Indeed, their glorious representations of what had happened to them in Argentina gained credibility partly as a result of the fact that those who returned often became the new caciques and political bosses of their villages. This image was further popularized in the novels and short stories of such revered writers as Francisco Grandmontagne and Benito Perez Galdós. Another image is the one designed by intellectuals who wanted to see in the returned emigrant an agent of regeneration or revolution, an anticlerical figure who would disrupt the status quo. But Castelao seeks to offset all these representations—the one that stresses success and the one that stresses social and cultural change—with another, equally archetypical image. His returned emigrants bear the face of failure, and the tuberculosis killing them represents the setback, perhaps the punishment, to which they are subjected for having left Galicia to search for their fortunes overseas. There's no emigration epic here, or if there is, it is decidedly negative.

The range of interpretations of tuberculosis among Galicians went from notions of heredity to notions of environmental conditions. The hereditary position was shared by essayists and lung experts on both sides of the Atlantic. It underlined the importance of innate predisposition to the disease. But while the Argentines believed that Galicia was the site of the predisposition, the Galicians blamed the disease on the immigrants' stay in Buenos Aires: when the emigrants returned, sick and weakened, they passed their recently acquired ills onto their descendants and spread the disease to rural areas.

Aráoz Alfaro, who, oblivious to nationalistically charged epidemiological explanations, was perhaps passionate only about the fight against tuberculosis; he avoided referring to innate dispositions and emphasized what he thought would make a difference in the life of Galicians, that is, improving the living and work conditions of the Spanish in Buenos Aires. Castelao, on the other hand, didn't intend to articulate his own epidemiological reasons; his interest lay in warning about the ordeals of emigration, and tuberculosis was one of its consequences.

As Aráoz Alfaro said, the supposed Spanish predisposition to the disease couldn't ignore the large number of Spanish immigrants working in the urban service sector and the connection between those jobs and the high rates of tuberculosis morbidity. The tendency to work in certain fields was attributable to informal employment networks that tended to concentrate immigrants from the same region in similar occupations; there was as well a kind of self-selection by which less healthy people looked for jobs that did not require great physical effort. These jobs were perhaps particularly attractive to individuals with lower defenses and incipient tuberculosis, whether brought over from Galicia or acquired in Buenos Aires. In the end, this occupation's profile proved key to defining the gross, crass, stereotyped idea of the Galicians, the Gallegos, as an ethno-cultural group with very distinctive characters: the clumsy, stupid, unsophisticated waiter or doorman for men, and, for women, the candid, gullible, ignorant young maid who sometimes turned into a seductress—sexually bold, unscrupulous, and lacking judgment or morals. Both characters were likely to come down with tuberculosis.

Part stereotype and part reflection of a real immigrant experience at the beginning of the twentieth century in Buenos Aires, these images largely occluded the existence of a well-established Galician elite. They were quite powerful figures in the import–export business, banking, trade, and insurance. This Galician elite was fully established in the last third of the nineteenth century, and later, in the late 1930s and early 1940s, it came to include intellectual and liberal professional exiles and immigrants, generally supporters of the Spanish republic. Some of them, particularly those who consolidated their positions in the first decades of the twentieth century, put together a glorious history of the "Galician race," celebrated in community activities and holidays. In its own way, this was an adaptation of the prevalent notion of inferior and superior races used by the Argentine elite to discuss the demographic future of the nation. The Galician elite spoke enthusiastically of a "Celtic race with Germanic touches," superior to other races, such as native Argentine criollos, Indians, mulattos, and Italians. This ancestry, they claimed, should be taken into account when dealing with the sometimes condescending look Castilian Spaniards gave Galicians and the stereotypes of Galicians articulated by sectors of Argentine society (both among the elite and other immigrant groups). It should also be considered in assessing the contributions made by each ethno-cultural group to the process of forging a modern Argentine race able to resist tuberculosis.[44] But for quite some time, these celebratory discourses on the Galician condition could not balance the strength of the derogatory ones, in which ignorance, simplicity, and tuberculosis tended to mark ordinary Galicians.

The Vigor of the Basques

The few statistics available on tuberculosis mortality and morbidity didn't differentiate between nationality groups or points of departure on the Iberian Peninsula. Although in Galicia tuberculosis was discussed in regional and ethnocultural terms, in Buenos Aires it was seen as a problem related to Spanish immigration as a whole. Broadly, this was owing to the fact that an enormous proportion of Spanish immigrants were from Galicia. Indeed, the term *Gallego* came to be synonymous with Spaniard. Calling Spaniards Gallegos was a common practice in an endless number of situations: in neighborhoods, in the working world, in comic strips published in the papers, and in the dialogues of popular theatrical farces like *sainetes*—humorous, generally one-act, verse plays largely based on satirical observations of ordinary people's lives.

Not infrequently, though, Argentine essayists interested in forging the national race came up with attributes, largely based on stereotypes, that defined the specific characteristics of certain supposed races. *Los baskos en la nación argentina*, a book edited by José R. de Uriarte and published in 1919, is an example of how some sectors of Argentine society celebrated the "Basque race." The editor of the newspaper *La Baskonia*, Uriarte sets the tone for these reflections, a tone passionately repeated by his many guest contributors. Uriarte says the Basque is a "race that never knew a moment of exhaustion or fatigue . . . nor the historical drowsiness of other races who slowly fade."[45] Manuel Gálvez wrote, "Basques are, in a way, the founders of Argentine energy, [the people who] helped to vanquish the desert" and created the large *estancias*, or cattle estates, that dotted the Pampas. Ayarragaray stressed that the Basques put aside their prejudices to become a part of Argentina, "though they untiringly maintained the greatest and most noble concern with the purity of blood." In so doing, they avoided "mixing and mingling" and kept their race pure. Sicardi said the Basques have good eating habits; they are, he went on, "hygienic and healthy, not greedy or inclined to crime, not psychotic, and very generous and honest." Basques were "muscular, gigantic immigrants," "the most vigorous ever to come to Argentina," and they, of course, "didn't bring any syphilis or tuberculosis."[46] Some responses to a 1919 survey on the most desirable immigrants organized by the Museo Social Argentino praised rural groups from the "Germanic and Slavic countries, the Basques, and the Latin Germans from northern Italy." The rest were undesirable and liable to bring "congenital racial ills or social types" that would "turn the country into an anarchist base camp or the universal house for public charity."[47]

In the eyes of several factions of the Argentine elite, the Basques were different from other Spaniards. Their celebrated reputation was largely the result of the success of the descendants of Basque merchants who had settled in the Río de la Plata region at the end of the eighteenth century. To a lesser extent, it was due to Basque immigrants with a background in shepherding who came to the Pampas in the nineteenth century and did well in the agricultural sector, eventually becoming *estancieros*, or large landholders. No wonder there are so many Basque surnames—the Anchorena, the Alvear, the Unzué, the Martinez de Hoz, and the Ortiz Basualdo, to name a few—among the founders of the Sociedad Rural Argentina and on the members' list of the Club del Progreso, the Círculo de Armas, and the Jockey Club, all of them exclusive social institutions of the turn-of-the-century Buenos Aires elite.

In the late nineteenth century and the early twentieth, the first waves of Basque immigrants were followed by another that had quite a different experience. In this case, it largely resulted from what they found in terms of employment in the Pampas cattle and agricultural export sector, in the urban work available in Buenos Aires, in the cultural preferences of both employers and employees, and certainly in the facilities offered by the community networks built by earlier immigrants. This massive second Basque emigration included people from the Basque coast and the inland areas, people with a long tradition of small rural property ownership, and working women. The immigrants were fairly representative of the whole Basque region and the whole of Basque society. In Argentina some of them worked on dairy farms or engaged in other rural activities. Others chose low-wage jobs in the urban world, mainly domestic labor. The jobs the Basques held in Buenos Aires were largely the same as the ones the Galicians performed. In the period 1894–1910, some 60 percent of the women in both groups who worked outside the house were maids, and more than 25 percent were seamstresses. From 1888 to 1910 the relative number of Galicians and Basques performing nonmanual labor was fairly comparable.[48] Nevertheless, these labor similarities were interpreted very differently as a result of both how well each group performed on the job, as well as their supposedly relative predisposition to tuberculosis.

The work situations of Galicians seem to have been key to the way in which Galician doctors explained how their countrymen contracted tuberculosis. They were also central to the way in which Argentine essayists, doctors, and social engineers discussed the notion of Spanish tuberculosis in the context of their efforts to define a national race. But where Basques were concerned, explanations for tuberculosis did not center on environmental factors or the Spanish predisposition to the disease. Indeed, in terms of the elusive category of race and its relation to tuberculosis, the Basques were considered an extremely vigorous ethnic group whose resistance to the disease mainly resulted from innate or racial conditions: a wholly ungrounded positive stereotype.

Curiously, the celebration of the innate physical and moral resistance of the Argentine Basques failed to take into account the impact of tuberculosis on the Basques in the peninsula. Across the Atlantic, in the Basque provinces of Vizcaya, Navarra, Alava, and Guipúzcoa, doctors and social critics like Francisco Ledo García and Gumersindo Gómez called tuberculosis an endemic disease and claimed that at the beginning of the twentieth century tuberculosis mortality in Bilbao was twice that of Madrid and Barcelona. They explained the presence of the disease in Basque society as an unfortunate consequence of rapid urban and economic growth in the late nineteenth century associated with the shipyard, iron, and steel industries as well as the fishing industry in coastal towns and mining inland.[49]

The assumed absence of tuberculosis among the Basques, then, confirmed the image that an Argentine elite with distant Basque ancestry wanted for itself. Thus, while Basques enjoyed the benefits of a mythical racial superiority, Spanish immigrants closely associated with the figure of the Galicians were perceived as a threat to the successful making of the Argentine race because of their supposed predisposition to tuberculosis.

Jews and Tuberculosis

The biomedical and sociological discourses that connect tuberculosis to race reveal more about those who articulated these discourses than about the groups described. In the case of Russian Jews, the predisposition question was quite peculiar. "Natural immunities" resulting from "ancestral urban experience and limited mixing with other groups" were mentioned.[50] That's why a report put out by the city government in 1909 indicated that Russian Jews didn't get tuberculosis, even when they lived in overcrowded environments.[51]

These natural immunities were not in keeping with the image of Jews held by traditional anti-Semitic discourses, which considered them an unclean and weak race, a threat to public health, and a group incapable of making a living and likely to become a burden to the state. The notion that Jews were physically weak persisted over time. It was often connected to the figure of the tailor or the textile worker, gawky and with very limited chest capacities. This stereotype was common in Buenos Aires as well as in other American and even European cities, where Jewish immigration was considerable.[52] The negative attributes associated with Russian or central and eastern European Jews were quite imaginative, and those who formulated them didn't make the least effort to back up their assertions. The Jewish predisposition to physical deformity and epilepsy was discussed as well as the tendency to moral perversion, madness, beggary, crime, anarchism, socialism, and maximalism. Their physical weakness was seen as innate, and their resistance to disease minimal.

Between the end of the nineteenth century and the early 1940s many spoke of the inadvisability of Jewish immigration. However, they consistently failed to tackle the question of how to deal with Jewish immigrants and had little relevance when it came to dealing with the Jews who moved to and actually settled in Argentina. In the early 1880s, before they were an immigrant group with some demographic relevance, La Nación called Jews an "eccentrically constituted race" that was difficult or even impossible to assimilate. Indeed, the newspaper stated, "any attempt at assimilation" might ultimately lead to the "decomposition" of a "national society in the making."[53] In his novel La gran aldea, Lucio V. López depicted conspiring Jews in myriad situations. This theme was taken up somewhat later by Martel in La bolsa, in which he made use of the commonplaces of French Catholic anti-Semitism, namely, the tropes of financial power, control of the press, greed, and the effort to take over the world or impose socialism. At the time, these stereotypes and prejudices seemed to express an uneasy recognition of the already overwhelming presence of foreigners in Argentina. In that context the alien condition of the Jews was used to articulate a vague and broader fear of social change as well as to resist it.[54] Some time later, in 1895, when Jewish immigration was becoming a more notable factor in the making of modern Argentina, José María Ramos Mejía, then president of the Consejo Nacional de Higiene, blamed Jews for introducing typhus.[55] Despite what shipping companies and colonization agencies involved in their arrival were saying in order to reassure Argentine immigration authorities, Jews became the only group of newcomers forced to undergo systematic "disinfecting" health inspections.

Many of these openly anti-Semitic views were intensified during the 1910s, when it was strongly believed that the improvement of the national race could be achieved only through a wise selection of immigrant groups. In 1913 the Catholic newspaper *El Pueblo*, commenting on the growth of Jewish immigration, warned about the "Jewish menace to Argentina."[56] Years later, the 1919 survey conducted by the Museo Social Argentino on the future of immigration in modern Argentina compiled the opinions of more than forty conservative, liberal, and socialist politicians and intellectuals. Their answers display a certain consensus on the importance of immigration as well as on the need to define some selection criteria, a common approach to the issue in many receiving countries in those years. The figure of the undesirable immigrant, detectable in almost every response, was articulated at times in relation to a spectrum of beliefs ranging from the notion of superior races to an idea of racial affinities, at times referring to employment issues, favoring immigrants with agricultural skills. Six people answered that Semitic groups, including Jews and Arabs, should be deemed exotic or inferior and therefore undesirable. According to these views, they were of no use to the agricultural-exporting system because of their long-standing urban history, and, consequently, they couldn't further the project of improving the "Argentine idiosyncracy and race."[57] Along with black Africans and Asians, Semitic groups were believed to conspire against the nation's ethnic homogeneity. There were also answers that voiced precautions based less on ethnic and racial prejudice against Russian Jews than on an energetic rejection of the revolutionary ideology Soviet Russian emigrants were supposedly carrying with them. Federico Stach, the only one who articulated an overtly anti-Semitic answer, concluded his remarks with the far-from-welcoming assertion that "there's no race living in Europe . . . as degenerated as the Jews."[58]

Throughout the 1920s, 1930s, and 1940s the anti-Semitic rhetoric continued. In 1924 Ayarragaray opposed Argentine openness to Jewish immigration stressing that Jews were a "decrepit and engrossed race" that could hardly contribute to populating the Argentine territory and forging a "homogeneous white national type." In stressing that Jews were an exotic, inferior racial type, Ayarragaray promoted an immigration policy that favored the incorporation of "agile, optimistic races that could be assimilated readily, peoples from Latin, Germanic, or Anglo-Saxon cultures."[59] In 1933 the profascist journal *Crisol* called the Jews a "seed of extremism," "a breeding ground" for "all antinationalist organizations," an "economic and social danger," "a nation's moral leprosy." Drawing on familiar themes from the nineteenth century, the journal saw Jews as "a threat even more vicious than tuberculosis." Between 1939 and 1945 the back cover of the journal *Clarinada* bore a summary of the Protocols of the Learned Elders of Zion and denounced Jewish Bolshevism and Jews' intentions to weaken the nation by spreading diseases.[60]

However, these extremist voices didn't set the tone of the discussion. Though many proposed attracting "racially superior" immigrants capable of generating a superior national type by means of Darwinian natural selection even as they supported impeding the entry of "inferior races," most people concerned with these matters merely expressed a preference for the Anglo-Saxon, Nordic, or European–Latin types. This was the clear tendency of most of the opinions gathered in the 1919 survey. Despite these opinions, though, attempts to effectively select immigrants were decidedly unsuccessful. Italians and Spaniards kept coming in, while Nordics and Anglo-Saxons were glaringly absent. Jews, too, kept coming. By 1900 Argentina had received around 15,000 Jewish immigrants; by 1915 that number had reached 116,000, by 1930 it was more than 190,000, and by 1940 there were over 245,000 Jewish immigrants. In 1919 in Buenos Aires alone—indeed, in a just a few of the city's neighborhoods—there were 150,000 Jews.[61] Even in the 1920s, when the immigration policies became more restrictive for certain groups, including the undesirable central and eastern European Jews, the proportional increase of Polish Jews was greater than that of Italians and Spanish.[62]

The experience of Jewish immigration during the first third of the twentieth century evidences, once again, the limited practical effect of discourses and policies aimed at attracting those believed to improve the growing Argentine population. The assorted anti-Semitic arguments that supported such discourses and policies—among them, those that stressed the congenital weakness of the "Jewish race" and its sinister role in the spread of disease and contagion—endured despite the relatively low rate of tuberculosis morbidity and mortality in the Jewish community of Buenos Aires. Along with this somewhat grotesque racialization of disease, there were more discerning interpretations, like the one offered by the Italian doctor José Sanarelli. Accepted in many Western countries and quite well known in the medical milieu of Buenos Aires, Sanarelli's argument affirmed that the "Jewish race" had achieved "progressive self-immunization" as a result of inbreeding, long-term residency in the urban world, and extended exposure to the bacillus. However, this relative immunity was doomed to disappear over time since it wasn't racially inherent, but acquired; hence, the Jewish race would soon become extremely sensitive to the disease.[63]

In 1936 Elías Singer's doctoral thesis criticized Sanarelli's argument, pointing out that Jews were not a race but a people. He also criticized other explanations based on religious and cultural particularities such as better hygiene habits, sedentariness, lack of interest in sports, and no inclination toward non-manual jobs. Against these idiosyncratic remarks Singer argued that "personal hygiene depends directly on personal habits and upbringing." Basing his opinion on 250 cases seen at the Liga Israelita contra la Tuberculosis de Buenos Aires, he concluded that Jews had a low rate of mortality but a high rate of chronic morbidity. They enjoyed, on the one hand, "inherited immunity" owing to sick parents with mild tuberculosis, and, on the other, "acquired immunity" owing to the large number of sick individuals with benign tuberculosis.[64] Independently of his conclusion, Singer's reading of the relations between Jews and tuberculosis sought to deracialize the question of who died and who came down with the disease. Most clearly anti-Semitic voices, however, saw in Jews an immigrant group that was expected to get sick and die of tuberculosis. The problem for them was that Jews were not dying of tuberculosis in significant numbers.

The Tuberculosis of the "General Roca's Indians"

Although the issue of determining which ingredients were best for arriving at the ideal racial and ethnic mix focused on the immigrants, it also touched on the native population. During the last third of the nineteenth century, the size of that population declined steadily, from more than ninety thousand in 1869 to eighteen thousand in 1914, according to the national census. Official explanations attributed the decline to assimilation through racial mixing. They also claimed it was the inevitable result of the natives' disgraceful behavior, from alcoholism and a lack of hygiene to infanticide and abortion. It was no coincidence, however, that the drastic drop-off occurred in 1879 and subsequent years, at the height of the so-called Conquista del Desierto, a military expansion over the Pampas and beyond as well as a war against its native population. The Conquista del Desierto unleashed pathological processes and sociocultural dislocations as well as accelerated the demographic decline of the vanquished native peoples of the Pampas. In a way, the war against the natives was not in keeping with the discourses and practices of the end-of-the-century Argentine elite, which was generally more enthusiastic about eugenicist strategies of improvement or incorporation of foreign immigrants than about the violent extermination of undesirables or the unfit.

Though this positive eugenics never doubted the need to select immigrants, it never considered annihilating them, particularly those perceived as inferior races, once they had settled in the country. This strategy of incorporation, assimilation, and improvement did not apply to natives, who by and large became the main target of an exterminating agenda and a clear evidence of a negative eugenics demographic policy. The Argentine military, intellectuals, and doctors did reflect on the conditions of the native people and their place in the project of making the national race. The army officer Federico Barbará, for instance, considered the disappearance of the native population similar to the one effected in the United States and a necessity. Indeed, he said, such a disappearance would serve to confirm the Indians' intrinsic weakness and natural inferiority.[65] Years later, at the beginning of the twentieth century, Carlos Octavio Bunge elaborated on the problem of race, which he called the engine of history. In *Nuestra América*, published in 1903, he discusses the physical characteristics of a particular race as the determining factor in their psychology and morality, concluding that all of them were hereditary. However, biological inheritance was not everything. Cultural experience and the environment also contributed to the formation of genetic capital to be passed on to future generations. Bunge was a Lamarckian and therefore trusted in the heredity of acquired traits. He acknowledged the existence of civilizing races that could progress indefinitely and advised against mixing dissimilar races, arguing that in the process only the defects and none of the virtues of the races involved were passed on. Therefore, he believed in the need to exclude certain racial groups in order to build a biologically fit society. On the basis of these assumptions, he discussed the "Latin American evils," echoing the ubiquitous process of miscegenation. Bunge believed that the mixing of the white Spaniards, the natives, and the blacks had set off a physically and morally degenerative process. According to his diagnosis, in Argentina the negative effects of this mix could be offset by encouraging the mass immigration of what he labeled progressive races. By intermarrying, they would eventually produce "a single Argentine type [who was as] imaginative as the tropical Indian and as practical as the inhabitant of cold climates; a complex, complete type."[66] In attempting to design the traits of the future, Bunge reviewed the traits of the recent and colonial past. He considered the conflictive encounters between natives and overseas races; between the rich, urban classes and the rural and semirural masses; and, finally, between the poor inland provinces, the Argentine interior, and the wealthier coastal provinces of the littoral. His assessment showed him to be an uninhibited social Darwinist, above all when he celebrated the beneficial effects of tuberculosis in the noble task of selecting and purifying the race. He stressed the fact that "the city and province of Buenos Aires received an ongoing flow of European immigration during colonial times, and due to its colder weather, coastal setting, and the meanness of the tribes from the Pampas, the city of Buenos Aires kept a fair distance from the Indian populations." According to Bunge, this auspicious beginning was followed by "alcoholism, smallpox, and tuberculosis, [which] God bless them! decimated the Indian and African populations in the city, purifying their ethnic traits and Europeanizing them."[67]

Samuel Gache, a hygienist, was less euphoric than Bunge about the connection between tuberculosis, the whitening of the littoral population, the disappearance of the natives, and racial improvement. In the early twentieth century, he wrote that the white man's Conquista del Desierto injected a "lethal poison" into the "Indian races," starting off a process of "progressive degeneration." Their disappearance would be "the logical, cogent result" of "the vicious circle of isolation brought on by defeat" and marked by the "unwavering persecution of the national army." This condemned the survivors not only to "a civilized life," but also made them easy targets for "tuberculosis, smallpox, alcohol abuse, and other ills brought by the white men."[68]

Tuberculosis was also seen as the inevitable result of an innate weakness, a weakness underscored by the natives' inability to ward off the Conquista del Desierto. In addition to the hackneyed arguments of social Darwinism, more specific explanations were offered for the natives' predisposition to tuberculosis. In a series of essays on the subject, José Mateo Franceschi, a military doctor who worked on the Indian frontier from 1871 to 1875, wrote that inbreeding, life in crowded shacks, and the lack of iron in the Pampas soil had undermined the Indians' health, affected the quality of water and food, and predisposed them to tuberculosis. This also explained, according to Franceschi, why the breast milk of Indian mothers was less nutritious than that of non-Indian mothers, as well as the abundance of anemic, physiologically weak Indian women. He was discussing tuberculosis in Indians as a "wasting disease" or a "disease of the worn out." This characterization, present also in Europe and the United States throughout the second half of the nineteenth century and the first third of the twentieth, not only permeated numerous medical explanations but also was a recurrent argument used to regularly advertise and sell iron-based "strengthening tonics" and elixirs to increase bodily resistance and to diminish innate weakness.[69]

In the early twentieth century some studies explained the high tuberculosis mortality rate among natives, blacks, and mixed-race populations in terms of their racial predisposition. The sudden disappearance of most of the so-called "Roca's Indians," natives captured during Gen. Julio A. Roca's Conquista del Desierto who ended up living in the city, reinforced the belief that natives were highly vulnerable to contagion. The argument stressed the "virginal nature" of their race and the very limited amount of needed antibodies city people had.

No wonder medical studies concluded that the Roca's Indians developed extremely acute and galloping tuberculosis.[70]

In the 1940s Antonio Cetrángolo discussed the issue in the larger context of tuberculosis as a hereditary disease. He pointed out that "Indian children abandoned in the Pampas when the elders fled, escaping from the national army troops," were "given to the families of colonels, army officers, and even soldiers" who lived in Buenos Aires. Some were able to make their living as servants or policemen. But many died of tuberculosis as a result of "the terrible change of weather and environment to which they did not adapt" and the "dreadful hygiene, work, food, and housing conditions" they had to endure. The few natives who survived their voluntary or forced incorporation into the life of modern Buenos Aires had astonishing resistance, both physical and emotional. That resistance allowed them to adapt to a new social and work environment, to survive infection, and to bear children who had the same resistance, maybe even more. Cetrángolo emphasized that the case of the Roca's Indians made it possible to affirm that "hereditary immunity doesn't exist; the decrease in the tubercular mortality of the Indians infected with the bacillus is due solely to an environmentally determined selection process." This distinguished specialist helped deracialize the issue, as Singer had done in the case of Jews, by stressing that the hereditary factor was not as important as many had believed. Cetrángolo pointed out that—even though in certain cases the hereditary factor couldn't be ignored—material, cultural, and emotional living conditions were actually the most important factors when it came to contagion.[71]

The story of Ceferino Namuncurá Ceferino, who later became *el santito de las tolderías*, a popular and enduring figure throughout the twentieth century both in urban and rural Argentina, illustrates what happened to many other, more anonymous Roca's Indians, who probably led even harder lives. The son of a captive white woman, Rosario Burgos, and the Indian chief Manuel Namuncurá, Ceferino was born in 1886 in Chimpay, Río Negro. He was a member of a Mapuche community, which, in 1879, decided to stop fighting the national army because of the thousands of deaths that had resulted from the Conquista del Desierto and the less violent pressure of Salesian missionaries. Soon Chimpay turned into an extremely poor Indian enclave whose survival depended on meager subsidies provided by the federal government, subsistence farming, begging, and occasional sales to the white population settled in the area. In 1897 Chief Namuncurá decided to take his son Ceferino to Buenos Aires, where he could learn a trade. An army general managed to get the child a scholarship at the Talleres Nacionales de Marina, where he had a very unhappy experience as a carpenter's apprentice. Then Ceferino's father contacted Luis Saenz Peña, the former president, to intercede with the Salesian fathers to admit the child to the Pío IX school. There, Ceferino seems to have adapted better than at the Marina workshops, but now he had to cope with the routines of city life and, most important, learn to accept being the only native child in a school attended by six hundred white boys. He spent the summer of 1898 at an agricultural school in the Buenos Aires province, where he was supposed to temper his character and strengthen his body. He failed his final exams that year at the school in Buenos Aires, so he went back to the agricultural school in 1899, where he became a catechist the following year.

In 1902 doctors confirmed that Ceferino had tuberculosis. At least in part he was repeating the story of one of his brothers who, ten years before, had moved to Buenos Aires and died two years later. In 1903 Ceferino moved back to northeast Patagonia to pursue a career as a priest and look after his health. His father tried in vain to convince him to return to the Chimpay community, but Ceferino was obsessed with the ideas of sin and the fear of losing his faith, so he opted to stay in the bosom of the Catholic community. He began avoiding his family and became a chaplain at the San Francisco de Sales school. There, he was overfed in an attempt to fight his disease. In 1904 Ceferino traveled to Italy, where it was thought he could recover and become a priest. He died there in 1905 at the age of eighteen.[72]

There are several similarities between tuberculosis in criollo, Argentine-born women, mainly women of mixed Indian and Spanish ancestry, and in the Roca's Indians. At the beginning of the century the tuberculosis mortality rate among criollo women was significantly higher than that among immigrant women. Between 1908 and 1917 statistics showed that criollo women died of tuberculosis at the same rate as Argentine-born men, while the mortality of immigrant women was considerably lower than that of immigrant men, roughly twelve per thousand among women and twenty per thousand among men. These figures were quite similar to the ones in North American and European cities. In trying to explain the fact that criollo women were dying of tuberculosis in higher proportions than immigrant women vis-à-vis Argentine-born or immigrant men, respectively, some studies underlined the fact that criollo women "spent a lot of time indoors in very unfavorable conditions; they are poorly fed, badly dressed, have too many children, are often unwed and abandoned by their lovers." Unlike immigrant women, criollo women had "habits, jobs, and a lifestyle that made them vulnerable to tuberculosis."[73] Their race, having too many children, and holding certain jobs were deemed to predispose them to tuberculosis.

In fact, the notion of racial mixing and the weaknesses of so-called colored peoples was discussed in the first decades of the century, though the results of this thinking were totally discredited in the 1930s. The fertility rate was higher among native women than among immigrant women. And although the connection between high fertility rates and tuberculosis had been questioned starting in the early 1930s, it was thought that the physical demands of frequent pregnancies in a context of poverty or hardship could undermine immunity in "poor mixed-race, criollo women." As for the jobs these women held, many, in addition to the nonpaid household work they did, were employed in factories. Criollo women also worked as maids and in the textile, food, printing, glass, and tobacco industries to offset the decrease in immigration, particularly in the years that followed the crisis of 1890 and those of the First World War, when the first phases of import-substitution industrialization were taking place. They were internal migrants themselves or the daughters of migrants. The relatively high rate of tuberculosis in criollo women, like that among the Roca's Indians, was probably owing to their having grown up in places with little or no exposure to the bacillus; furthermore, their new routines, the pressures of city life, and the vertiginous pace of work, quite frequently piecework, both in and outside the home most certainly affected their resistance.

From the 1940s, when there were no antibiotics, to the 1950s and 1960s, when there were, many migrant women's experience of the disease didn't change. It is the story of many young women who arrived in the city from the hinterlands, the Argentine interior, with low immunity levels and ended up catching the disease. Jorgelina S. recalled growing up in the mountains: "When my dad died, my mother started giving us away. I had to go with a family from Buenos Aires. They took me to the city, I believe it was in 1942, with a lot a fantastic promises. I was fourteen. . . . But I didn't even go to school. I worked as a maid for three years. And there I got sick. The lady of the house urged me to eat because I was getting sick. But I didn't want to eat. Once she threatened me. 'If you don't eat,' she said, 'I will send you back to your mother.' And that was exactly what I wanted, so finally I got my way. At that point, the lady of the house where I was working took me to a doctor and that's when they told me I had tuberculosis. I had to be admitted to a hospital."

The situation of drafted soldiers was also similar to that of Roca's Indians. An article published in 1899 by the *Anales de Sanidad Militar* pointed out that those who "join the army are from the lowest social class, and the change of routine just worsens their situation." The low standards of hygiene, the agglomeration of the troop, fatigue, changes in diet, the rigors of instruction, and the psychic disorders of sadness and nostalgia were "all responsible for the etiology of tuberculosis among soldiers." In this context, "the recruited young man becomes sick with worry, as does his blood."[74] Thirty years later tuberculosis in soldiers was seen as a pathological manifestation of the experience of young men who "came from rural areas that were untouched by tuberculosis" and lived in the "garrisons of Buenos Aires most prone to the disease, where they caught it, usually in its active form."[75] According to a military doctor, once soldiers were identified as tubercular they "left the precinct of their own free will or they were sent back to their places of origin," where they became "active foci of contagion."[76]

In times of biomedical uncertainty about tuberculosis, the cases of the Galicians, the Basques, the Jews, the Roca's Indians, criollo women, and soldiers from the provinces reveal that, in the effort to order an urban world saturated with occasions and opportunities for mixing, the discussion of degrees of predisposition—of individuals and of groups—to the disease was quite often articulated around prejudices, preconceptions, and stereotypes. The explanations for the disease were rarely based on solid studies, and the fact of belonging to a certain national, ethnic, or racial group ended up overriding other dimensions of the individual experience. Vague stereotypes were used to explain predisposition to the disease, simplifying a very complex etiology. Depending on the case, what mattered was the risk presented by the work or home environment, questions of lifestyle, levels of income and education, diet, general health, and the degree of exposure to the bacillus. If race played a role at all—an issue still debatable nowadays, even when framed in genetic terms—it is clear that the ways in which it was articulated, in a time of profound biomedical uncertainty, reveal the many uses tuberculosis had in talking about other, strictly nonbiomedical issues.

CHAPTER EIGHT

A Female Disease

During much of the nineteenth century tuberculosis was shrouded in mystery; little or nothing was known about its origin or its victims. In medical and scientific circles it was seen as the disease of a thousand causes, all explained by weak medical theories. Beginning in the 1860s with Jean Antoine Villemin's research into the contagiousness of the disease, and especially with the rapid emergence of modern bacteriology and the discovery of the Koch bacillus two decades later, the aura of mystery began to dissipate. Nevertheless, the need not merely to explain contagion and susceptibility to contagion, but also to find an effective cure, greatly spurred attempts to explain the disease. These ranged from interpretations based on notions of heredity to those stressing psychosomatic and social dimensions. Associations and metaphors abounded. Whether fleeting or enduring, these theories and imageries gave rise to a sort of tuberculosis subculture. In Buenos Aires, literature, film, and theater, popular magazines and newspapers, medical and health journals, tango lyrics, poetry, and sociological essays all made reference to tuberculosis, treating it both as an element of reality and as a metaphor or ideologized way through which to speak of other topics and concerns. It was also very often feminized.

The feminized portrayals of tuberculosis were partial representations of the subculture. Both men and women caught and feared catching the disease. But between 1880 and 1950, men died of tuberculosis at a greater rate than women, and, though in the late 1920s the mortality rate of both sexes was declining, it declined more sharply among women than men.[1] However, in most of the written and visual narratives that circulated in Buenos Aires during those seven decades, tuberculosis was seen as a female disease. Men were not totally absent, but women consistently tended to be at center stage.

In Eugenio Cambaceres's novel *En la sangre*, the issue for Genaro, the leading character, is his mother's "damned cough, [which] doesn't let him rest." In his sick mother Genaro sees "a laughingstock, a burden . . . that fills him with shame." The mother is also a source of unease when it comes to his mingling with elite social circles, which he wants to join. In the end, the mother, along with her tuberculosis, is sent back to Italy; rid of her now, Genaro is convinced he can also rid himself of his humble past and everything he considers the cause of his personal and social awkwardness. From then on Genaro pretends to be someone he's not. He learns to be a pretender, a character that the essayists José Ingenieros and José Ramos Mejía have discussed extensively as a distinctive feature of the social dynamics of Buenos Aires around the beginning of the twentieth century. Within a few years, after successfully gaining control of an estate that once belonged to a patrician family, Genaro becomes a large landowner.[2]

In *Los derechos de la salud*, a play written by Florencio Sánchez in the early twentieth century, tuberculosis gradually dehumanizes Luisa. She is very conscious of her deterioration: "For the past year, my senses and faculties have weakened. I've become an idiot. I've lost the ability to ponder things and facts. I can't see, touch, feel, or understand. I'm being attacked by a disease that has brought me to the gates of death."[3] In *La gallina degollada*, a story by Horacio Quiroga written in 1925, tuberculosis is bound to the phantoms of heredity. In a desperate moment, the story's leading man and woman blame each other for the children they've raised, who have been "diagnosed [as] idiots." The husband calls his wife "a consumptive little viper!," and tells her to ask the doctor "who's to blame for the children's meningitis, my father [who had died of delirium] or your crappy lungs."[4]

Though tuberculosis affects men in Nicolás Olivari's poetry, women bear the burden of the disease. Olivari's collection of poems entitled *La musa de la mala pata*, dated 1926, depicts women with tuberculosis who not only live in the city but are truly part of it. Indeed, the city has made them "monstrous and sickly." And perhaps for this reason they are destined at some point to share their lives with a penniless poet, who proposes that he and his beloved "unite our physical wretchedness / my worthless, aching airs / your incipient tuberculosis / and my metaphysical restlessness." In Olivari's tubercular women, disease is not punitive or terminal, but an embodiment of the social margins, of urban desolation and sorrow. Olivari's seamstresses, typists, prosti-

tutes, lovers, *Estercitas*—young women of the neighborhood—and adventurous women, *milonguitas*, who dare to leave their homes and neighborhoods
for the lights of the city center, all of them are burdened by wretched bodies
and dismal souls. They are "sick and extremely skinny" or "consumptive and
asexual . . . with large, lifeless eyes." They are also impossibly vulgar, with an
extreme, yet ordinary, ugliness that can never hope to become a menacing or
feared beauty.[5]

Only a few narratives centered on male characters with tuberculosis. In
a highly naturalistic style, in which surfeits, pedagogy, denouncements, and
fatalism abound, the writer Elías Castelnuovo, through the character of Lázaro
and his disease, narrates the pain of the "proletarian writer." Lázaro is convinced that, in working at a city newspaper's editorial office, "a dark, unhealthy
place," he has lost two things he will never recover: his health and his intelligence. Lazaro's disease combines heredity and social explanations—he's the
poor son of a servant and an "unknown consumptive man"—with a sort of
romantic reading of tuberculosis: he is a journalist whose sensitivity to the
evils of the world predisposes him to sickness. Castelnuovo uses tuberculosis as a way to reconstruct, without any aestheticized pretensions, a sick person's decline and death in a narrative steeped in horror and pathos.[6] In *Camas
desde un peso* by Enrique González Tuñón, a young artist, the narrator of a
collection of shorts stories on urban outcasts, is portrayed as a social victim
with a refined sensibility: "I speak as a penniless intellectual who's dying of
consumption and cannot even count on a bowl of soup every day."[7] Writing
stories either during or set in the 1920s to 1940s, Roberto Arlt, Ulises Petit de
Murat, and Manuel Puig also wrote in a literary subgenre centered on sanatoriums in the foothills and rest hotels and boardinghouses. Rather than delving
into the refined sensibility of the tuberculars or the social injustice that con-
demns them to a life of disease, these works center on the characters' inner
worlds, affections, alienations, peculiarities, and obsessions, as well as on their
nostalgia for the past and a life outside the enclaves of the rest cure.[8]

But tubercular women dominated the tuberculosis narratives of the late
nineteenth century and early twentieth. Three female characters seem to re-
cur: women who are sick from passion, a narrative that, at the beginning of the
twentieth century and particularly after 1920, became connected to neurasthenics and thereby to psychology; working women whose sickness is caused
by their extremely long workdays; and neighborhood *costureritas*, young
seamstresses who go astray, move downtown, become milonguitas, frequent
the cabarets, get involved in the world of prostitution, and wind up catching
tuberculosis.

From Passionate Consumptives to Neurasthenic Tuberculars

In her book *Peregrinaciones de una alma triste*, Juana Manuela Gorriti discusses tuberculosis as "a disease of the soul." She uses it as a vehicle to relate the transgressions of a woman who seeks to achieve personal freedom and dares to question masculine medical knowledge.[9] Dated 1876, the text audaciously undertakes to speak of masculine issues, often questioning and challenging men's opinions. Gorriti presents herself as a writer who tells stories of women in order to forge a place for them in the construction of the nation and to criticize the narrow domestic chores to which they were usually confined. Her stories depict women's private lives in order to reexamine official public history. She underscores the differences between what she sees as the intuitive, personal discourse of women and the rational discourse of men, which, in the late nineteenth century, was heavily informed by scientism and positivism.

The daughter of a soldier in the war for independence, Gorriti married a mestizo military officer when she was fifteen. Her husband would eventually become president of Bolivia. She had lovers and gave birth to several children, some out of wedlock. She made a living by teaching and writing. By the age of forty, she was a highly respected public voice. A tireless traveler, Gorriti toured South America at a time when most Argentine intellectuals traveled to Europe. She lived in Lima, La Paz, and Buenos Aires, where she died in 1892 at the age of seventy-four.[10]

In *Peregrinaciones de una alma triste* there are plenty of similiarities to Gorriti's own life. It's a travel journal in the format of a novel that starts off as a dialogue between two young women, childhood friends who separate and meet again after a long time. Laura tells her friend about her trips across Argentina, Brazil, Chile, and Peru: her story is full of incidents, people, and places; it includes Indians and their captives, bandits, attempted rapes, life in a convent, civilized men who embody barbarism, and women disguised as men in order to "avoid the infinite difficulties that befall skirts everywhere."[11] Laura, the traveler, is apparently the only common thread running through the stories, which glorify disorder, chaos, and rebelliousness.

Laura's journey begins when she decides to run away from home, a despotic doctor, and the city where she lives. She's consumptive, and running away represents a young woman's aspiration to escape the suffocating attention she receives from her family in the hope of finding individual freedom. This is a woman who distrusts medical knowledge and medical doctors and who is willing to wander the continent looking for "the air that the lethal atmosphere of the city [is taking away from her]." In fact, her treatment is the story's turning point: taking daily "drops of arsenic," wearing "light and loose dresses," and behaving "calmly, avoiding fatigue, desires, [obeying] the doctor, and nothing else." Her doctor tells her about an exceptional young male patient who recovered by "subject[ing] his lungs to the fatigue of endless journeys." However, the doctor specifically states that "this remedy can only work on a subject," an autonomous individual. And since Laura the woman is not considered as such, she should not entertain this as a possible treatment.[12]

But Laura disagrees. She thinks of herself as a subject capable of making decisions and suspects that in the long-journey therapy, rather than in the confinement of home, arsenic-based concoctions, and submission to her doctor's orders, she will find a cure. She conjectures that, like the young male patient cured by travel, she has contracted a "disease of the soul [that] has caused a disease of the body." She becomes convinced that her doctor "attacks the pain without attacking the cause." In her journey Laura seeks the "only medicine" that will save her: a "variety of scenarios for my life, and a variety of scenarios for my lungs."

The therapy Laura chooses, the one her doctor prescribed for the young male patient but not for her, was hardly exceptional. A number of doctoral theses from the late nineteenth century maintained that tuberculosis could be caused by "sorrow and sadness" and, along with tonics, rest, and silence, cautiously prescribed "a change in setting." The popular science manual *Medicina Doméstica*, written in 1854 by D. J. Pérez, recommended "natural tonics against consumption" and warned that "when consumption is suspected, it is advisable to travel for a change of setting and climate." By the end of the century, in discussing the passions from a medical and social point of view, Lucas Ayarragaray warned that the "effect of medicines depends as much on the patient's spirit as on physical disposition," and traveling produces a "change in the state of mind and speeds up recovery."[13]

Laura decides to leave; she sneaks out, evading the strict surveillance at her house and wearing "voluminous overskirts" to hide her "slimness" and high heels; she lets her curls hang down under a "coquettish little hat" with a "shadowy, yet transparent veil" dangling over the makeup she has daringly put on. On her way to the station she runs into her doctor, who doesn't recognize her, an attractive young woman, as the patient he used to advise. The doctor does not hesitate to start flirting with her but soon realizes he has no chance. He says goodbye and attempts to discredit and demean the young woman who has so impressed but ignored him. Mockingly, he says, "Farewell, tiny sugar pie. Have a nice trip, and try not to melt down!!"

Once she's rejected this man both as her doctor and as her lover, Laura begins her pilgrimage. Soon, her intuition is confirmed: once she has begun her travels she can, despite the doctor's advice, eat, drink, run, play the piano, sing, and dance "with the zest of a recently released prisoner." She finds that "each of these vital acts is like a health certificate, completely forgetting about fevers, the coughing, and the sweat." Later in her journey Laura writes a mildly ironic letter to the man who unsuccessfully tried to seduce her at the station: "Dear Doc, this tiny sugar pie body is actually quite far from melting down: it is growing stronger by the hour."

At the time, doctors and patients speculated endlessly about the causes of pulmonary consumption. They largely concluded it was a disease of fatigue, "the result of the excessive workings of body and spirit." The possible causes included "life in the city and urban excesses" and "weakness and emotional suffering, disappointments, headaches, depression, and troubles."[14] In Gorriti's novel, the doctor believes Laura's disease is a consequence of her innate weaknesses, while Laura finds it a "disease of the soul" that has come to affect her body. The doctor's explanation and recommended course of therapy reaffirm the role of women in the nineteenth century: she is told to limit herself to the female realm of the household; since she is fragile, she must be subject to strict control, permanent seclusion, and obedient submission to her inborn disability. Laura, though, attributes her disease to her intense and troubled inner world, and the therapy that finally cures her, the invigorating journey, entails questioning her doctor's recommendations.

During much of the nineteenth century, in Europe and other places far from the Western world, tuberculosis was related to a romantic vision of the world, a metaphor for delicacy, impotence, and grief. Riddled with double meanings, tuberculosis was both a curse and a sign of refinement, a disease of waning energy and of exacerbated sensibility, an illness connected to vulnerability and spiritual elevation.[15] In Gorriti's account some of these notions are juxtaposed with both the ups and downs of Laura's struggle with and eventual triumph over the disease and her self-assertion as an independent woman in the face of medical knowledge articulated by men.

At the beginning of the twentieth century, despite a growing awareness of the social nature of the disease, the idea of tuberculosis as a disease of the delicate, distinct, and sensual soul hadn't completely vanished. An article published in the magazine PBT in 1905 read, "Consumption has degenerated into the mild indisposition that many girls claim to have caught out of sheer coquetry; soon, for the sake of elegance and distinction, we'll all be cultivating the sport of tuberculosis."[16] However, as the century progressed, the allure of the archetypical, romantic consumptive girl was challenged by the manifold images of the modern woman as well as a new paragon of beauty that praised healthy, fit bodies. In 1931 an advertisement for cod liver oil published in the magazine *Para Tí* clearly evidenced this shift: "Such poor little sick women, with pale skin and skinny ugly bodies! Why look terrible when you can easily obtain a magnificent youthful body brimming with health?"[17] In 1937 an article published in the magazine *Viva Cien Años* suggested to its readers to have fun, be active, and smile because "backward nations are the saddest ones, with effeminate boys and shy, judgmental, and lifeless girls who are the neurasthenics or tuberculars of the future."[18]

The connections between neurasthenia and tuberculosis were nothing new; they were grounded on metaphors of deterioration, loss of strength, and fatigue, the last of which was used to explain a myriad of illnesses that, one way or another, involved exhaustion and the wasting of an inborn resource. The symptoms of nervous exhaustion included irritability, excessive sensitivity, tension, and decay, and it suggested both a physical and an emotional state. This decrease in energy—a sort of disability that, according to the doctors, could sometimes impede the proper regulation of passions—was connected to neurasthenia, chlorosis, and tuberculosis, especially in the case of upper- and middle-class women.[19]

Neurasthenia and chlorosis became objects of new medical concern during the last third of the nineteenth century, but interest in them waned after a few decades. Quite often, as a result of their highly imprecise symptomatologies, many doctors confused these maladies with other sicknesses, particularly with consumption in the nineteenth century and with tuberculosis until well into the twentieth. Whether deliberate or not, the confusion meant that, at the turn of the century, popular publications contained a great many ads for strengthening tonics. In 1898, for instance, the *Grageas del Dr. Hecquet* were pills advertised as "the best ferruginous medicine against anemia, nervousness, chlorosis, consumption; the only one that rebuilds the blood, calms the nerves, and doesn't cause constipation." A decade later, in 1908, advertisements for the *Preparación de Wampole* promised "swift, certain relief from blood impurities, nervous dyspepsia, and consumption," while *Ovo-lecitina Billon* claimed to "put an end to anemia, chlorosis, neurasthenia, rachitis, and tuberculosis."[20] By the end of the 1920s nothing seemed to have changed substantially, and the tonic *Virol* offered a solution for "waning energy, nervousness, fatigue, neurasthenia, anemia, exhaustion, and tuberculosis."[21]

Starting at the end of the nineteenth century and through the 1930s and 1940s, the notion of mental fatigue became important to the understanding of the connections between neurasthenia and the psychology of people with pulmonary tuberculosis. A series of articles spoke of "the tubercular personality." These articles maintained that certain personality traits were the result of "toxemias," or poisons produced by toxins. Some doctors connected dementia praecox, psychosis, and states of "mental confusion" with "tuberculosis toxemia."[22] An article written by León Charosky and Antonio Dalto, published in 1934 in *La Prensa Médica Argentina*, supported this connection with references to an extensive specialized bibliography—in some cases century-old studies—as well as observations made by the authors themselves, who examined hospital and private medical records of women with active and inactive tuberculosis. For the former, they noted a strong correlation with specific psychological disturbances such as "acute delirium, mental confusion, manias, melancholy, exhibitionism, dreamlike delirium, erotomania, mystical, and persecutory hallucinations." In the case of women with inactive tuberculosis, Charosky and Dalto observed "fear, irritability, depression, exaggerated optimism, and eroticism"; in the case of women admitted to the hospital, they noticed "selfishness and exacerbated envy," and, for those who were able to manage their disease at home, "intellectual excitement, pessimism, neurasthenia, and dyspepsia." In their conclusions the authors attempted to narrow down the too-broad and fragmented set of symptoms, suggesting that the most prevalent psychological alterations were related to "disturbances of affectivity and irritability." They saw a prevalence of "tuberculosis among schizophrenics" and stated, "It is undeniable that tuberculosis engenders, by means of toxins, not only neurological and psychological disturbances, but also other psychopathic disorders."[23]

By the early 1940s Charosky's and Dalto's interpretations were being criticized by Gregorio Bermann. He argued that their conclusions were the result of a "mechanistic, narrow, and materialistic medicine" that believed disease to be "caused by external factors" and ignored "the personality of those in pain." Grounding his views in Sigmund Freud and others, Bermann called for acknowledging the weight of the "reaction of the Self to the disease." He affirmed that "psychic problems are not a faithful reflection of pathological processes" and that the psychology of the tubercular had to be approached in terms not of adaptation to a certain illness or environment, but of toxins.[24]

During the first four decades of the twentieth century psychology endeavored to further define the "personality of the tubercular" in an attempt to make it possible to diagnose the disease and distinguish it from others with similar symptoms. For example, it was said that euphoria, optimism, sexual appetite, and creativity were common in people with tuberculosis, but not in those with pneumonia, bronchitis, and asthma. The effort to define with certainty the personality of the tubercular ultimately gave rise to a list of behaviors: nervousness, propensity to lying and crying, hostility, demanding and arbitrary behavior, fickleness, irritability, and intolerance. Bermann noted that "almost every adult with tuberculosis has acute neurasthenia." Nonetheless, he was very cautious in this respect because, like the tuberculosis expert Antonio Cetrángolo before him, he was trying to avoid simplifications that coupled "certain psychologies" with pulmonary tuberculosis. He rejected the idea that the tubercular possessed an "exalted sensibility, intelligence, genius, and profound eroticism" or was "cowardly and evil." He recognized that, like other chronic diseases, tuberculosis took hold of a patient's "body and soul." Though Bermann did venture some generalizations, he urged professionals to keep in mind that different stages of the sickness generated different states of mind and that social class, age, religion, gender, and nationality were all important variables; he warned against the notion of grouping all tubercular patients in a single, dominant psychological type.[25]

The attempt to link certain personality traits with tuberculosis—that is, to connect mental behavior with somatic manifestations—continued well into the 1950s, though it never became a cogent theory. It did, however, contribute to an increasing recognition of the importance of individualizing the psychology of patients, both men and women, in sanatoriums and hospitals. Ultimately, the myriad connections among fatigue, neurasthenia, and tuberculosis in patients served to feminize a number of characteristics that had been defined as masculine for much of the nineteenth century. The notion of manhood at that time was largely based on the idea of an inborn tendency to action. Exhaustion and disability were naturally unmasculine: a weak man with tuberculosis was the antithesis of the masculine ideal. When connected with neurasthenics, tuberculosis feminized sick men, though it did give them creative and intellectual power. These shifts, at least in part, reveal how modern psychology drew from the romantic idea of consumption as it was articulated by medicine and literature, that is, a disease which, though many men might have it, focused on women and their delicacy, voluptuousness, softness, weakness, and sensitivity.

Tísicas *and Working Women with Tuberculosis*

The poet Evaristo Carriego created the literary barrio of Buenos Aires; he was also "the first observer of the *arrabales*, the city's outskirts, their discoverer, their inventor."[26] In his poems the barrio becomes the emotional geography of the poor. It is also a refuge, a friendly space strongly imbued with the hospitality of home, motherly warmth, and the tranquility and safety of childhood. In Carriegos's barrios stroll hurdy-gurdy players, tenement kids, midwives, tavern-goers, drunken husbands, frustrated brides, blind men, and dying old ladies. *Tísicas*, consumptive young women, and costureritas were the women Carriego used to develop his story of tuberculosis in the barrio.

Tísicas and costureritas are not the same. Tísicas live and die in the barrio in a process of deterioration and destitution. Costureritas, on the other hand, are good barrio girls who go astray and decline because they succumb to the temptations of downtown Buenos Aires nightlife, which inevitably leads to a tragic end. If the tísica suggests that tuberculosis is a disease born of over-work and barrio sadness, the costurerita embodies an existential adventure in which tuberculosis is deeply bound up in mundane passions, social mobility, degradation, guilt, and moral rebuke. Years later, tango lyrics reinvented this character in the figure of the milonguita.

Tísicas were a call to compassion and empathy. In *Residuo de fábrica* the on-set of tuberculosis is brought about by factory routines: "The workshop made her sick, and thus defeated [she was] / at the age when girls blossom, she may not know / the beautiful joy that may ease / her endless, incurable suffering." The tísica leaves the workshop to move back home, where she tries to adjust to family life only to be rejected: "She's coughed again. Her little brother / who sometimes plays in her room / is suddenly serious and silent, as if there's one thought in his mind . . . / Then, he rises and leaves, abruptly / ponder-ing something, as he moves / with a little pity and much disgust: / the piglet, again, is spitting blood."[27]

In *El alma del suburbio* Carriego re-creates the romantic depiction of the disease and the extremely sensitive and passionate female characters found in many nineteenth-century European novels: "the tísica next door" bemoans her unrequited love and ponders the burden of the "sweet melancholy of a forgotten, yet beloved, verse that a gallant troubadour sang to her once." In *El ensueño* something similar is hinted at: the young girl with tuberculosis tries to ignore the shouts of her drunken father while thinking about the "gratify-ing, unreal dream she had when thinking about that boy she saw next to her neighbor's bed, one Thursday afternoon at the hospital." In *Las manos* the poet deals with "the romantic hands of the tísica who, / in the agonizing voice of an arpeggio, like an anxious, anguished spell, / called on Chopin, as she lay dying." This romantic depiction is even more apparent in *La viejecita*. Here, Carriego's tubercular female characters are in the austere, plebeian settings of the Buenos Aires barrios: "Such heroines, so poor and obscure, in those dra-mas! / So many Ophelias! The barrios and city outskirts have their pure and consumptive Ladies of the Camellias." Tísicas are citizens of a world of work; they belong to the universe of sadness, humility, and misfortune anchored to the barrio. They're not necessarily or shockingly poor; indeed, the hands of the tísica playing Chopin reveal that at least some of them had access to an object, a piano, that would soon become quite important to any home aspiring to the values, icons, and habits of the incipient middle classes. Indeed, these women with tuberculosis have no connection whatsoever to bohemian life.

Tísicas were barrio women. Remarkably, Carriego places them not in the tenement, but in the humble barrio homes. In keeping with this mise-en-scène, they are characterized not by indigence, promiscuity, and crowded dwellings, but by work. The association between excessive work and tuberculosis was not invented by Carriego. It was first suggested in the late nineteenth century and continued well into the 1950s. Though sickness was deemed the result of excess, overwork was not comparable with other excesses—too much sex or drink, for example—in which individual responsibility and personal life choices may explain contagion. According to doctors, hygienists, essayists, union leaders, and journalists, tuberculosis could be caused by environmental factors in workshops, factories, piecework performed at home; by a specific kind of labor, a precedent of what would later lead to reform in labor medicine and definitions of occupational disease; or by capitalist exploitation, which was blamed for creating the existent social system. Indeed, tuberculosis was brought up, directly or indirectly, in any and all discussions of shortening the workday, night work, home wage work, piecework, fatigue, industrial hygiene, workers' rest, and the pace of production.

By the end of the nineteenth century Ingenieros had found in the criticism of overwork and work-related fatigue a vehicle for an agenda concerned with the "rights of social forces over those of individuals."[28] Elvira Rawson de Dellepiane spoke of "humble women workers, machine-women mercilessly exploited at the sewing and ironing workshops where they often catch tuberculosis."[29] In 1910 Augusto Bunge furthered this argument in a report commissioned by the federal government in which he alluded to "diseases of overwork" caused by the "intensity of labor and excessively long workdays" and "a lack of fresh air, [time spent in] crowded places, dust, the lack of ventilation, and sunlight."[30] Carriego is part of this climate of ideas that explained tuberculosis among working women not as a punishment for those who dared to leave domesticity behind, but as evidence of social injustice. In the 1920s tango lyrics like *Obrerita* and *Fosforerita* furthered this view.[31] In *Camino al Taller* work and disease lead to a fatal end: "On the way to the workshop, on the way to death / under a bundle of clothes you're taking to sew / who knows, will I ever see you again? / poor little seamstress, on the way to the workshop." In *Muñeca de Percal* the tone is similar: "Early in the morning, you go to the workshop / where the hellish noisy machine / shatters your every womanly dream . . . / faith punishes you with a harsh cross / you're the girl who, in a miserable attic / suffers from incurable and cruel tuberculosis / until death comes looking for you in a big funereal car." In *Cotorrita de la Suerte* tuberculosis is born of overwork and unrequited love: "Oh, the factory girl is coughing at night / coughing and suffering from the cruel realization / of how her life extinguishes while the pain / never leaves her tender heart respite . . . / She's waiting for her beloved, eagerly / and on the very afternoon she died, poor thing / she asked her mommy, 'Hasn't he come yet?'"

Though less so than poetry and song lyrics, the literature of the time also depicted working women as possible victims of tuberculosis. Josué Quesada and Julio Fingerit wrote short stories, published in *La Novela Semanal*, in which the image of seamstresses and female shop workers is in keeping with Carriego's depictions. Álvaro Yunque worked along the same lines, further accentuating the association between disease and overwork. In *La muchacha del atado*, one of his celebrated short stories about urban life, Arlt explored the work lives, misadventures, and hardships of these young women and how they worked both in and outside of their homes.[32]

Women had been a part of the world of work from the beginning of the twentieth century.[33] A report issued by the National Department of Labor in 1901 called women working at home for wages a "convenient supplement" to a household income, though there were also "female-headed households" in which women were the sole breadwinners. However, it seems that wage work done by women at home was largely complementary to other jobs, including prostitution, that were temporary and random and could be adapted to a flexible schedule, thereby making it possible to coordinate work and household responsibilities. Tuberculosis was not unusual among women who worked on their own or for somebody else but who didn't have to endure the arduous work of the factory. In addition to factors that could predispose anyone to tuberculosis contagion — namely, poor working and living conditions — women working at home also had to deal with the trials of piecework and a sedentary lifestyle. Piecework was typically unstable; it could entail dangerous physical efforts when attempting to make deadlines and meant a fluctuating monthly income. In that context it was frequently said that overworked seamstresses tended to have poor posture; their repeated movements and monotonous work routines hindered the proper functioning of the respiratory tract.[34]

Despite what some medical doctors and journalists said again and again, a study from 1915 indicated that seamstresses' predisposition to tuberculosis was not due to the closed environment of the tenement—after all, most of them worked in a backyard or next to a door or a window. Carriego had suggested something similar in his poems when he refered to modest barrio houses as the places where most of his tísica seamstresses lived and worked. The real problem was the seasonal nature of the work and the badly paid overwork it entailed.[35]

In literature and tango lyrics, therefore, barrio tísicas crave pity and compassion. They live hard, honorable working lives, but tuberculosis appears to be their final burden. Over and over again, the barrio seems to honor them with poems and tangos which, like commiserative, elegiac orations spoken in honor of deceased or almost deceased young tísicas, stressed the labor and social dimensions of their disease.

Costureritas and Milonguitas in the World of Tango

Unlike the tísicas, pained souls who became sick from excessive work without ever leaving the friendly barrio, the costurerita "who went astray" because she dared to leave her domestic world in the barrio, and the milonguita, the young barrio women who becomes a downtown cabaret girl, are the leading players in a tragic tale of social mobility and high expectations. The costurerita is Carriego's character and the central figure of perhaps his best-known poem. The milonguita is a quintessential female character in tango lyrics from the 1920s and 1930s. Both cases tell the sad story of the young, ingenuous barrio girl from a humble yet dignified home who, after a brief visit to the world of the night, falls into prostitution and illness. The innocent, virtuous barrio world is where this melodramatic plot begins. The tone is marked, predictably, by moral polarization: there are no in-betweens, only great joy or terrible sorrow. The departure from the barrio, whether out of deception, ambition, or love, is the moment that interrupts a common life that should have gone on without great changes or surprises. The departure from the barrio is also the moment at which roots, home, and maternal love are betrayed. The setting shifts, and in the process the identity of the costureritas and milonguitas changes: they are doomed to wander the strange and cruel world until their inevitable fate, disease, befalls them. Unlike other melodramatic tales, this journey, commonly articulated by poets like Carriego and the many male authors of tango lyrics, lacks suspense and is no more than an organizing motif of a predetermined decline.

The figure of the costurerita combines preoccupations with daily work, social ascent, and nightlife. In his poem *La costurerita que dió aquel mal paso* (that is, the story of "the seamstress who went astray"), Carriego gave a local flavor to a female journey firmly established in the history of Western literature. Of this poem, Jorge Luis Borges wrote, "It is the biography of the splendor, exhaustion, decline, and ultimate darkness of a woman shared by all men."[36] In Carriego's account, the seamstress's decline underscores the sweetness of the barrio. On the one hand, the narrator wonders why the "little red riding hood" is tempted by the city lights when the barrio has almost everything a girl can ask for. The journey downtown is, then, a leap into the void, an unnecessary pilgrimage. On the other hand, both the barrio and the family home are loyal and sheltering to those who leave for no good reason. "Going astray" is not forever because one can always go home again. The barrio offers the compassion given to prodigal sons and daughters and serenely understands, rather than punishes, those who return from the land of doom: "Come on in, do not fear, sister; we won't say a word / the little ones still miss you, and the rest will see in you the lost sister who returned / you may stay, you'll always have a place at our table."

Elements of this decline are also seen in Andrés Cepeda's poetry. Though no longer read, in his time Cepeda was a popular poet who roamed the arrabales; he was arrested several times for robbery in the outskirts of the city and became somewhat famous when some of his verses and songs were set to music and performed by Carlos Gardel, the most venerated tango singer of the early decades of the twentieth century.[37] Cepeda was murdered in 1910. At least two of his poems involve costureritas and milonguitas. In *Marta, la tísica* the narrator runs into Marta, the woman who left him for one of his friends and was later herself left for a younger girl. Marta gets sick, begs for food in the streets, and, before dying, receives the empathetic lament of the man who once loved her "with all his soul," the man she abandoned a long time ago. Though the man in the poem suffers the loss of love, he doesn't get sick. The abandoned woman, however, catches tuberculosis and dies. In another poem, *La tísica*, the narrator is betrayed both by the false friend and by the ungrateful woman he once loved "the way one can love only at twenty." In time, "she lost her sight" and "sank into vice." "Left alone in the storm," she "cursed her seducer" and "fell prisoner to consumption"; now, she "lies dying in a hospital." At this point, the abandoned boyfriend comes back as a sympathetic, considerate, and compassionate man, capable of forgiving, forgetting, and standing by her in death.[38] In Cepeda tuberculosis is a sickness of women who circulate at the margins of a geographical and social order, far from the friendly barrio. It's a disease of passions, of women adrift who end up tubercular and abandoned by men capable of pardoning.

In the 1920s and 1930s Carriego's legacy was taken up by tango lyrics, film, and literature. The style was less sentimental, though certainly more nostalgic, largely because some of Carriego's barrios had undergone or were about to undergo modernization. Samuel Linnig, José González Castillo, Héctor Pedro Blomberg, Enrique González Tuñón, Celedonio Flores, José A. Ferreyra, and many others cultivated what was then called the romantic legend of the other world, the journey of those who were Estercitas—young women of the barrio—but at some point launched themselves into the cosmopolitan maelstrom of downtown nightlife, where they became milonguitas and prostitutes."[39] To a certain extent it is the same journey that, ten or fifteen years earlier, Carriego's costureritas made. What is new is not the stories but their emphasis and setting, as well as the authors writing them: tango lyricists, filmmakers, journalists, and fiction writers who saw the milonguita not only as a character in need of understanding and compassion, but also as someone embodying traces of their own urban experience. The emphasis was on the milonguitas rather than on the Estercitas, that is, on the young women of the night who frequented the city center rather than those with a barrio life.

By the 1920s, downtown was a symbol of leisure time to Buenos Aires residents. Statistics from 1923 show that that year over seven million people attended some sort of entertainment. On Friday, October 9, 1925, for instance, *La Nación* and *La Razón* contained more than seventy ads for operettas, vaudeville and variety shows, comedies, dance events, plays, music halls, zarzuelas, and movies.[40] In addition to these attractions, downtown nightlife included brothels, dancing academies, cafés with female waitresses doubling as prostitutes, and cabarets. Though some barrios had some of these features, much of the erotic appeal of these night places lay in the fact that they were located downtown, where the supply of such amusement was abundant and accessible to a broad range of budgets. Downtown, men from all walks of life enjoyed the adventure of entertainment offered by young women from the barrio now working as barmaids, cabaret girls, and prostitutes.

The powerful erotic charge of the downtown developed over time and was greatly influenced by tango. A hybrid cultural artifact born on the city outskirts, tango drew on *candombe* choreography and other dances from the black population living in the Rio de la Plata region; it also reflected the massive presence of immigrants in the city's social and cultural fabric. The early years of tango are obscure, though it certainly developed on the city margins.

Between 1870 and 1880, dance events near military barracks were organized by prostitutes who knew how to dance the convoluted steps of *milongas, habaneras,* and *tangos.* In the late nineteenth century, tango reigned not only in brothels and dance halls, where it served as both simulation and stimulation to entertain the men waiting their turn for commercial sex, but also in dance academies, vacant lots, and barrio streets where improvised dances were performed to the tune of the hurdy-gurdy. It was also played in men-only cafés. In these original settings, tango lyrics were very simple and mainly focused on the joys and pains of the arrabales, where the cult of courage and the skillful use of knives were combined with the workings of local political bosses and the police. The main characters were *guapos,* or tough guys; prostitutes; pimps; and *compadritos,* men who imitated the tough style of pimps and guapos yet most of the time worked for a living.

Tango was danced by men and women in pairs but also by men alone as they waited their turn in the brothels. It was, above all, a dance of the margins. By the beginning of the twentieth century, however, tango was no longer limited to the outskirts, and it was becoming accepted in broader social circles. Young upper-class men, many of whom occasionally ventured to the outskirts, brought tango first to the more exclusive brothels and later to their homes. By then, more and more Buenos Aires residents could see people dancing tango at sainetes, open-air dances, and carnivals. Carnivals were a perfect occasion to explore a dance that was still connected with prostitution and frowned upon or regarded with suspicion. At around the same time, the first tango recordings were released. Tango became increasingly decent and ultimately a respectable cultural form. On the one hand, popular and emerging middle sectors could identify with the urban themes of tango lyrics, music, and dance, now stripped of their initial erotic charge. On the other, largely owing to tango's success in Europe and the United States, the Buenos Aires elite enthusiastically embraced it. Once certain unsettling features of tango had been overcome, it was no longer necessary for those who wanted to show off their dancing to make more or less secretive visits to the brothels on the outskirts, or to participate more openly but far from home in the world of Parisian salons while on their long European vacations.[41]

It didn't take long for tango to become an ultimate Buenos Aires form of expression. It gained ground in respectable dance halls, reputable tearooms, and downtown and barrio cafés. It was also accepted at family gatherings, and tangos were played on the pianos increasingly found in middle-class homes. Tango and the stories communicated by song lyrics could be heard in the theater and at the movies. Often a tango written to be included in a sainete, if successful, offered the story line for another sainete based on the lyrics of that tango. Many movies not only re-created tango stories in images but also took their titles from them. The development of the music, radio, and recording industries; the consolidation of theater as a popular form of entertainment; the increasing professionalization of musicians and singers; and the birth of trios, quartets, and orchestras left less room for improvisation in tango. These changes also affected tango lyrics, which became more important and focused on narrating stories constructed around strong moral dilemmas with which the *porteño*, the Buenos Aires resident, could easily identify. Tangos became more melodic and turned into an urban narrative in which the epic of the arrabales, along with their real-life guapos, pimps, prostitutes, and compadritos, began to fade away. This epic never disappeared entirely, though, and new or revamped characters were quick to arrive. Among them was the milonguita, the 1920s and 1930s version of Carriego's costurerita, a young woman who came to embody some of the anxieties and tensions attendant on modern relations between women and men.

Tango was cabaret and dance music par excellence, and cabarets were the places for unbridled sexual fantasies and a prelude to paid sex. It was, accordingly, associated with modern threats to morality, to the cult of domesticity, and to formal dancing.[42] The first cabarets flourished in the Palermo and Belgrano neighborhoods, not downtown. Like Parisian cabarets, these clubs were usually located near parks, and during the summer they functioned as restaurants where people could dance at night and listen to an orchestra. Cabarets and restaurant-cabarets became more common in the 1920s; they were now open year-round and located downtown as well as in some barrios. At least twenty such cabarets were quite lavish and elegant. They became social centers where rich men spent their time and money and less rich men, who had to wake up and go to work the next day, amused themselves at early evening shows.[43]

Tango musicians were attracted to the better salaries offered at downtown cabarets, where they earned more money than at brothels on the city margins. Mirroring the social and geographical journey of the musicians, milonguitas connected downtown nightlife and cabarets with an opportunity for rapid social mobility. Nevertheless, the milonguita's journey, whether real or imaginary, didn't begin at the city margins, in the obscure world of misfits; it began in the barrio. It was the narrow-mindedness, humbleness, and hard work and routines of the barrio they desperately wanted to leave behind. Unlike monotonous work at a sewing machine, cabarets whet these girls' appetites for luxury, easy living, fast social ascent, and perhaps an artistic career.

Cabarets were populated by three types of women: *coperas*, or bar girls, who indulged in conversation, drinking, and dancing with the customers and, after a long and patient ritual, sold themselves for sex; *queridas*, the lovers of wealthy customers who enjoyed the permissive and intimate atmosphere of cabarets; and *artistas*, professional singers of some repute.[44] Whatever their status, all these women had bet on a life away from the domestic barrio ideal. Their choice for a more autonomous life was perceived by many men as a threat to the existing gender order.[45]

The milonguita's journey is a recurrent topic of movies, plays, and tango lyrics written by men during the 1920s and 1930s. *Delikatessen Haus*, a sainete written by Linnig and released in 1920, included the tango *Milonguita*, which was highly acclaimed and responsible for enshrining the milonguita character. Two years later José Bustamante shot the film *Milonguita*. José Agustín Ferreyra—a sort of Carriego of Argentine film in that he was a pioneer in bringing to the silver screen a realistic picture of the barrio and its humble people and their misfortunes and illusions—described the milonguita's journey in numerous films: *El Tango de la Muerte* (1917), *La Muchacha del Arrabal* (1922), *Melenita de Oro* (1923), *Corazón de Criolla* (1923), *La Maleva* (1923), *El Organito de la Tarde* (1925), *Mi Último Tango* (1925), *La Costurerita que Dio Aquel Mal Paso* (1926), *Muchachita de Chiclana* (1926), *Muñequitas Porteñas* (1931), and *Calles de Buenos Aires* (1933).[46] These movies (some silent, some talkies) repeated the characters, themes, and scenarios of the tangos, namely, working young women, Don Juans who make false promises, understanding humble boyfriends, alcoholic fathers, generous mothers, ambition, innocence, social inequality, the barrio, the downtown, and the cabaret. Unlike tango lyrics, which typically were fatalistic, these movies, in the spirit of Carriego's costurerita, emphasized the inborn purity of women and the redeeming nature of the barrio, both of which offer milonguitas the opportunity to escape from the traps and illusions that have led them to confusion in the first place.

But it was in tango lyrics that the milonguita's journey downtown was fully revealed. In *Mano a mano*, the decision to go downtown is apparently motivated by poverty. Similarly, the lyrics of *Margot* explain, "You were born in a miserable room on the outskirts." Yet in this case poverty is merely a prelude to personal ambition: "Your rambling was your own fault, you didn't do it innocently / the whims of a rich girl came into your head / since the day a collar-stud tycoon romanced you; . . . I remember, once you didn't have a thing to wear / and now you're dressed in Chinese silk and roses; . . . you're no longer my Margarita, now they call you Margot." And if in *Flor de fango* (1914) and *Galleguita* (1924) ambition is manifested in "jewelry, fashionable clothes, and champagne nights" and "the obsession with . . . making a lot of dough," in *Milonguera* (1925) and *Percal* (1943), on the other hand, the issue is existential: "A nutty girl / who dreamed of pleasure and grandeur" or a young girl "who wants to go downtown and triumph / and forget the percale and cheap clothing." In *De tardecita* (1927) the milonguita's drive becomes plain; it's the search for economic well-being and a glamorous lifestyle removed from the narrow confines of the barrio: "Downtown lights made you believe / that the joy you were looking for / was far from your home. . . . and you wore silk, not percale / lavish dresses and great luxury bewitched you with ambition."

The sojourn in the city center, the promised land, sooner or later turns into decadence. In some cases this appears as an inevitable outcome. *Mano a mano* tells of the "poor, short-lived triumphs" of the milonguita. In *Pobre milonga* (1923) night in the city center is a punishment from which there is no possible salvation: "You'll be milonga till the day you die . . . / what a dreadful ending that'll be." And in *No salgas de tu barrio* (1927), the author, a man, uses a didactic female voice to express his concerns: "Like you, little girl, I, too / was pretty and I was good; / I was humble and I worked, / like you, in a workshop. / I left the fiancé who loved me . . . / for a young man with slicked-back hair / who brought me to the cabaret; / he taught me all his vices, / he trampled on my hopes, / he turned me into this garbage, / little girl, that you see before you."

The cabaret is the decadent setting that appears most often. There, tuberculosis, while exemplifying the dangers of the woman's fall, also connotes the eroticism and sexual heat, the disillusionment, estrangement, coldness, and degradation of her situation. Often it is depicted as a disease of the soul, a malady related to the passions. In one of the short stories written by González Tuñón for *Tangos*, his first book, it is connected to deception, high expectations, and, finally, insanity. Probably in order to stress the romantic aspect of the disease, the author calls it *tisis*, which is phthisis or consumption. In the story, a "lovely consumptive girl has deranged" two melancholic cabaret regulars: a "Yony," a North American Johnnie, and a man from Buenos Aires.[47] This "lovely consumptive girl" has very little in common with the ill-fated barrio girl. On the contrary, she provokes intense, disturbing, almost obsessive love affairs.

In *Carne de cabaret* (1920), tuberculosis is connected with disillusion and deception. It is a disease of the soul and the body: "Poor doxy . . . / sick, lost little soul / who falls into the clutches of a clumsy sugar daddy / . . . her illusions die at the cabaret . . . / and in her haggard, yellow little face / one can see the traces of untrue love . . . / she found no one who would show her compas-

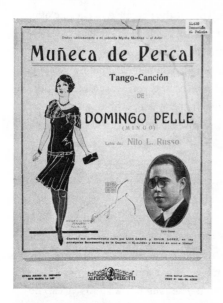

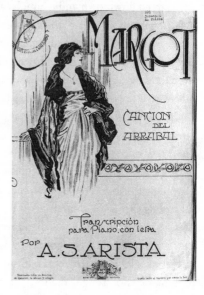

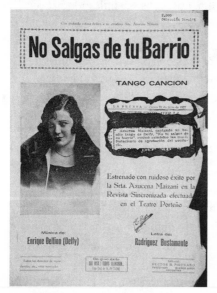

Sheet music covers of tangos
written mainly in the 1920s and
1930s in which the topic is the
milonguita's journey from her
neighborhood to the city center.
(Courtesy of Biblioteca de la
Academia Porteña de Lunfardo,
Buenos Aires)

sion / and she was left alone, to suffer / to let her aspirations die / and thus she rolled over . . . / falling from the cabaret into the hospital." González Castillo linked tuberculosis to estrangement. Written in 1924, the tango *Griseta* tells the story of an innocent French girl who arrives full of hope in a city that offers her the dark life of the cabaret. In this journey, the final destination is again downtown Buenos Aires, though the trip begins in Europe, not in the barrios of the Argentine capital. The figure of Griseta is reminiscent of the consumptive characters in *La Bohème*, the opera by Giacomo Puccini, and in *The Lady of the Camellias* by Alexandre Dumas Jr. It reaffirms the idea of tuberculosis as being connected with bohemia, passion, frailty, and excess: "A rare mixture of Musette and Mimí / caressed by Rodolfo and Schaunard. / She was the flower of Paris / brought by a novel-like dream to the arrabal . . . / Little Frenchie . . . / who would have said your Grisette poem would have only one stanza / the silent agony / of Margherite Gauthier . . . / Lulled by the deadly humming of a bandonion / poor girl, she fell asleep / just like Mimí, just like Manón."

Tricked, trapped by ambition, or goaded by circumstances, many European girls like Griseta arrived in Buenos Aires and wound up in cabarets. In *Madame Ivonne* (1937), "the doll of the Latin Quarter" falls in love with an Argentine man who deceives her, "between tango and *mate*," and convinces her to leave Paris. Ten years later "she's no longer a humble fleur-de-lis" but a "gray skylark . . . who drinks champagne with sad eyes." In *Galleguita* sadness becomes sickness: after her first date, "the divine girl / who arrived one April afternoon / on Argentine shores" ends up in a cabaret. The narrator takes pity on the girl who couldn't survive: "And now I see you / darling Galician girl / seated all alone, so sad and sorrowful / . . . and the grief / that is killing you / is clearly painted in your deadly pallor. Your sadness is endless . . . / you're no longer the lovely Galician girl / who arrived on an April day / with no treasures and belongings besides / your black Moorish eyes / and your gentle little body." In *Pobre francesita* (1924) tuberculosis means deception, and failure: "I arrived in Argentina dreaming of treasures / yet even the poor call me 'Hey, you' / all I have are my golden locks / and the treacherous evil announced in my cough . . . / I'm not happy anymore / I would give anything to go back to Paris." Estrangement and tuberculosis ultimately kill the leading character of the tango *La que murió en París* (1930), a "dark-eyed Argentine girl" who left her family home and traveled to the unknown and idealized Paris. The coughing begins "when she arrives," announcing a life full of nostalgia for the world left behind—"the happy barrio"—and imminent death in a country of strangers: "Paris and the snow . . . were killing the darling flower of the arrabal."

Whether leaving Buenos Aires neighborhoods or arriving in European capitals, the milonguita embarks on a journey that is always melodramatic. Moving from barrios to cabarets, from innocence to degradation, milonguitas are beautiful, coquettish, sensual, selfish, self-confident, and, most of all, determined to leave behind the barrio's humbleness and the narrow confines, both social and geographical, of the barrio. Tango lyrics and the masculine perspective behind them spell out the risks, even the mistake, of daring to consider a life beyond the barrio, the dangers of succumbing to the downtown city lights, because suffering, sorrow, anguish, loneliness, and tuberculosis must follow the inevitable loss of youth. In the end, the milonguita is abandoned by the rich, unscrupulous man who took advantage of her when she was young.

Included in the portrait of the milonguita and her deceitful seducer is the narrator, a man who knows the downtown world from within and is a regular at the barrio cafés. He is usually a victim who can't do anything to prevent the sinister alliance between the wealthy Don Juan or pimp and the milonguita with her ambition and beauty. In the narrator's eyes, this alliance corrupts the very essence of romantic love. In this context of abandoned men, tango lyrics settled into their most familiar strains: those of misogyny resulting from the ever-present threat of the cabaret women.

There are, however, other visions as well. Some reveal the ambiguous and varied forms of masculinity in tango lyrics.[48] In a tone not unlike Carriego's, in De tardecita the barrio and its people are loyal to those who have left: "And even if you come back defeated / you'll know the old gang / still has faith in you." In Mano a mano, the abandoned barrio boyfriend tells the milonguita that "when there is no more hope in your heart / . . . please remember this friend who will risk his neck / to help you in any way at all, whenever you need him." The tone is not mere pity. This is a weathered man who is willing to take the milonguita back because he has set his hopes on another sort of love, motherly love, an unconditional and boundless love beyond the temptations of materialism and money. It would seem that mother's love is the polar opposite of the oscillation between love and lovelessness that characterizes the milonguita's life. If in many tangos tuberculosis is a punishment for the milonguita's wrongdoings, disease is absolutely absent in the mother figures, who are faithful and wholly devoid of eroticism and sexuality. Unlike milonguitas, mothers never fall into temptation or shirk their domestic duties; mothers don't get involved in fleeting romances or have sex; they are brimming with a vital strength that protects them from tuberculosis. Thus, the image of tuberculosis in tango lyrics, as well as in certain works of literature and film from the first decades of the twentieth century, is grounded on a moral economy in which men and mothers don't get sick, while young women who dare to leave the barrio do.

The milonguita is convinced she can conquer the future by means quite different from those of the young barrio woman, whose happiness is based on the pillars of home, maternity, and marriage. The milonguita's life choices and her relationships are diametrically opposite to those of women in other narratives, such as the reading material in elementary school textbooks, sentimental novels, and home economics manuals.[49] The milonguita's life also contradicts the doctoral theses, essays, and articles written by doctors—a few of them women—that connect women's health to the forging of the national race, the consolidation of domesticity, and reproductive obligations. Moreover, these visions deem the domestic scene the only place capable of materializing this eugenics agenda. Outside the home, women's fragility, inborn weaknesses, and dubious physiological balance—along with their nondomestic physical and spiritual demands—make them, from puberty to menopause, easy targets for disease.[50] By showing their concerns with the milonguita's daring attitude and predicting the tragic end of the journey downtown, tango writers, mostly men, added another voice to a group populated by journalists, educators, and doctors who defended the home as the natural place for women to live their lives.

However, the milonguita's life choice was part of its time and did not always have an unhappy ending. Her journey makes plenty of sense in early twentieth-century Buenos Aires history, a society in which differences between social groups outside the elite were blurry and shifting. The journey downtown embodies the risks of the adventure of social mobility in a country where a partial reconfiguration of gender relationships had started to become visible. In 1926 a law reformed the Civil Code, allowing women to look for employment without their husband's consent. The reality not just of milonguitas but also of women working in workshops and factories, of upper-class women being active in philanthropy, of women employed in downtown department stores, of women doctors and typists, and of women riding the tram afforded them a new place on the public scene, a new role based on realities, not discourses. In the face of these changes, men in the world of tango—or at least the men writing most of the tango lyrics—couldn't hide their unease. It is this ethos that explains the reproachful tone and "dreadful ending" to the barrio girl's journey downtown.

Though many of them responded to these changes in gender roles, only a few works by men openly acknowledged them. *La hija del taller* by Fingerit offers a different account of the many young women's trajectories shaped by aspirations of a rapid rise in society: Anita leaves her mother's workshop, marries three times, and becomes a property owner; Juanita, a former costurerita who, after indulging in a few luxuries, catches the "cruel disease" and is admitted to the hospital; Pepa, "the girl who ran away with the boy with the Ford"; Manuela, "who became an old man's concubine"; and the ironing girl, who declares, "I'm gonna have my kicks . . . these hands will never ache from ironing again."[51] Olivari's poem *La costurerita que dio aquel mal paso*, whose title is similar to that of Carriego's reference to the seamstress who went astray, ironically suggests that had the costurerita not gone astray she would now be a tísica dealing with consumption. In the end, Olivari lists ample evidence, including a "small apartment [she has] in a distant neighborhood," an "old man who doesn't bother her much," and a "string of pearls," that "she didn't really do that bad" in her journey downtown.[52] In the newspaper *Crítica*, González Tuñón celebrated in a series of short stories how an "eighteen-year-old proletarian beauty" conquered the city, a feat that will keep her from the "resignation" of a "retired worker."[53] And Ferreyra's film *La chica de la calle Florida* portrays the universe of a young woman who not only works at a downtown store but also finds in her work and consumerism ways of gaining a certain independence from traditional patriarchal society.

From the margins of the tango world and mainstream literature, two women developed a different reading of the milonguita's search for upward mobility. In *Se va la vida* (1929), a tango written by María Luisa Carnelli under the male pseudonym Luis Mario, the narrator invites the young barrio woman to take chances if a wealthy man offers her a promising life: "Listen to me: here's a piece of advice for you / if a tycoon promises to set you up / don't hesitate, just go for it . . . / don't water the garden of unhappy dreams / because maybe / if you're lucky enough / if you make up your mind . . . / Don't think about gloom or virtue / live your life and youth!" For her part, the poet Alfonsina Storni, a controversial and subversive voice in Argentine literature of the 1920s, celebrates the newly acquired public role of working women, though she is ironic about the results. On the one hand, she makes fun of the "languid poets" who insist on the "unavoidable stumble" of the costurerita willing to leave the neighborhood and the domestic world. On the other, Storni mocks the young women courageous enough to imagine their lives beyond the marital and maternal horizon of the barrio, but only to dream of "artificial paradises" in which they picture themselves as middle- or upper-class women once again confined in the domestic world.[54]

Nonetheless, this was not the prevalent tone. The "dreadful end" and fragility of the milonguita indicate how tuberculosis—female, whether in reality or in the imagination—embodied the uneasiness and anxiety felt by men in the world of tango. Unable to ignore the growing presence of women outside the domestic realm, they depicted the journey of the young barrio woman downtown as a transgressive adventure, too independent, threatening, and unnecessary. In the 1940s, as tuberculosis mortality declined, the figure of the milonguita faded away because, among other reasons, tango lyrics tended to emphasize a melancholic tone and because the issue of social mobility during the first Peronist administration—regardless of Eva Perón's individual journey downtown—would become more collective and framed within a discourse of enhanced dignity in the home and the workplace. By the 1960s the idea of the milonguita and her life were a thing of the past. Horacio Ferrer, in his tango *La última grela* (1967), not only calls the young barrio women venturing downtown "proletarians of love" and "Madame Bovarys" from Buenos Aires barrios, but also stresses the fact that both the melodramatic trajectory and the character of the milonguita are no longer features of the Buenos Aires reality. Rather, they are topics of the history of tango, the history of gender relations in the city, and the history of tuberculosis.

CHAPTER NINE

Forging the Healthy Body

Physical Education, Soccer, Childhood, and Tuberculosis

"I am convinced that tuberculosis cannot enter a sound thorax that bespeaks a healthy athletic condition."[1] Dated 1937, this statement is part of a discourse, one that endured for seven decades, articulated by a diverse group of politicians, doctors, educators, and essayists. They deemed the strengthening of bodies a guarantee of health and disease prevention. Domingo Faustino Sarmiento was a major proponent of the discourse. In 1885, when he noticed "many lung diseases originated in the tightness of the ribcage containing the respiratory instruments," Sarmiento recommended "educating the body."[2] In 1916 an article published in *Anales de la Sociedad Militar* encouraged "physical culture" as a way of avoiding "the tuberculosis-inducing sedentary nature of modern life with its cinemas, nightclubs, and theaters." In the article, physical culture was also said to ensure health and education, form character, and provide individual and collective strength.[3] Moreover, in the early 1940s, the *Primer Congreso Nacional de Educación Física* as well as many doctors and educators found physical education to be "an anvil to forge a high-quality, strong, enterprising, and capable race" and "a decisive resource in the fight against tuberculosis."[4]

One of the recurring themes in "the body's education" of which Sarmiento spoke is breathing. In the early twentieth century any pamphlet on tuberculosis prevention addressed the advantages of what was then called respiratory exercise for those on the way to recovery, as well as for healthy people who sought to avoid the disease. It was said that "anyone who breathes poorly, especially women, is predisposed to pulmonary tuberculosis." And health magazines like *Viva Cien Años* promoted, time and again, "good, natural breathing from the diaphragm and balancing the use of the thorax and the abdomen as is done by children and savages."[5] Recommended to men, women, and children, respiratory exercise was one of many resources, practices, and discourses that privileged physical activity as a form of prevention.

During the last third of the nineteenth century many social reformers enthusiastically supported male participation in classical gymnastics and began to consider the practice of individual and group sports of English origin. But it was not until the new century that an idealized vision of physical culture had really taken hold. According to the socialist newspaper *La Vanguardia*, physical culture would "keep the organism strong, offset serious concerns by providing a cheerful note of play and pleasure," and combine "health, beauty, flexibility, dexterity, and virility."[6] In addition to these qualities, others added the virtues of "discipline, which builds character and prepares it for the struggle for life," "the stimulation of healthy ambition, solidarity, mutual respect, and self-regulation," and, finally, "cooperation, emulation, and self-control."[7]

But not all physical activities were equally encouraged. While hygienists, enlightened businessmen, and working-class and community leaders passionately recommended physical exercise, they did not embrace all sports.[8] Swimming, rowing, tennis, cycling, and track and field enjoyed a certain degree of respectability, not only in the middle and upper classes but also among unions and leftist political groups dedicated to the physical and moral uplifting of workers. There were announcements in anarchist magazines of family picnics that offered "swimming lessons on grass" for children and adults, and articles in the socialist press that celebrated the spread of track and field among the poor.[9] Boxing, on the other hand, gave rise to harsh and ongoing debates between those who deemed it basically virile and those who deemed it an act of barbarism.[10]

Despite the debates and recognition of the potential value of physical activity, sports and gymnastics had limited impact on the life of common people in Buenos Aires. Among men, though, soccer was another matter. Soccer started out as a male sport played in institutions and schools connected to the British community, but by 1907 it was being played in more than three hundred mostly neighborhood clubs.[11] The game took an even firmer hold in the following decades thanks to a vast network of neighborhood, trade union, parish, and business associations in which amateur soccer was played and to its emergence as a professional sport with paid players, large crowds, and modern stadiums. Pickup soccer games in streets, parks, and vacant lots were also increasingly common.[12]

As a result of the vertiginous growth of professional soccer, the discourse on the strengthening of bodies became bound to a criticism of the "professionalism of physical culture" and "sport as a spectacular display." Many people, among them businessmen excited by new, capitalist, American ideas about well-being, sought to channel "the enormous crowds at the stadiums toward the personal practice of exercise and sport." Others pointed out the danger of promoting sport as an end in itself: "One does not play sports to become stronger but rather one wants to become strong only to triumph in sports; when this is so, life ceases to be a road and becomes a stadium, with the ball at the center of the universe."[13] Most anarcho-syndicalist and libertarian workers' groups vehemently rejected soccer, arguing that "you cannot fight against exploitation while kicking a ball." But sectors connected with socialism and communism made an effort, especially in the 1920s, to construct an alternative sports culture, one removed from the traps of professionalism as well as from "bourgeois and boss-controlled clubs." The socialists praised "healthy workers' sports," and the communists "red, liberating sport."[14] With the arrival of the first Peronist government in the mid-1940s, the place of amateur soccer was reinforced by the strengthening of professional soccer, the recently created municipal fitness centers, and the efforts by organized labor to encourage after-work activities. Beyond the undeniable importance of preaching on physical exercise and the wide range of personal motivations that encouraged young men to practice certain sports, it was soccer—either organized soccer played by teams affiliated with amateur leagues or pickup games on Sundays in neighborhood clubs, streets, and parks—that provided most of the opportunities to do something that vaguely resembled the respiratory and antituberculosis exercise recommended by educators and doctors.

In the last third of the nineteenth century "the outdoors, physical activity, exercise, and cold water" were considered resources which, if employed from the start, in childhood, would allow "women from the working classes or the elite to improve their health and thus avoid falling into the hysteria and chlorosis that lead to tuberculosis."[15] But the idea of respiratory gymnastics for women swiftly became bound to their reproductive functions and their decisive role in the birth of a renewed Argentine race. Dated 1892, Arturo Balbastro's thesis, one of many in that era that discussed "the woman question," aimed to critically reconsider a feminine ideal that discouraged gym classes in schools for girls. Instead, he believed in physical education in primary schools in order to fortify the bodies of future mothers and thereby diminish the dangers of racial degeneration.[16] Justino Ramos Mexía's thesis, dated 1898, maintained that the social role of men and women was determined by evolution and that females ought to focus on ensuring the "quality of the race." Since "womanhood lies in nothing other than motherhood, and maternity must be the central axis of woman's feelings and health," it was necessary to develop a special curriculum for them, a parallel program aimed at enhancing their "intellectual aptitudes" that would "irradiate over cradles and domestic chores."[17] The innovative idea of women doing physical exercise reflected the determination to improve their condition as mothers, an agenda that hardly questioned traditional notions of how women should use their bodies. This was the driving force behind the discussion of the most appropriate type and intensity of physical exercise for women.

By the late nineteenth century the debate was restricted, not only because of the lack of civil rights for women and their limited access to education but also because of very specific and daily restraints like tight corsets that hindered breathing and long, heavy dresses that impeded rapid movement. In the twentieth century, fashions changed somewhat, making physical exercise possible. Nonetheless, the changes tended to reaffirm rather than challenge the established and essentialist maternal focus. In 1919 a treatise on hygiene pointed out that "exercise is more necessary for women than for men" and that the strengthening of the female body called for "fitness of the abdominal and pelvic zones in order to develop muscles to keep blood circulation active in the areas where the sexual organs are located." It also spoke of "respiratory exercise," which "fosters the development of the lungs and the mammary glands."[18] This treatise warned against "the exercises performed by certain women who adhere to an absurd feminism," exercises that would eventually turn them into "hybrid human beings, tomboys with all the defects and none of the virtues of both sexes." Gymnastics that aimed to strengthen the female body in ways that had no direct link to motherhood or reproduction was perceived as a transgression. This kind of physical exercise was practiced by many women in Mediterranean countries as well as in English-speaking Europe and the United States. There is some evidence of its presence in early female track and field clubs in Buenos Aires, at whose meets in the 1920s, according to a journalist, "many young women could abandon [their] anonymity." Further evidence is found in the circulation of Spanish translations of texts such as *Amor y gimnástica*, a very successful novel written by Edmundo de Amicis that celebrated physical exercise for women precisely because of its ability to facilitate liberating sensations that went beyond the demands of fashion and motherhood.[19]

During the 1920s and 1930s sports gained a place in some women's lives. Próspero Alemandri, an educator and active member of the club Gimnasia y Esgrima de Buenos Aires, encouraged women to practice "in moderation tennis, golf, horseback riding, cycling, skating, swimming, basketball, and dance," while avoiding "fencing, soccer, obstacle courses, and boxing," since they went "against women's nature."[20] The reasons for accepting some sports and rejecting others were vague, if not arbitrary. Some of the explanations, however, acknowledged that "outdoor life, liberal education, and the demands of contemporary society have transformed women both physically and psychically, providing them with more endurance when it comes to facing the double task of the home and the duties women impose on themselves." At a time when modern life promoted an ideal of beauty that encouraged health and vivacity as opposed to the nineteenth-century ideal of delicacy, sensitivity, and coyness, the relationship between women and physical activity underlined a "hygienic practice" targeted not only at "avoiding sickness and keeping the natural figure," but also at producing a "legion of strong mothers, not women athletes."[21] This point of view was expressed in *Viva Cien Años*, a magazine with a largely middle-class readership, at the end of the 1930s, as well as in *Revista Grafa*, a monthly publication of the early 1940s sponsored by the owners of one of the most important textile factories in the city, where more than 50 percent of the workers were women. Both publications associated physical exercise with the ideals of motherhood, skilled work, and the future of the nation.[22]

This increasingly sophisticated notion of physical exercise was also evident in *Gimnasia para la mujer*. Written in 1938 by a female gym teacher employed at a public hospital, the book celebrates the biological particularities of women.[23] It contained recognizable turn-of-the-century feminist ideas about health that questioned the supposedly natural weakness of women, pointing out that socially assigned roles generated and reinforced this weakness. These discourses implicitly encouraged broadening civil rights for women by emphasizing preventive medicine, a balanced diet, and changes in clothing and exercise.[24] *Gimnasia para la mujer*, along with some articles published in *Viva Cien Años*, admitted that gender differences had a biological basis, but they had more to do with "the structure of the tissue, impregnated by chemical substances emitted by the ovaries" than with "the particular forms of the sexual organs."[25] According to the authors of these articles, ignoring these truths led former feminists to advocate the same education for males and females. They, however, affirmed that the idea was not to "imitate men," but "to develop women's skills according to their nature." Mechanical exercises and sports were discouraged, while physical activity that involved the whole body and varied according to a woman's age and type of work—whether housewife, office employee, or factory worker—was encouraged. This female exercise combined Swedish gym and rhythmic and relaxation routines; it strongly recommended "respiratory reeducation," since "99% of women breathe badly . . . and it is not normal for a woman to choke when she climbs stairs or waltzes." These are "signs of partial breathing, and they're much more troublesome than the first signs of age." Learning how to breathe properly entailed an attempt to recover a natural "diaphragmatic breathing" that, besides "balancing the thorax and the abdominal zones," "constitutes a powerful healing and preventive resource, particularly against tuberculosis." To breathe this way, it was necessary to avoid "restraining clothes which cause thoracic respiration."[26]

It is difficult to assess the extent to which these suggestions were put into practice. This is true of the last third of the nineteenth century recommendations centered on the need to improve the Argentine race as well as those of the first decades of the twentieth century, emphasizing the importance of certain forms of exercise that were in keeping with the female nature and provided a respiratory re-education, while questioning others for creating tomboys. Regardless of the real impact such discourses had on women's daily lives, by the 1930s the relationship between sports, physical exercise, and women's health was different from what it had been at the end of the nineteenth century. Despite its limitations and disciplinary nature, the new relationship between women and physical exercise must have contributed, along with other factors, primarily antiseptic improvements, to decreasing the rate of puerperal mortality at the beginning of the century. But these novelties should not invite too exaggerated evaluations, such as the one articulated by Enrique Romero Brest, a key figure in the history of physical education in Argentina, when he indicated with enormous enthusiasm that tennis was monopolizing women's interest in sports. Nothing indicates that women's fondness for tennis was remotely like the importance of soccer in the lives of the men of Buenos Aires.[27]

The concern with respiratory exercise and physical activity was especially significant in the effort to prevent tuberculosis in children. By the mid-nineteenth century certain medical texts pointed out that gymnastic exercise in childhood fostered the development of "the muscular system, particularly the chest and the arms," "bringing forth the vital energy" needed to avoid disease.[28] Half a century later, this association became more sophisticated and began producing very specific initiatives.

Children and the Future of the Nation

In the mid-thirties an article published in *La Doble Cruz*, the magazine of the Liga Argentina contra la Tuberculosis, discussed the topic of healthy childhood in terms of a larger debate on the future health of the nation: "The most efficient way to combat tuberculosis is through initiatives geared toward children. By saving them from perilous contact, feeding them, making them strong, we are building stronger and more resilient generations. . . . It is in childhood that most cases of tuberculosis occur, and it is the body's reaction during those years that determines victory or defeat for the rest of children's lives." Fear of contagion and notions of prevention shaped the figure of the so-called pretubercular child, a child whose "delicate countenance, weakness, anemia, or depression" made him a potential victim of the disease.[29]

The image of the pretubercular child took shape in the second half of the nineteenth century in Europe and the Americas, and by the twentieth century it played a crucial role in most of the antituberculosis campaigns as well as in the growing concerns for children's mortality and health. In conjunction with a new ideal of motherhood, the preoccupation with children promoted specific daily practices designed to protect women's and children's health. A new field of expertise was emerging. In France it took the name of *puericulture*, in Spain of *maternología*, in Italy of *nipiología*, and in Cuba *hominicultura*. The Anglo-American world also embraced the movement for children's care and health, at times even framing it along with the then-called sanitary home sciences.

These new disciplines, which were sometimes informed by eugenic or hereditary ideas that stressed the importance of race and ethnic background, largely shared an agenda, regardless of their country of origin. They encouraged the use of Louis Pasteur's antiseptics in deliveries, aimed to increase the birthrate and to strengthen the national race; they also acknowledged children's role in the economy as potential human capital for the industrialization and support of the expansion of the city's sanitation infrastructure. These disciplines encouraged outdoor, open-air schools and education on hygiene; established primary health-care units; and developed modern strategies designed to facilitate the incorporation of new practices regarding personal and home hygiene. One way or another they all nourished the triumph of a modern ideal of motherhood based on the effort of raising children scientifically; that is, according to medical notions aimed at improving the quality of the offspring. They also gave a new, enhanced relevance to traditional maternal love by making children, rather than husbands, the central object of so much female attention.

In Buenos Aires worry over child mortality and health was present during the last third of the nineteenth century. In 1887 Emilio Coni advised creating small maternity wards to aid poor women. In 1892 the municipal Patronato y Asistencia de la Infancia was created. In 1899 *El libro de las madres: Pequeño tratado práctico de higiene del niño con indicaciones sobre embarazo, parto y tratamiento de los accidentes* (which translates to "The book for mothers: A small practical treatise on children's hygiene with suggestions on pregnancy, birth, and treatment of accidents") was published. This was the first edition of a work by Gregorio Aráoz Alfaro that would be reprinted in many editions until well into the 1930s.[30]

However, it was not until the early twentieth century that these subjects constituted a specific field of scientific knowledge. This meant, among other things, that in 1919 the clinical pediatrics department at the University of Buenos Aires Medical School changed its name to Clínica de Pediatría y Puericultura. The growing importance of the field is also evident in legislative projects of the 1920s and 1930s that led to the creation of scientific institutions such as the Sociedad Argentina de Nipiología and the Sociedad de Puericultura. The interest in healthy children also led to the creation of hygiene home visitors associated with neighborhood antituberculosis dispensaries and registered wet nurses. In 1908 the Sección de Protección a la Primera Infancia was formed as a division of the municipal Asistencia Pública specifically geared toward protecting children. Together, these innovations and institutions expanded the health care network available to children and mothers, a network that, by the 1920s, was grounded in state agencies borne of initiatives that were fueled by municipal reformism as well as by the work of more than fifty organizations of various types.[31]

The contents of these maternalistic concerns were mostly defined by male doctors, though women were responsible for enacting and spreading them. Health visitors and elite women involved in philanthropy propagated the new credo and practices in society at large but particularly among women of the popular sectors. They were in charge of applying them in the more or less precarious households of the underprivileged. In primary schools, teachers incorporated personal hygiene as a topic to be taught to all pupils, and *puericultura* was included in the curricula of girls' high schools. At national and international symposia focused on medicine, children, and women, the issue of motherhood and child care received increasing visibility.

Women's groups with an array of ideological tendencies came to focus on modern child rearing. They included elite women of the philanthropic and quite traditional Club de Madres; feminists and socialists who gathered in the Unión y Labor association; organizations that launched periodical awareness campaigns such as La Semana del Nene (or children's week); and the Consejo Nacional de la Mujer, which designed and organized specific courses to educate young women interested in working in the area of child care.[32] This maternalistic agenda shared a common field of concerns and concrete initiatives, although not necessarily ideologies, that legitimized and justified women's presence on the public scene and allowed them greater personal and political autonomy.

The initiatives gained ground in the 1930s and 1940s. The increasing professionalization of government agencies, along with the presence of more women in the workplace, accelerated the definition of rudimentary state policies. The first labor law to address women and children was passed at the beginning of the twentieth century; it was followed by laws and decrees that prohibited women from working before and after delivery and also established free medical care, maternity subsidies, and the right to longer breaks at work for women who were breastfeeding. In 1936 the Dirección de Maternidad e Infancia, a division of the Departamento Nacional de Higiene, was created; in 1946 the Secretaría de Salud Pública de la Nación was restructured to include a number of agencies specifically involved in school hygiene.

In addition to undertaking ventures in preventive health and maternal child care, the initiatives addressed the declining birthrate and the need to preserve the ideal of motherhood among female workers. Child mortality had decreased dramatically, particularly in the periods 1875–1904 and 1930–49. Between 1870 and 1874 perinatal mortality in Buenos Aires was about 120.6 per 1,000, and the postneonatal mortality rate was 146.2 per 1,000. Between 1945 and 1949 perinatal mortality had decreased to 17.9 per 1,000 and postneonatal mortality to 20.0 per 1,000.[33] In spite of these changes, by the 1930s and even later, people still spoke of the need to take greater care of small children for "humanitarian reasons" and to protect them as "the future moral and material capital of the nation."[34]

In this climate of ideas, legislative and awareness initiatives, consolidation of professional groups, and decreasing trends in infant mortality, the problem of childhood tuberculosis played a significant role, though its impact on children's mortality was decidedly less than that of, say, gastrointestinal diseases. Between the 1900s and the 1930s, the rate of neonatal mortality caused by tuberculosis was about 14.5 per 10,000 inhabitants, and 4 per 10,000 for those under fifteen.[35] These numbers indicate that the impact of tuberculosis on childhood and puberty was quite limited, even admitting, as Aráoz Alfaro did in the late 1920s, that many cases of bronchopneumonia and meningitis were actually tuberculosis and should be treated as such.[36]

Given the figures, the zealous efforts to control children's tuberculosis apparently reflect something other than its actual impact on child mortality and morbidity. At the beginning of the twentieth century this concern was a result of the growing use of tuberculin tests, at the time justified as a key instrument in a broader discourse on childhood as the promise of the future of the national race. The test identified children infected with the bacillus who, though not ill, could easily get the disease. By 1915 some studies of apparently healthy children reaffirmed this susceptibility, revealing that more than half of the inoculated reacted positively to the tubercle bacillus, that is, were infected but not ill, and that in fifteen- and sixteen-year-old children the proportion climbed to 75 percent.[37]

The figure of the pretubercular child formed around this population of infected-but-not-yet-ill children. Pedro Guerrero, a specialist in respiratory diseases, discussed the topic at great length in one of his books. He affirmed that the causes of the predisposition were "multiple and varied," but exceptionally vulnerable were "those born prematurely, those . . . who live in unclean, humid places, the emaciated, the chlorotic, the scrofulous, the lymphatic, the anemic, the arthritic, those with near relatives who had or have tuberculosis, asthma, gout, and other diseases which contribute, directly or not, to the degeneration of the race."

Guerrero also indicated that measles, whooping cough, frequent flus, and endless colds could be read as "signs of predisposition in children who are still healthy."[38] This vague, imprecise etiology, current between the beginning of the century and the 1930s, led some to estimate that this "weak infantile population" constituted 10 percent of all children, while others considered it 31 percent.[39] The wild discrepancy explains why, in 1918, Coni warned against confusing weak children with "the wretched." Two years later a study reported that "many weak children don't actually have tuberculosis and cannot be considered inclined to get it." Neither "paleness nor skinniness with salient shoulder blades," physical features frequently associated with childhood tuberculosis, was related to positive testing for tuberculosis. It was said that, when it came to defining a tuberculosis policy, the goal should be to protect only "the weak, already infected children," leaving the others to the protective actions of the school.[40]

The welfare initiatives on behalf of weak children were carried out by the

Sección de Protección de la Primera Infancia de la Asistencia Pública Municipal, the Sociedad de Beneficencia, the Patronato de la Infancia, the Cantinas Maternales, religious associations, immigrants' associations, and certain hospitals. But it was the city government that led the efforts in this instance, namely by sponsoring clinics for breastfeeding babies, the control and inspection of wet nurses, special dispensaries offering in- and outpatient care to children and mothers, and instruction for pregnant women on hygiene and nutrition. The statistics released by the Sección Municipal de la Primera Infancia are very eloquent. In 1929 the total number of children under state care rose above 22,000, an enormous increase from the 232 of 1908. The rate of medical visits to homes with breastfeeding babies jumped from 2,214 in 1916 to more than 27,000 in 1929. The visits to care units increased exponentially from 2,709 in 1908 to almost 213,000 in 1929, and the visits of breastfeeding mothers to special kitchens from 390,000 in 1916 to 411,000 in 1929.[41]

Three of these initiatives became vital in the fight against tuberculosis: the family placement system for babies and children; physical education in primary schools and summer camps; and schools for so-called weak children.

A Healthy Place for the Newborn

As the idea that tuberculosis was not a hereditary pathology became more widespread, efforts aimed at strengthening resistance in children supposedly inclined to contract the disease began to stress the decisive role of the environment. The goal of these efforts was to diminish the risk of contagion in a population that was not presently sick but might be in the future. It was recommended that pretubercular children, those who lived with sick people or bore the vague signs that went with this label, be taken out of their homes in order to live with supposedly healthy families. In the mid-1930s the well-known expert in respiratory diseases Alejandro Raimondi asserted the benefits of this practice: "It is a demonstrable fact that the child of an ill mother who is separated from her at the moment of birth and placed under properly hygienic conditions can grow perfectly, just like the son of a healthy mother."[42]

This practice, called the relocation of the newborn, originated in France at the beginning of the twentieth century. The idea was that the home environment in small, rural, bourgeois families could fortify the bodies of the weak children born in the city. In the neighboring rural areas of the city of Buenos Aires property was in the hands of a fairly small number of families, which made it impossible to replicate the French model. So newborns were relocated within the city. As a department of the municipal Sección de Protección de la Primera Infancia, this service worked closely with a maternity ward exclusively for pregnant women with tuberculosis, with a pediatric preventive health care unit, and with a lactarium.

In the mid-1920s, health care for babies born to women with tuberculosis began with their immediate relocation to a unit adjacent to the maternity ward. In this room the newborns received the BCG vaccine and a wet nurse breast-fed them during their stays, which continued until a substitute family was found. The relocation system entailed previous inspections of the receiving homes and did not involve households with large families or poor living conditions. No family was allowed to receive more than one child, and the staff of the breastfeeding wards or the antituberculosis dispensaries made follow-up visits for each child. After two years with a substitute family, the child was brought to a preventive health care unit, where he or she lived until the age of ten. According to Raimondi, the relocation of newborns was the reason for the decline in child tuberculosis mortality in Buenos Aires between 1925 and 1934—a decline of around 45 percent, five points more than the general child mortality figures.

Raimondi's interpretation made some sense, considering that this strategy, unlike others, did have a quantitatively significant effect on the targeted population. On one hand, between 1928 and 1935, the Asistencia Pública Preventorio (that is, the specific municipal unit dealing with pretuberculars) admitted more than one thousand children of sick mothers, none of whom got the disease. The figures are probably similar for other preventorios managed by the Liga Argentina contra la Tuberculosis and the Sociedad de Beneficencia in the outskirts of the city. On the other hand, starting in 1925, the BCG vaccine was massively given to children of mothers with tuberculosis admitted to hospitals and, starting in 1933, to those born in maternity wards that were part of the Asistencia Pública. By 1935, the total number of vaccinated children surpassed twenty-one thousand.[43]

Physical Education and Soccer in Primary School

The new sensibility about children that was in the making by the end of the nineteenth century and the beginning of the twentieth entailed a subject of reflection and concern for both the state and civil society. Two discourses recognizing the existence of a fragmented childhood emerged around this time.[44] One dealt with the child–pupil figure, that is, the child of a nuclear family and a pupil at a public school. The other focused its attention on the figure of the minor, who was associated with orphans, abandoned and working-class chil-

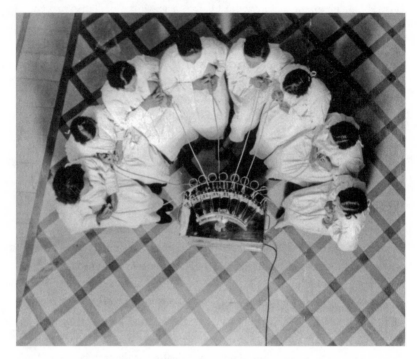

Wet nurses in charge of babies born to tubercular mothers at a municipal hospital lactarium. (Archivo General de la Nación, ca. 1930)

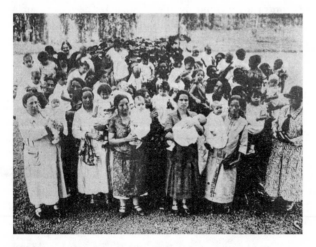

So-called pretubercular children leaving the hospital in which they were born, ready to spend their first years with supposedly healthy families. (*Archivos Argentinos de Tisiología*, 1928)

dren who needed the care of special institutions since the educational system couldn't incorporate or retain them. The two discourses were taking shape as the state consistently moved forward in its effort to school children. Other initiatives in this realm were encouraged by an array of organizations, some of them stressing ideals of self-management, mutual aid, and positivist regeneration. But they were quite modest and had little impact. By 1910 it was apparent that the state had become the most important actor in the process of childhood schooling. Although uneven and with limitations, above all when school retention levels are taken into account, the increase in the number of pupils and teachers at free public schools was remarkable.

In the 1920s and 1930s the official educational program was incorporating new ideas stressing rational, secular, and noncoercive models. These emphases associated with the new and active school movement produced an even more complex educational matrix—one already informed by Kraussian spiritualism; fragments of end-of-the-century pedagogical innovations associated with the rationalism of libertarians, liberals, socialists, and freethinkers; and moralizing, quasi-religious ideas reactive to the growing role of the state and adamant as to the reestablishment of the family as the main institution responsible for a child's education. In the 1940s this range of approaches to education set the stage for the educational initiatives of the first Peronist government, initiatives which further expanded formal schooling for children and also included extracurricular programs on a previously unthinkable scale.

Public schooling became a crucial part of children's lives. It played an active role in building a common, unified, patriotic, democratic, and republican culture, a culture both scientific and spiritualist in which Catholicism and secularism coexisted and both were subordinated to the state. Public schools conveyed a variety of knowledge, values, disciplines, and daily habits as well as a defined notion of respectability, both cultural and material, that entailed the individual discovery of being part of a nation. It emphasized the importance of hard work, moral righteousness, and personal hygiene.

School was the place to strengthen the body, preserve collective and personal health, and prevent diseases, tuberculosis among them. Concern with hygiene encouraged the creation of specific school agencies like the Cuerpo Médico Escolar in 1888 and the Visitadoras de Higiene Escolar in 1929. In schools, the issue was associated with physical exercise. Early in the twentieth century, *La Higiene Escolar*, a supplement to the official journal *Monitor de la Educación Común*, praised gym classes along with urban hygiene, fresh air at home and school, outdoor activities, and summer camps as some of the most "effective contributions to the prevention of tuberculosis."[45] Almost four decades later, the relation between physical strength, immunity, and schooling was still being commented on. *Viva Cien Años* pointed out that "in order to turn weak schoolchildren into healthy citizens . . . it is cheaper and more advisable to encourage a program of physical exercise and personal hygiene . . . than to waste money on hospitals and primary care units."[46]

For several decades, in numerous books and articles, Romero Brest spoke of the importance of physical education in the fight against tuberculosis. In 1917, as the director of the Instituto de Educación Física, he reminded an audience of primary school teachers of what he considered the value parents placed on physical education at school: "At the start of every year, I hear parents at the entrances to schools saying, 'Here's my boy, give him health and open up his chest.'"[47] A couple of years before, in an article in *El Monitor de la Educación Común*, Romero Brest had pointed out that gym classes at primary schools should consist of "a series of systematized physical exercises and outdoor games [aimed at] producing hygienic, esthetic, economic, and moral effects on the pupils. . . . Hygienic effects result from respiratory exercises [which must be practiced at the end of class] that serve to normalize the various bodily functions, leaving the subject in perfect physiological and hygienic condition."[48] In the 1930s Romero Brest emphasized the necessity of "breathing and thoracic exercises" in the physical education of children under twelve; he also discussed the appropriate intensity and duration of exercise, taking into account "age, previous training, history of lung diseases, and general condition." If done properly, Romero Brest stated, the "strengthening of the lungs offered biological energy and the joy of life [as well as a] culture of the spirit, the true aim of physical education."[49]

Yet systematized and respiratory gymnastics was just one of many influences on the modeling of children's bodies during the first four or five decades of the twentieth century. Others included military gymnastics, strongly focused on rigid formations and discipline, and sports aiming at teaching competitiveness and fair play. Military gymnastics was practiced at school and in official parades. Sports, on the other hand, began in schools run by the English community, and only some of them ended up being part of the public school curriculum. In the case of soccer, though, its spaces since the beginning of the twentieth century have been the street, abandoned city lots, squares, parks, plazas, and soccer fields at neighborhood clubs. Only occasionally, and not openly until at least the late sixties and early seventies, soccer had a recognizable, accepted place in school life.

By the late nineteenth century and early twentieth, the physical education curricula in primary schools were based on games (whether traditional, athletic, or unplanned) and gymnastics (military, natural, or systematic). Sometimes it combined music with physical movement as well as outdoor excursions and similar activities.[50] During the last two decades of the nineteenth century the prevailing form of physical education was military gymnastics. In the first decades of the twentieth century, systematized gymnastics became more important. In the forties and fifties group games were encouraged.

As the foremost advocate of physiological and systematized gymnastics, Romero Brest designed the Sistema Argentino de Educación Física. It defined the curricular contents of physical education while relentlessly questioning military gymnastics and competitive sports, notably soccer. Romero Brest's negative depiction of military gymnastics, usually practiced in situations of potential warfare or nationalist celebrations, succeeded in marginalizing it in the school curriculum by the mid-twentieth century. In regard to soccer, the success of the Argentine system was less apparent. By the end of the thirties and into the forties, educators had to acknowledge, more resignedly than enthusiastically, that playing soccer was an undeniable part of children's lives outside school, and this affected the contents of the curriculum as well as the kind of physical activity performed by students in gym class.

In the 1880s efforts were made to prove the legitimacy and value of physical education at school. There was an attempt to depict it as a resource for the ambitious project of modeling the national race and improving future generations, that is, the ethnically mixed offspring that characterized the Argentina of mass immigration. Public Education Law 1420 cited the need for daily mandatory gym classes for children between six and fourteen; these muscle-developing classes were to be based on routines, marches, and formations typical of military gymnastics. Broadly, the legislation advocated an integral approach that combined physical, moral, and intellectual aspects, individual willpower, practical education, and control of the fatigue resulting from daily instruction. However, the application of the law was in the hands of teachers who knew little about physical education. As a result, physical education was limited to the then-dominant military gymnastics, and in 1887 so-called school battalions were created. Child battalions trained by military personnel held exhibitions, performed maneuvers, and paraded in parks and squares. These activities were deemed instrumental to "strengthening the body and the spirit [and to facilitating the awakening] of nationalistic feelings." The Consejo Nacional de Educación made the activities part of the official curriculum the next year, evidencing the major role of military gymnastics in physical education at schools.[51]

By the turn of the century, the discussion of physical education became more complex. Some were trying to define its supposed scientific bases, discussing alternatives to military gymnastics, and disseminating manuals of nonmilitary exercises and games for boys and girls.[52] Such attempts at change were temporarily interrupted, first in 1892, on the occasion of the celebration of the quadricentennial of the discovery of America, and then again in 1895, when fears of a possible war with Chile reinforced the connection between school gym, military instruction, and patriotism. And so school battalions returned. Nonetheless, it was under this threat of imminent war that the first serious effort to create a rational program of physical education took shape. In reaction to the saber rattling, in 1898 a number of initiatives—including regulations, organizational plans, syllabi, and decrees, all originated by the Ministerio de Instrucción Pública—announced the arrival in the school curriculum of systematized and physiological gymnastics as an alternative to acrobatic gym, to competitive sports and track and field, and, fundamentally, to military gymnastics. The ministerial plans held that such activities were "at odds with the individual development of children as individuals, at odds with pedagogical philosophy, historical evolution, social morale, international loyalty and fraternity, social and local economy, and the findings of medical science and hygiene."[53]

At the time, short courses and pedagogical conferences were given to primary school teachers to train them to teach physical education. In 1906 a teaching school specifically designed for this purpose was created. In the following years there was widespread debate about including physical education as a mandatory part of the primary school curriculum, as well as about its role in recreational parks, summer camps, schools in the countryside, and schools for weak children. The debate focused on specific topics, though it touched on broader issues, such as the importance of physical education to modeling a national race, the correct administration of individual exertion; the forging of vigorous future citizens; and the control of vice, immorality, and crime. Yet again the discipline issue renewed the discussions between advocates of military gymnastics, which exalted a passive obedience based on hierarchies, and backers of systematized gymnastics, which emphasized discipline while aiming to develop individual responsibility, self-control, and the building of the future "citizen of the Republic."[54]

Meanwhile, Romero Brest promoted his Sistema Argentino de Educación Física in educational circles. He criticized French gymnastics for being antinatural, athletic, acrobatic, antihygienic, and aristocratic, since it could be practiced only by strong, talented children. French gymnastics was also deemed hazardous to children's health because it led to excessively labored breathing. Romero Brest condemned English gymnastics as well because it was based on games and sports, emphasized competitiveness, and had negative effects on the lungs. He did approve of its contributions to the moral and social education of children. Owing to its physiological and scientific nature, he heartily endorsed Swedish gymnastics, which paid particular attention to breathing. The Swedish system was thoroughly "democratic, as it was not interested in producing super athletes"; instead, it aimed to "perfect all people, the strong, the weak, the child, the adult." Nevertheless, Romero Brest thought it incomplete because it did not address human emotions or connect games with systematized exercises.[55]

Drawing on elements from most of these European traditions, Romero Brest pointed out in 1909 that strength and health were, in the Argentine system, the means, not the end. Its ultimate goal was, instead, a "psychomotor education" able to channel effort and willpower, build character, and teach social values. And in order to achieve those goals, the system emphasized methodical gymnastics, free and organized games, and marches and races that did not make use of fitness equipment, because the body was deemed the one and only exercise machine.[56]

Although in 1924 and 1934 there were efforts to bring back military gymnastics, by the 1920s systematized and physiological gymnastics was, at least in theory, the prevailing model in public primary schools.[57] This kind of gymnastics was largely fostered by the state, at least partly with the creation in 1929 of the Instituto de Educación Física. At the same time, the state imposed drastic budgetary restrictions, which impeded the development and growth of the institute. By the late 1930s Romero Brest himself seemed thoroughly aware of these limitations. He not only acknowledged that many schoolteachers did not take part in the physical education courses given at the Instituto de Educación Física, but also wondered what they would be teaching.[58] Romero Brest also learned about his own limitations in shaping the state agenda vis-à-vis physical education when an athlete who knew nothing about teaching or the spirit of the Argentine system was named coordinator of the recently created Dirección Nacional de Educación Física in 1938.[59] Moreover, illustrating the legislative paralysis of the interwar years, various law projects on physical education that Romero Brest and his team had designed were not even debated, let alone passed.[60]

Romero Brest's doubts that physical education teachers were actually teaching the gymnastics he fervently espoused were well grounded. On one hand, the Argentine system recommended exercise routines: daily classes for

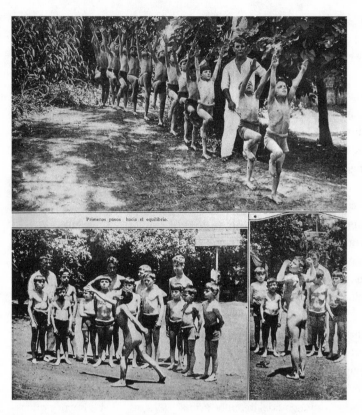

Primeros pasos hacia el equilibrio.

Respiratory gymnastics for boys in summer camps, ca. 1920.
(Colección Caras y Caretas, Archivo General de la Nación)

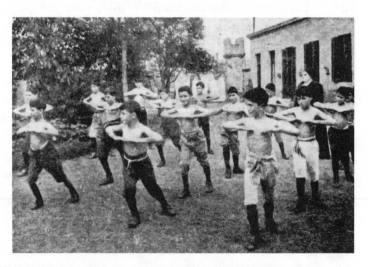

Respiratory gymnastics for boys in day schools. (Enrique Romero Brest,
*El instituto nacional superior de educación física: Antecedentes, organización
y resultados*, Buenos Aires: Cabaut, 1917)

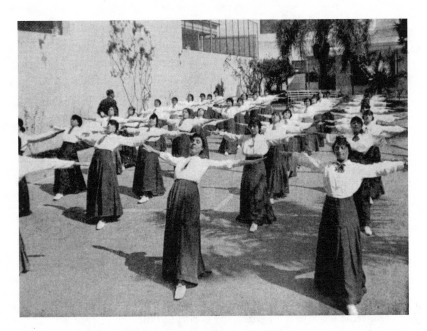

Respiratory gymnastics for young women. (Enrique Romero
Brest, *El instituto nacional superior de educación física: Antecedentes,
organización y resultados*, Buenos Aires: Cabaut, 1917)

half an hour in the lower grades of elementary school, and one-hour classes
every other day for the higher grades. In practice, this was no more than two
hours per week. On the other hand, according to the recollections of students
at primary school in the 1930s, 1940s, and 1950s, each teacher seemed to have
done what he or she was willing or able to do. Clara G., a primary school student in the 1930s, recalls that some teachers "took the class very seriously and
told us to have races or do exercise with hoola hoops." Others, however "used
the class time to rest and chat with the other teachers, checking in on us every
once in a while to make sure we were under control." José R. remembers that
most of his teachers used to say, "Boys need to burn energy," which explains
why "they pretty much let us do whatever we wanted. We could have fun as
long as we were not out of control."

The playful nature of physical education classes became a topic of increasingly heated debate in the first half of the twentieth century. Even in the late
nineteenth century it was said that "exercise is not hygienic if the child doesn't
feel happy."[61] In 1919 a doctor claimed that Swedish gymnastics was "extremely
methodical and not very attractive to Latin American children, who have a
vivacious and undisciplined nature." This doctor also suggested that "the best

respiratory gymnastics against tuberculosis" entailed "physical games that stimulate children's boisterousness, shouting, and joy."[62] By the late 1930s *Viva Cien Años* asserted that "pleasure is an indispensable component of sport," and "making school gym a mandatory subject like Latin, mathematics, and history under the pretext of improving the race only takes into account the serious side of the issue. Exercise cannot be truly hygienic unless those practicing it are happy while doing so."[63] These comments suggest a debate of which the Argentine system seemed largely unaware or at least unconcerned. The Argentine system was barely influenced by the tradition of natural gymnastics and the ideas of the Modern School movement. It was still very focused on the physiological and hygienic sides of school gymnastics, while slighting its more playful aspects. It deemed recreational activities a way of increasing discipline, not a means of having fun.[64] However, when individual memories of school gymnastics are taken into account, the picture is more nuanced: though Rosa L., who was a student in the early 1930s, remembers her gymnastics classes as being "very agreeable," Bernardo A. saw them as a sort of break from school, "not particularly boring or fun."

According to Ernesto S., a primary school student in the late 1940s, physical education class was related to the controversial role of soccer in the Argentine system of physical education. He says, "We were forced to play games that were not much fun when all we really wanted to do was play soccer. We were allowed to play soccer only very occasionally." Everything indicates that this is a faithful description of the place soccer occupied in the minds of physical education experts. Indeed, by the mid-1930s Romero Brest was already becoming aware that sports, including soccer, were "a necessary part of physical education" since they "imparted hygienic, social, aesthetic, and moral values."[65] Such recognition arrived, however, after decades of intense resistance. For instance, in 1905 soccer had been excluded from the national physical education program because it was deemed a vehicle of moral corruption, bodily violence, and dubious values that belonged on the streets, not in school. The next year, an article published in *La Higiene Escolar* suggested that the Ministerio de Instrucción Pública should call for a "competition to reward a new type of outdoor exercise which, in the form of a game, would replace soccer, a game anachronistic, noxious, and connected with the barbarism of primitive eras."[66] Even as late as 1938 Romero Brest had not tempered his reservations about the role of soccer in the physical education of children; he maintained that "without educational guidance, even the willful child who grows out of playing in squares and streets cannot become the energetic adult of the future."[67]

Children's soccer was only for boys. It was entirely irrelevant to girls, whether in school or elsewhere. For them, the Argentine system had invented *pelota al cesto* (literally, the ball in the basket), a school game similar to the Dutch *korfball* and the Anglo-American netball. Pelota al cesto is played with a soft ball that does not bounce, and hoops without backboards that sit on top of two posts, one at each end of the court, within a semicircular shooting circle. The purpose of the game is for players to pass the ball to a teammate within the opposition's shooting circle and score goals. Blocking, tackling, and holding are not permitted, and the rules prevent players from dominating the game through sheer physical strength. In the 1920s and 1930s this new game was central to the Argentine physical education curriculum. By 1950 it was played in most of South America, and in the 1960s some countries included it in their official curricula as girls sport.

In the early 1920s boys were also encouraged to play pelota al cesto. In the 1960s some primary schools for boys even had it in their curricula. But, by and large, the effort was not very successful. Boys were mainly interested in playing soccer, and there were adult voices who did not share the militant opposition to soccer displayed by Romero Brest and his group. Among politicians, Congressman Tomás le Bretón of the Unión Cívica Radical stated in 1915 that soccer facilitated "physical and moral development" and should be played in schools.[68] Ten years later the Consejo Deliberante defended soccer, asserting that it was important to have fully equipped plazas with well-defined areas "to play ball"; it also considered soccer a useful way to keep children off the streets and away from their perceived threats.[69]

Nonetheless, soccer was far from being a part of the school curriculum, least of all in primary school. Still, by the early 1940s *Viva Cien Años* spoke of "school inaction" when it came to providing children, especially boys, with entertaining games and sports. It claimed that inaction was "the cause of the mighty prevalence of soccer, a sport that was born almost spontaneously and that, in time, has acquired the volume and intensity of an avalanche."[70] This was an accurate description of the role of soccer in the streets and neighborhood plazas in Buenos Aires. At school, though, soccer was barely recognized. Bernardo A. recalls that some teachers, eager to rest for a while or to show how attuned to the students they were, "let us play small soccer matches as long as we kept it cool." And Raúl R. remembers that several times physical education class consisted of "going to the neighboring square with the teacher and playing a pickup game." Other teachers, faithful followers of the Argentine system doctrine, opposed soccer with varied and elaborate arguments, claiming it was responsible for bringing the moral code of the street into the schools or discarding it because it lacked educational value. Another reason that probably factored in was that women teachers, the majority of those in charge of primary education, could teach boys very little about soccer. And not all of them were ready to accept that fact, which altered and even undermined the traditional student-teacher relationship.

During the first Peronist government children's soccer became somewhat accepted as a potential pedagogical resource. This didn't actually happen in schools but outside of them, through an array of initiatives that included inter-school competitions, the well-known Campeonatos Evita, organized by the Fundación de Ayuda Social Eva Perón. An extension of the Peronist state, the foundation took charge of building the athletic side of "the new Argentine." To this end, it was first geared toward boys; girls were incorporated later. The foundation sought to combine playfulness and competition in an ambitious "integral education" project in which soccer and, to a lesser extent, other sports served to improve the school population "physically and morally."[71] Accordingly, hygienic and health concerns were explicitly acknowledged, and tuberculosis hovered over these issues since every player in the Campeonatos Evita had to undergo not only periodical physical examinations but also tuberculosis tests and chest x-rays.[72]

Summer Camps and Schools for Weak Children

In 1934 a study evaluating the performance of the city government in terms of tuberculosis prevention at schools was presented at the Primera Conferencia Nacional de Asistencia Social. The study indicated that 2,113 children attended six schools for so-called weak children, 15,767 children attended 8 summer camps, 1,587 attended summer camps by the sea, and some 7,000 children ate at 22 school cafeterias.[73] Some found these figures modest given that 20 percent of the 300,000 children in the school system allegedly had a weak constitution. Others, however, considered this information solid evidence of the success of an institutional network for pretubercular children based on summer camps and special schools run by the city government. The network was even vaster if similar programs fostered by the federal government and by private organizations are included.

Construction of this network began in the late nineteenth century. In an article published in 1892 in *Revista de Higiene Infantil*, Coni praised summer camps. Years later, in the summer of 1895, the Consejo Nacional de Educación organized, in the resort city of Mar del Plata, the first summer camp for six hundred boys and girls between the ages of eight and fourteen. At the beginning of the twentieth century, the state, the city government, and half a dozen private organizations set up summer camps for weak children. In 1902 the Liga Argentina contra la Tuberculosis ran a summer camp in Claypole, and the Sociedad de Damas de Caridad ran another in San Miguel, both in Buenos Aires Province and only an hour away from Buenos Aires. Starting in 1907, the Sociedad de Damas de Caridad (a very traditional women's charity society) admitted more than a hundred girls on a regular basis. The Compañía de Tranvías Anglo Argentina (which translates to "streetcar company of Anglo-Argentina") started a summer camp in Quilmes in 1916, an initiative that was quite exceptional in that few private companies joined in the efforts of the state and the welfare and charity institutions.[74] In 1925 the Sociedad de Escuelas y Patronatos issued a report stating that in its almost two decades of existence, its summer camps in Bella Vista and Santos Lugares, both near Buenos Aires, and in Río Ceballos in the foothills of Córdoba had hosted more than forty-seven thousand children. At that time the national government, through the Consejo Nacional de Educación, was running summer camps in Mar del Plata, Tandil, Carhué, Ciudadela, and Mina Clavero with a total attendance of around five thousand children.[75] In 1938 *El Monitor de la Educación Común* reported that the state-run summer camps in the mountains and on the plains had taken in more than eleven thousand children, most of them from Buenos Aires, for twenty-five-day stays.[76]

The development of schools for weak children was similar to that of summer camps. At the beginning of the twentieth century, they had been endorsed by the Cuerpo Médico Escolar as well as by distinguished experts in hygiene like Coni, Genaro Sisto, and Augusto Bunge. Years later José María Ramos Mejía, the president of the Consejo Nacional de Educación, also backed the idea. In 1912 a study based on the schools at Parque Lezama and Parque Avellaneda stated that, as time went by, the total number of children at the schools varied from seven hundred to one thousand. In 1933 the journal *La Semana Médica* estimated that more than two thousand children attended the four existing outdoor schools.[77]

During the first three decades of the twentieth century, there was both criticism and praise of this growing network for disadvantaged children. Some pointed out problems of organization and criteria in terms of the climate of the sites chosen for summer camps, for example, or the poor state of school buildings or, on the contrary, their striking monumentalism, which stood in stark contrast to the children's modest, simple homes. Others said that, comparing the total number of children attending schools and summer camps to the perceived number of weak children in need of attention, not enough had been done.[78] Undoubtedly, the vague definition of infantile weakness led to these divergent opinions, making it more difficult to assess whether the initiatives were achieving their goals. In any case, this concept was firmly established in the state's discourses on mass schooling, and summer camps received funds from the city government and logistical and financial support from the Consejo Nacional de Educación. They were also widely accepted by the people.

The stays at summer camps were shorter than those at schools, which could last from September to May. Whatever the length of stay, both focused on strengthening the body, supervising nutrition, providing access to fresh air and sun, and developing discipline, personal hygiene, and correct behavior.[79] Formal instruction was not a priority because it was assumed that the intellectual development of children would be possible only once they were in better physiological shape. The emphasis was on practical education, especially for very young children, as well as an effort to develop individual recovery strategies, which were, most likely, seldom carried out.[80]

The topic of outdoor restorative education appeared regularly in *El Monitor de la Educación Común*. Articles by foreign specialists were reproduced as well as original texts written by Argentine doctors and educators. These texts were the local version of a movement championed in Europe starting in the 1880s and supported in North America and Latin America as well. The movement was, undoubtedly, influenced by the antituberculosis campaigns that underlined rest, nutrition, and fresh air. Unlike the antituberculosis medical units and hospitals, which were targeted at adults and whose restorative and disciplinary intentions did not significantly change over time, the schools and summer camps ended up being an educational, recreational project. From the beginning, these projects set out not only to broaden the ribcages and increase the weight of children, but also to study how this was done. These studies were never statistically very convincing, but, according to many hygienists, they offered convincing evidence of the benefits of summer camps when it came to strengthening weak, pretubercular children.[81] As early as 1904 the physiological restoration of children was a priority of Sisto, one of its most enthusiastic advocates. He declared that "hygiene was more important than pedagogy" at summer camps.[82] His words, however, didn't serve to alter a tendency that was well established by the 1920s. In practice, the emphasis on remedying children's weaknesses was becoming only a part of a broader educational agenda in which prevention and hygiene were equally important, as in almost every educational project, whether aimed at weak children or not.[83]

All the descriptions of a typical day at summer camp, whether day camp or overnight camp, evidence a clear effort to organize routines that combined good nutrition, rest, recreation, gym, the development of new intellectual and manual skills, and personal hygiene. In the summer camps on the coast, heliotherapy and the benefits of fresh air were stressed. The summer camps on the plains offered a varied list of educational and recreational activities, including animal farming, agriculture, and building of sheds as well as theater, reading groups, drawing, arts and crafts, and "occasional classes in geography, history, morality, and geometry." Some activities were exclusively for boys or for girls, though both sexes were encouraged to do anything that entailed "airing and strengthening the lungs," from songs and rounds to "methodical, regular, and orderly exercises," which might cause "slight fatigue but strengthen the organism." There were also sports and group games, not only those recommended by the Argentine system—such as pelota al cesto, tug of war, and swings and slides—but also soccer, though some deemed it violent and unhealthy for pretubercular children.[84]

Both schools and summer camps constituted an early effort at social engineering. They combined the agendas of established professional groups, such as doctors and educators from various traditions, and new professional groups, such as physical education teachers and social workers, wealthy women active in philanthropy, socially concerned Catholics, socialists, liberals, libertarians, Masons, and freethinkers. All of them were concerned with the consequences of urban life, and children were thought to be at spiritual and physical risk; more generally, they were concerned about the future of the Argentine population. As was true of many other social engineering initiatives, their meanings were many. For example, as a reaction against the figure of the weak, pretubercular child, the summer camp might be seen, from a Catholic perspective, as an institution for spiritual recovery that facilitated physical strengthening. On the other hand, its secular rendering entailed an institution that improved physiological resistance by developing values associated with individual freedom and responsibility. In the context of the independence centennial celebrations, nationalistic rhetoric praised the summer camp as a "laboratory to build the civic spirit, to make children familiar with their native landscape," and to model the "patriotic soul" and create a "national type."[85] Striking a hygienist and social welfare chord, Coni later considered the summer camp the optimal place to forge the "strong child with a vigorous mind [who would be] the man [and Argentine] of the future." No matter where the emphasis was placed, the tone was decidedly positive, one that was confident the needed changes would ensue if the right improvement measures were appropriately applied.[86]

The summer camp project was part of the city government's early twentieth-century reformism and consequently was bound up in a broader problem of the rights of urban residents as consumers. In their way, the summer camps expressed a political vision of childhood, one in which the city government was an active investor in the society of the future, as well as a facilitator of strengthened fraternal bonds and mutual support. Municipal reports of 1926 attest to this project, stressing that summer camps "bring children closer to the sun and air" while at the same time "giving them the chance to live a life in common that entices intellectual development and feelings of solidarity which are so important to the future."[87] These were devices for urban planning and social reformation, parts of a network of institutions and initiatives aimed at regenerating and improving living conditions while nourishing children with an optimistic outlook on life. As their pedagogical functions were replacing their original hygienic–sanitary functions, summer camps for pretubercular children became an effort to foster the harmonious development of children. They provided an education of the body, the mind, and the feelings. They taught ethics and sociability and the more or less free exercise of the imagination as a way of learning. And all of this in close contact with nature. These concerns, along with the shift from strictly hygienic questions to questions of education and recreation, were quite apparent in other, broader initiatives aimed at the life of children outside school. As might be expected, leftist and Catholic groups fueled some of these initiatives. But others originated in the Anglo-American world and were adapted somewhat to the Argentine context; for example, the Boy Scout movement and its emphasis on learning by doing, on soft militarism, self-confidence, collaboration, good citizenship, and a confident attitude vis-à-vis the outdoors.[88] Starting in the 1920s this tendency and these experiences in after-school informal education would be reinforced by a renewed and relatively successful effort to equip the city's green spaces with "playgrounds and physical culture plazas" as the "best places for recreation."[89]

Like regular school, summer camps and schools for pretubercular children extolled the virtues of the outdoors. They should, according to the *Revista del Monitor de la Educación Común* in 1924, exercise "a great influence at home, at the workshop, and in society as a whole."[90] Generally speaking, this "great influence" was grounded in the dissemination of a battery of daily habits that entailed disciplinary, socialization, and assistance contents. More specifically, summer camps and schools for weak and pretubercular children were a manifestation of one of many so-called civilizing missions that tried to deal with the complex problem of morbidity and infant mortality. Owing, perhaps, to its association with the salience of tuberculosis as a public issue of the late nineteenth century, the figure of the weak and pretubercular child was pivotal to that mission. As such, it facilitated the articulation of concerns about childhood with those about poverty. If, as some thought, the predisposition to the disease had to do with a compromised immunity resulting from poor living conditions, the strengthening of children's bodies became an urgent need to be faced in every household, with the help of the state and civil society institutions. In this context, particularly when scant material and symbolic resources made it difficult to face the prospect or the reality of having someone with tuberculosis in the family, parents seem to have been inclined to follow the advice of visitors from the antituberculosis neighborhood dispensaries or hospitals and to send their children to summer camps or schools for weak children.

Parents were not forced to send their children to summer camps or schools, and their consent was required. The persuasive skills of medical visitors and the parents' conviction that such places were beneficial mattered when it came to making this decision. Indeed, it was apparently common for working-class (not necessarily poor) families to strive to send their children to summer camp, where, among other things, fun, organized recreation, and good food were available. In fact, this very positive perception of the camp was already in the making by the mid-1910s, when several doctors working at summer camps warned that well-to-do families were sending their children to a place for supposedly weak, pretubercular children. The remark was intended to attract the attention of municipal authorities and stress the fact that the popularity of the camps among families that were not precisely poor was taking resources away from those who really needed them.[91] In the 1930s getting a spot at a summer camp or school was not easy for either weak children or healthy ones. Clara G., who grew up in a working-class neighborhood, recalls with envy that one of her neighbors, a healthy girl like her, managed to go to camp every summer. She even managed to go to the one in Córdoba because her parents "knew whom to talk to in the city government."

By then, and even more so from the 1940s on, attending urban day camps was a eugenicist initiative that involved not just pretubercular children but also thousands of ordinary children, who were looked upon as the beneficiaries of the state's effort to "physically improve the coming generations."[92] The Sección de Lucha Antituberculosa Municipal enthusiastically notes in its annual reports the massiveness of the summer camp effort. In 1934 those of the city's Dirección de Educación Física likewise indicate that almost 750,000 children took part in the activities offered by nine day camps.[93] It is quite apparent that summer camps and schools did not stigmatize those who attended them; they were not regarded with suspicion or fear. Promising greater strength and

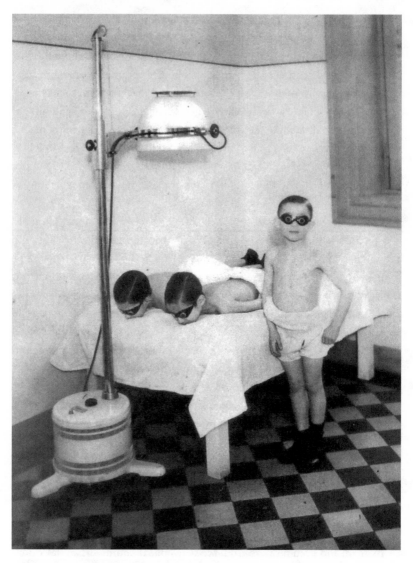

Pretubercular boys getting x-ray examinations in summer camp.
(*Archivos Argentinos de Tisiología*, January–May 1940)

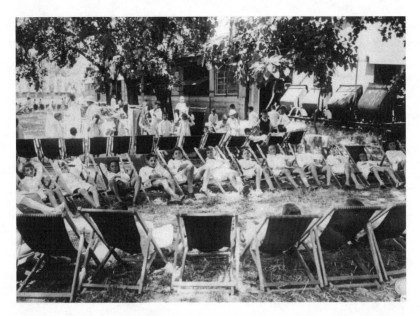

Rest time at a day camp, ca. 1930. Participants were no longer perceived as weak, pre-tubercular children but as children who deserved to experience an organized outdoor urban vacation. (Parque Avellaneda, Archivo General de la Nación)

leisure activities, these organizations were mainly concerned with children's welfare and socialization. In terms of welfare, they offered access to a better diet than the one available at home as well as frequent medical examinations. Socially, both summer camps and schools in the countryside offered a practical education unavailable at regular day school: students learned to brush their teeth before going to bed, to eat in a group, to change clothes in front of others, and to sleep in a dorm, away from home. Operating on very strict schedules, daily life at summer camps conveyed routine and discipline, which implied the growing importance of agents outside the family—above all, the state—in modeling children and their habits. In these routines, learning from one's own body was steeped in morality. These efforts, aimed directly at children and with no intermediaries, likely ended up creating household tensions and unknown disruptions in the relationship between children and parents, who were at times protective and careful, at times negligent and abusive.

In a way, summer camps and schools for weak children were one of the finest resources in the fight against tuberculosis. No other program or institution combined prevention and recreation so effectively. Summer camps became more important as the twentieth century progressed, although they never turned into a real alternative for the masses. For this reason, even if camps could be proven to be an effective way of increasing children's immunity, their impact was perforce limited. On the other hand, seeing summer camps and schools as a refined, elaborated strategy of power used to model children's bodies and souls seems excessive. They were, rather, part of an inevitably disciplinary, socializing, and educational project that, according to the memories of students, offered a stimulating entry into the modern world of education and organized leisure.

CHAPTER TEN

Tuberculosis and Regeneration

Imagined Cities, Green Spaces, and Hygienic Housing

Progress, crowds, order, and welfare were crucial components of an urban ideology that, starting in the last third of the nineteenth century, had a major impact on Argentine sociological thought. In the context of a future challenged by the problems inherent to the modern metropolis and, to a lesser extent, to industrial growth, the discourses on degeneration and regeneration, reform, and deep social change were defining their scope, priorities, and limitations. From the beginning, hygiene was at the core of these discourses, whether as an exercise of power; a preventive technique concerned with environmental issues in the urban world; a way to manage the modern city; or a social policy bound to the production of technologies to be used in different settings, such as family homes, neighborhoods, schools, factories, and workshops. Hygiene was the great counselor, an expert in the art of observing, correcting, improving, and reinventing the health of the social body as a whole. In its vastly ambitious agenda, hygiene persistently focused on tuberculosis as a social plague, clear evidence of degeneration, a disease born of the physical and spiritual decline of individuals and society. At the same time, hygiene was also instrumental in imagining alternative urban scenarios in which progress and science would facilitate the envisioning of reformed or radically different worlds. The connection between tuberculosis and urban change—a change strongly shaped by ideas of regeneration—made it possible not only to imagine a life in places where tuberculosis was, if existent, largely controlled, but also to underline the benefits of some kind of social order, the outdoors, fresh air, and hygienic housing.

Imagined Cities

In Argentina utopian narratives were not a prolific literary genre. Nonetheless, certain ideas and visions, found mostly in journalistic articles and academic essays, revealed a strong tendency to envisage and somehow model the future. Written in the late nineteenth century and early twentieth, four works that envisioned cities discussed hygiene and tuberculosis. In *Buenos Aires en el Año 2080* Aquiles Sioen imagined a city with a monument that celebrated the defeat of tuberculosis in a sort of hygienic urban paradise. Pierre Quiroule conceived his Ciudad de los Hijos del Sol as an urban setting surrounded by a greenbelt located in a radically different and disease-free world. Emilio Coni acknowledged the impossibility of eradicating tuberculosis, and his *Ciudad Argentina ideal o del porvenir* (which translates to "The ideal or future Argentine city") offered an institutional network of medical care and prevention in which the state played a decisive role. Finally, an article published by the newspaper *Crítica* depicted Buenos Aires in the year 2177, when vaccines had guaranteed individual biological resistance, and the Argentine capital was a place where no disease, not even tuberculosis, would be a threat or cause of fear. These four imagined cities are largely local in that their projects were directly influenced by the real Buenos Aires where the authors lived. Only Quiroule's ambitious city tended to imagine a brand new society with different roles for individuals, family, women, production, leisure, and land use.

These ideal constructions diverged from and were better than reality. They were also quite close to a state of happiness. In them, the city was no longer a source of human misery nor tuberculosis one of its more dreadful consequences. Their authors believed that the correct use of science and technology, the virtues of healthy living, and a largely egalitarian society would make it possible to materialize such envisioned urban worlds. With more or less intensity, these imagined cities were influenced by the classical myth of Hygeia, a symbol of healthy life in a pleasant environment, as well as by eighteenth-century practical *sanitarismo* (as early concerns for urban health were described in Spain and Latin America), which announced the need for an active state responsible for public health. Also, as might be expected, the cities had the imprint of late nineteenth- and early twentieth-century social hygiene shaped by biomedicine, social science, positive eugenics, prevention, regeneration, and the strengthening of individual bodies.[1]

These imagined cities made use of the idealism commonly found in utopian literature as well as of the pragmatism of a planner's agenda; radical discourses aimed at reorganizing society as a whole; and reformist projects focused on intervening by means of hygiene, urban sanitary works, and welfare. None of these utopias managed to go beyond a rudimentary, all-encompassing urbanism born of excessively simplistic and conscientious planning. They all envisioned urban societies imbued with a sort of harmony and discipline typical of humanitarian asylums, where assured well-being had defeated disease or, at least, managed to control it.

The Clean City

Buenos Aires en el Año 2080: Una historia verosímil was published in 1879. The book begins with a giant ship, one capable of traveling over twenty-five hundred miles a day, arriving at Buenos Aires harbor on one of its frequent intercontinental trips. The travelers enter the dazzling city with its 2.8 million inhabitants and "take pictures" with "pocket camera[s] that produce color photographs."

The first snapshots show a series of "wide, spacious, and well-ventilated avenues," including a 160-meter-wide avenue flanked by leafy trees and government offices: "Large carriages propelled by electricity are constantly and automatically watering, sweeping, and cleaning the dust and mud off the streets and boulevards."[2] Remarkably, cleanliness is key to this utopia, where hygiene is deemed absolutely necessary to protect the city's health and morality. Indeed, in this vision, health and morality begin in public spaces and ultimately blossom in people's bodies, especially those of the poor.

The city imagined by Sioen, a French journalist who lived in Buenos Aires, is coeval with other sanitary utopias such as *Les Cinq Cents Millions de la Begum* by Jules Verne and *Hygeia: A City of Health* by the English author Benjamin Richardson.[3] To a certain extent all of these books epitomize a decade in which the miasmatic as well as Pasteurian theories strived and competed to explain recurrent urban epidemics. Water was the most decisive purifying element. It was believed to be effective against the miasmas from which infectious diseases allegedly sprang and against the germs that, as modern bacteriologists argued, caused the diseases. In Sioen's Buenos Aires, water and green spaces guaranteed a healthy urban environment. A woody greenbelt around the city and a park overlooking the Riachuelo River served the densely populated southern areas. The park was spacious and useful for hygienic, aesthetic, and leisure ends. Sioen imagined a metropolitan park, a "green lung" with leafy trees to facilitate the "city's breathing" and provide recreation. Combining technical innovation and traditional ways of spending free time, Sioen's image of the cosmopolitan park entailed free access to "all sorts of entertainment: dancing, concerts, circuses, libraries, soaped poles to climb and slide down, exercise machines" as well as "German giants, Laponian dwarfs, aerostatic ascensions, magnetizers, and recreational physics cabinets."[4]

A "triumphant avenue" connected the park to the geographic and administrative center of the city, where a secular pantheon celebrated the men who had contributed to forging "modern civilization." The pantheon was not an attempt to reaffirm nationhood; Argentina's founding fathers, civil war soldiers, and politicians were not mentioned. Instead, the statues celebrated "the ones who stored solar energy in order to use it for everyday needs," "the ones who applied platinum technology to mark cattle, raising the value of Argentine livestock for millions a year," and "the ones who converted 30,000 Andean Indians to Catholicism and civilization."[5] In this pantheon the sun was considered an energy source and a guarantee of health; technology was serving a pivotal sector of the Argentine economy; and persuasion was the means of civilizing and evangelizing Native Americans. The statues weren't memorials to the Argentine past, nor did they aim to forge a collective memory; they honored, rather, science and technology, social and economic progress. The pantheon also included a statue celebrating "the doctor who discovered the cure for consumption."

Sioen's imaginary city is in tune with the attempts to curb urban growth by means of "hygienic greenbelts" in a city whose boundaries were still undefined. Throughout the nineteenth century, this initiative gave rise to many projects, such as the early boulevard system that connected Entre Ríos and Callao streets in 1822; the Plan de Lagos of 1869; the "boulevard around the old town" designed by Felipe Senillosa in 1875; the boulevard created by Mayor Torcuato de Alvear in 1882 in an attempt to control the size of the city itself; the 1887 waterway proposed by two French engineers; and, finally, today's General Paz Avenue, built in 1888, which ultimately set the legal boundaries of what became the Argentine capital city.[6]

Similarly, the wide roads and avenues, like the Avenida de Mayo, built in the 1880s, were designed in an attempt to order and consolidate the urban grid. When Sioen called attention to ample, spacious streets and the "triumphant avenue flanked by trees and government offices," his imaginary city is reminiscent of the large avenues that appeared in projects aimed not at renovating but at ordering late nineteenth-century Buenos Aires. These projects, including Sioen's, were part of a tradition geared toward regulating urban space; only rarely did the projects reveal the radical and transformative influence of the Parisian urban reformer Baron Georges Eugène Haussmann.

Instead, the great avenues were devised to facilitate circulation, improve hygiene, beautify the city, define its social geography, and determine its civic and ceremonial axis.

As for parks, Sioen's utopia was ahead of the report of 1882 on a multifunctional urban park for Buenos Aires written by the city official Juan de Cominges. Sioen's "great park" was designed mostly for "the city's southern area," where yellow fever epidemics had caused major disasters a few years earlier; it served sanitary, recreational, aesthetic, educational, and contemplative ends, and it was accessible to everyone regardless of social class. The park imagined by de Cominges in his report was part of a wider project involving the design and construction of the Parque de Palermo. His report extols the same virtues Sioen cited in his book when he imagined his great park, and, similarly, its author was as emphatic as Sioen when it came to defining the park as a public space able to serve the elite as well as common people.[7] Both Sioen's and de Cominges's parks reveal the strong influences social and hygienic reformism had on them, not only much more apparent and profound than on most of their contemporary liberal thinkers and political actors of the conservative republic, but also on the projects and practices advocated by emerging professionals and municipal functionaries trying to impose some order on the city layout.

If Sioen's greenbelt and the parks and avenues intersecting it were part of the intellectual climate that marked the last third of the nineteenth century, the secular pantheon celebrating civilization entailed a critical reading of the official position on the indigenous question. Instead of validating the massive extermination of the natives in times of the so-called Campaña del Desierto, one of the statues of the pantheon pays tribute to the person who converted them to Catholicism and facilitated their assimilation into modern Argentina. Dedicated to "the one who discovered the cure for consumption," another statue in the pantheon makes it clear that the Frenchman Sioen observed the present and imagined the future as an optimistic American would. Only a few years before Koch's discovery of the bacillus and seven decades before the coming of antibiotics, Sioen dared to predict a world without tuberculosis in spite of the fact that he was living in a period marked by medical uncertainties and ineffective therapies.

Buenos Aires 2080 imagines a tranquil, benevolent city that successfully combines the advances of hygiene and scientific progress with the benefits produced by an agricultural-export economy. Social inequalities remained—after all, Sioen envisions a city, not a society—though the state has taken over certain welfare functions, among them granting free access not only to certain goods and services but also to plenty of fresh air and leisure. Sioen conceived of a city that had become a metropolis without major conflicts in the context of an improved and very humanitarian capitalism. The sun was worshiped as a source of both life and energy; water as a guarantee of cleanliness, green spaces, and hygiene; and exercise as the way individuals could strengthen their bodies. In his city, tuberculosis was finally a thing of the past.

The Anarchist City

Published in 1914, *La ciudad anarquista americana: Obra de construcción revolucionaria* is probably one of the most outstanding pieces of utopian literature ever written in Argentina and the one most influenced by the tradition of Western utopian urbanism. Quiroule, a French typographer, was an active anarchist in Argentina in the late nineteenth century and early twentieth and one of the movement's most prolific intellectuals.

La Ciudad de los Hijos del Sol was the name of his urban anarchist utopia. A rejection of modern urban life, this imagined city entailed an ideal urban space where nature and society combined in unprecedented harmony.[8] Quiroule imagined a small city of around twelve thousand inhabitants; its size made it possible to balance the demands of production, consumption, hygiene, and well-being. He rejected the "capitalist city" and proposed instead communal life on new social grounds. This world was organized as a network of communes and characterized by solidarity, noncompetitive relationships, the dissolution of family, rationalized productive processes tied to moderate consumption, collective property, equal access to goods and services, a short workday, and a lot of free time. Abundant fresh air and sunlight offset the ruling austerity, which, according to Quiroule, was widespread yet not tedious. In large part La Ciudad de los Hijos del Sol was an antimodern city: there was no room for the "torturous concern about getting someplace exactly on time" or for "those dreadful iron towers" or for the "progress that exalts the modern city and is actually just a pretext for more and more regulation and taxation."[9]

In Quiroule's city, urban space is less dense and the boundaries with the rural world blurred. Aspiring to economic self-sufficiency, the city, in Quiroule's vision, had to be small because this was the key to harmonious connections between nature, science, and technology. While its design was derived from the tradition of urban settings in the countryside, it lacked the paternalist utilitarianism and social hierarchies of that tradition. In this sense, La Ciudad de los Hijos del Sol's similarities with Buckingham's Victoria Town layout published in 1849 are as striking as the ideological differences of their authors.[10] Quiroule's city was a reaction against the metropolitan world, characterized by a "diabolic mingling of all the things that can hurt man: dirtiness, disease, corruption, degeneration, criminality, oppression, poverty, . . . a receptacle of sadness, tuberculosis, and death." He invites his readers to "run away from the big cities [in order to] breathe fresh air, to live under the glory of the sun, to give humanity new lungs and thereby regenerate the species." In La Ciudad de los Hijos del Sol "glass blowers who work until they catch consumption" and "bakers who knead the nutritious paste with their hands day after day and night after night until murderous tuberculosis turns them into corpses" were unthinkable. So were retail employees, seamstresses, and typographers who, overwhelmed by work, persistently had the highest rates of tuberculosis mortality.[11]

The few health centers in this city simply saw to "minor accidents or surgery." This paucity was due not to a shortage of infrastructure but to a population that had "enriched its blood rationally and naturally" and had "rejuvenated their organisms" thanks to the freedom and happiness of the world in which they lived. This population had learned "the art of taking care of itself and of being healthy, [and] had gotten rid of almost all former ills." In Quiroule's world, "diseases have been practically eradicated." It was a disease-free world, a tuberculosis-free world: "The city's inhabitants were healthy in body and mind because they led simple lives; they were dutiful and adamant vegetarians, they were not forced to perform exhausting and unhealthy tasks, and they had no vices." They never knew of "dreadful tuberculosis, horrific smallpox, appalling typhoid fever, [diseases] that devastated—and continue to devastate—unfortunate peoples on the old continent who were weakened by abuse and excess: lethal workdays, orgies, bad diet, hardships, alcohol, prostitution, treacherous respiratory and organic intoxication, or the poisonous impure air and toxic waste of industrial exploitation."[12]

This was also a world in which the common man was his own doctor, thanks to "the rebuilding power of natural agents [such as] the air and the sun." "Cures," Quiroule maintained, "depended on vital oxygen supplements," and so he rejected "infamous serums, vaccines, and other despicable inventions raucously celebrated by ambitious swindlers and quacks exploiting the science of Asclepius." Indeed, Quiroule questioned the very existence of the medical profession, which in his city was a secondary, part-time profession, and affirmed that "the art of healing [was no longer aimed at] indefinitely prolonging the sickly state of a patient."[13]

The anarchist city was a wonderful setting for the rational use of free time.

Each neighborhood had a swimming pool surrounded by trees where people could swim and do exercise routines, the most important activities in an agenda geared toward strengthening bodies rather than having fun. Outdoor schools prioritized a practical education that sought to balance manual and intellectual skills while teaching daily hygiene habits. These habits included individual hygiene and public manners and behaviors, for example, the inadvisability of spitting, "that habit dangerous to both the body of the person who spits and to public hygiene and health." Schools offered instruction on proper ways of sleeping, indicating that people should sleep "lying south to north, aligned with terrestrial magnetic currents." This recommendation was based on warnings about the loss of individual vital energy owing to terrestrial magnetism, a conviction that was in keeping with what some anarchists thought about masturbation as a waste of strength in men, a habit that weakened the reproductive capacities in women, and a cause for predisposition to tuberculosis in both.[14]

In La Ciudad de los Hijos del Sol home and housing were transformed in more than one way. On the one hand, the home-family unit was no longer a crucial part of social reproduction since the monogamous couple and the nuclear family were swept away by free love and communal child rearing. At the same time, houses were "elegant glass chalets" of various shapes, colors, and dimensions, apt for "individuals, couples, and families." Set in a healthy, natural environment, the houses were austere inside, mainly because there was a deliberate effort to avoid the accumulation of dust—a recurrent topic in antituberculosis campaigns as well as evidence of the impact modern bacteriology was having on matters related to home cleanliness. The glass furniture Quiroule imagined was an integral part of the house; it had no "impossible-to-clean moldings and ornaments" and was "elegant, impermeable, and hygienic."[15] Like the European avant-garde artist Paul Scheerbart, the author of *Glasarchitektur*, published the same year as *La Ciudad Anarquista Americana*, Quiroule and his liberating aesthetic embraced the moral possibilities of forms and materials and extolled their ability to transform the environment and the metropolis. Through his glass chalets Quiroule sought to maximize contact with the therapeutic, strengthening rays of the sun without sacrificing aesthetics. His city had little in common with what he called the "bourgeois city": "the distribution of the anarchist houses was more poetic and rational, . . . the chalets' architecture, a happy combination of Etruscan and Japanese styles," consisted of "small enchanted castles" with ceilings like "luminous firmaments," where "sunlight and moonlight penetrate glass walls, instead of simple windows."[16]

La Ciudad de los Hijos del Sol is the negation of the "bourgeois metropolis"; its physical space facilitates the coming of a new social order in which tuberculosis and disease no longer exist. Quiroule's socially equalitarian new world was capable of guaranteeing the full development of healthy, happy, and creative individuals; it also entailed a rational use of modern technology at the service of hygiene and health as well as an aesthetic based on a modernist exoticism that purportedly differed from naturalist illusionism. In this utopia, the combination of humans' essential goodness and the harmony of nature and science made it possible to imagine progress not connected to an ethos of productiveness but at the service of creative leisure. As for Quiroule, his utopian imagination suggests a militant intellectual active in both the aesthetic and the political avant-gardes, a quite unusual combination in modern Argentine history.

The Hygienist City

La ciudad argentina ideal o del porvenir epitomizes the reform vocation that informs most of Coni's prolific academic, technical, and professional writings.[17] The author of this imaginary city was perhaps the most distinguished and sophisticated voice of Argentine hygienic reformism in the late nineteenth century and early twentieth. Coni's main concerns were with ordering a fast-growing, changing urban world. Just like Sioen's utopia, his ideal city was influenced by Richardson's *Hygeia: A City of Health*, published in 1876. In fact, as the editor of the *Revista médico quirúrgica*, Coni was instrumental in the publication of a Spanish translation of *Hygeia* the same year it was published in English. The timing illustrates the early participation of this group of Argentine physicians in an international network of hygienists, its center in Europe but with already well-established connections in the periphery.

Written in the late 1920s, *La ciudad argentina ideal o del porvenir* treats issues that only partly coincide with those in the work of Richardson and even with Coni's hygienist agenda of the late 1870s. In *Hygeia*, social problems related to urban and industrial growth are reduced to sanitary problems; by and large, this is also the emphasis of *Progrès de l'hygiene dans la république argentine*, a detailed study Coni wrote in the early 1880s focusing on urban hygiene, sanitary infrastructure, and environment as collective and urgent problems.[18] By 1920 the city Coni attempts to reform has new problems and presents new challenges that he defined as part of a broad, ambitious, welfare-oriented agenda. In other words, if in the 1880s Coni was a tenacious advocate of the expansion of the potable water and sewage systems, in 1920 he became an unfaltering organizer of public health care institutions dedicated to prevention, moralization, and individual improvement.[19]

The city depicted in *La ciudad argentina ideal o del porvenir* is an attempt to accommodate and contain the social and urban problems that had sprung up in the framework of the agricultural-export economic expansion. Its priority was to assist and moralize the popular sectors that had grown exponentially thanks to massive transatlantic immigration. Like most social reformers of the time, Coni's social regeneration project was very concerned with housing. In his city there were no tenements, ruined boardinghouses, or shacks: public authorities and private companies built houses and neighborhoods where the "physical and moral contamination of workers' houses was something of the past, and prevention of contagious diseases was optimal." Educating the working masses created "a worker drawn to his hygienic, cheerful house, with children who will not fall into vice precociously. The race will be physically and morally improved, and collective housing will be only an embarrassing memory."[20]

The idea of hygienic, decent, modern housing defines Coni's city. *La ciudad argentina ideal o del porvenir* looks like an impeccable, extended, model working-class neighborhood. In this presentation the influences of the North American City Beautiful movement and the British Garden City movement are unmistakably apparent: the grid as a way to organize urban space, a construction style purposely egalitarian, the pursuit of beauty not for its own sake but as a social control device for creating moral and civic virtue among urbanites, and the belief that beautification could provide a harmonious social order that would increase the quality of life and help to eliminate social ills. This is an urban world inhabited by homeowners who have fully assimilated the rites of hygiene. They are mainly first- and second-generation immigrants in addition to some internal migrants, all of whom venerated home life and understood the advantages of having a vegetable garden to ease the transition from the rural world to the modern urban world.

This is not a radically utopian world. At the time, many discussed the increase in homeownership that went along with the expanding urban grid. Socialists had reservations about the process in which urban tenants were moving to new, still not fully consolidated neighborhoods with many fewer services and less infrastructure. Instead, they promoted building big collective tenant houses. Likewise, many foreigners who visited Buenos Aires early in the twentieth century considered the "outdated" urban grid backward and unsuitable; unable to make good use of the then-fashionable picturesque architecture and urban design; and inclined to use variety, irregularities, and asymmetries. But according to much public reformism, personified at that time by municipal functionaries like Domingo Selva, Francisco Cibils, and Benito Carrasco, the market was already turning workers into homeowners. This view was in keeping with the literary and journalistic work of Manuel Gálvez and Enrique González Tuñón, as well as with the hygienic reformism of which *La ciudad argentina ideal o del porvenir* is a prime example. These authors considered homeownership not only the private alternative that would eventually alleviate the crowded working-class dwellings downtown, but also a way of transforming workers into citizens in their neighborhood homes.[21] Not surprisingly, though Coni's city does not reflect the real city as a whole, it does give a sense of the emerging neighborhoods that came with urban expansion. Inhabited by immigrants and Argentines, workers and craftsmen, merchants and public employees, those neighborhoods were a sort of sea of family houses punctuated by a few large and medium-sized industries, a throng of barely mechanized workshops, and small corner stores.

But welfarism is the most peculiar topic of *La ciudad argentina ideal o del porvenir*. It is not merely a discourse aimed at guaranteeing basic living conditions in the city; it is also a tight network of prevention and therapeutic institutions, managed and coordinated by doctors, architects, and sanitary engineers, all of them urban professionals to whom the modernization process was legitimating their own areas of expertise. According to Coni, municipal authorities had to control all the initiatives related to both social philanthropy—namely, "protecting and aiding children, the sick, seniors, the mentally ill, the defenseless"—and public hygiene concerns, particularly "general prophylaxis, disinfection, food, and veterinary inspection." An information bureau was in charge of coordinating and expanding these tasks, channeling individual charity efforts into a modern, centralized state philanthropy.

Coni's city entailed an exhaustive classification of therapeutic and welfare actions according to age, gender, and type of disease. Protecting children was a prime concern; children and mothers received the diligent support of numerous state-run institutions. For pregnant women, maternity wards offered services like home deliveries, private gynecology offices, and maternity cafeterias. For single mothers, Coni suggested asylums where they could raise their children while receiving financial support. For children, there were breastfeeding wards; neighborhood maternity wards; doctors' offices dedicated to prevention; homes for orphaned, indigent, and abandoned children; and summer camps and year-round camps for weak children. For workers, there were private doctors' offices and pharmacies in factories, technical schools, and arts and crafts schools. For the impoverished, night asylums, and, for the homeless and delinquents, there were asylum-workshops featuring compulsory work regimes.

La ciudad argentina ideal o del porvenir had a central hospital connected to a network of neighborhood clinics and dispensaries to fight diseases, especially those that affected the poor sectors of society. Medical care for tuberculars was delivered through the "Asistencia Nacional a los Tuberculosos Pobres," a state institution in charge of controlling social hygiene dispensaries; anti-tuberculosis medical wards; suburban hospitals; sanatoriums in the country-side and mountains, and at the seashore; and summer camps for recovering tuberculosis patients. Summer camps for normal and weak children with tubercular parents complemented this arsenal of measures against tuberculosis. Acute cases of chronic diseases—mainly tuberculosis and leprosy, mentally deranged patients, the blind, deaf, mute, and people with speech defects—were sent to asylums or special colonies.[22]

Coni rendered the city into a sanitary unit in which prevention, surveillance, and fair compensation for individual efforts reigned. La Ciudad Argentina Ideal o del Porvenir is a modern city that managed to control not only its geographical growth but also its movement, one in which the pace of urban life was, in fact, that of the neighborhood. Coni's city explicitly aspired to building a healthy space. And he is particularly thorough when discussing housing, residence patterns, and problems related to daily life reproduction. By and large, issues of production and productivity are absent. His main concern was trying to control and regulate an urban world that had burgeoned astoundingly quickly. And in order to achieve those goals people must follow hygiene norms, adjust their eating habits, organize their impulses, and transform the population, above all its poor sectors, into a sort of clean child.

Coni's city was not free of disease. Thanks to a biological and social equilibrium ensured by welfarism, his city managed to control tuberculosis and, to a lesser extent, infectious diseases in general. La Ciudad Argentina Ideal o del Porvenir entails a realistic hygienism borne of both the recognition of a conjunctural medical impotence when it came to controlling certain diseases and the acceptance of disease as a fact of human experience. It is an attempt at social regeneration. It didn't attempt a radical transformation of society, but emphasized reform and improvement by means of prevention and state philanthropy. Coni's position lay between pragmatism and utopianism. He dealt with the problem of the urban masses by segregating degenerates and the acutely sick in order to protect and help those labeled as healthy and thus guaranteed to continue functioning. His is an urban vision mostly concerned with populations and the city, not with the reproduction of the workforce. More than anything else, Coni's city was an institutional network geared toward assuring health and well-being.[23]

Coni's humanitarian approach superseded the classical, repressive, and reclusive criteria with which disease, abnormality, indigence, and criminality had been discussed and confronted. In his city, hospitals and asylums were no longer places of banishment. By intervening in both public and private spheres, with social sensibility, paternalism, and sometimes rigor, the state was supposed to be the great social agent not only in the fight against tuberculosis, but also in the effort to keep the population from physical and moral deterioration. Social engineers—among them, first of all, hygienist doctors—were the state specialists responsible for governing and handling the conflicts and difficulties resulting from the adjustments of immigrant masses, who were frequently perceived as being unstable and even dangerous. In this sense, Coni's city seems to be in conversation with the classical figure of the "guardians of order" in Plato; or the scientific, technical elites who control everything, like those conceived in the utopias of Francis Bacon, Marie Jean Condorcet, and H. G. Wells; or especially in Theodor Hertzka's *Freiland*, in which doctors strategically positioned in many state agencies dominate the narrative.[24] *La ciudad argentina ideal o del porvenir* expressed the strength of public reformism as embodied by professionals and experts in key positions in state bureaucracies who advocate philanthropy and welfare initiatives aimed at guaranteeing progress and social harmony, transforming people's habits at home, broadening social citizenship to a point at which none will be left out, and facilitating the emergence of new social actors.

The Technological City

On October 23, 1927, the newspaper *Crítica* published an extensive article entitled "Buenos Aires en el Año 2177."[25] It is one of the most accomplished pieces of anticipatory journalism from that time. Its writing style is agile, direct, profusely illustrated, and very representative of the renovation, innovation, and expansion of print media in the 1920s. Like other newspapers and magazines, especially the newspaper *El Mundo* and somewhat later the weekly magazine *Ahora*, *Crítica* sought to provide high-impact news. *Crítica*'s agenda focused on social, scientific, and technological concerns as well as on forward-thinking stories. In denouncing poverty and social inequality, *Crítica* expressed a type of welfare philanthropy rich in sensibility and solidarity. It aimed to become the voice that not only spoke for and about the people but also channeled their needs. In fact, it quite frequently attempted to play the role of health care provider by running free clinics with doctors, replicating a practice of institutions like local parishes, mutual aid and sports associations, and even more traditional newspapers like *La Prensa*.

Crítica's scientific and technical journalism was vast, ranging from discussions about the theory of relativity to how to fix a radio or whether there was a specifically Argentine branch of medicine. It contained articles on biology and disease as well as parapsychology, fortunetellers, clairvoyants, quacks or healers (which the paper could defend or abhor with equal enthusiasm), and medical miracles, including lung grafts and x-rays. It featured fields of knowledge that were frowned upon in academic and professional milieus and unorthodox cures for pains that the medical establishment didn't know how to deal with. In its cutting-edge journalism, *Crítica* featured articles about utterly revolutionary means of transportation, robots that were part of daily life, interplanetary travel, and the possibilities of creating artificial life.

The prefiguration of the future city in "Buenos Aires en el Año 2177" combines science, technology, and social solidarity. It is a "fantastic city hundreds of stories high" where electricity had greatly simplified industrial processes and transformed social life. An "almost total technical perfection" made factories' "smoke crests" a thing of the past. "The truly amazing speed of locomotion" and "radiotelephony" facilitated the emergence of a new political system, one in which states were simply "provinces administered by a universal council." Widespread access to incredibly fast transportation had transformed the cities into "administrative centers and territorial granaries." Electricity had thoroughly changed "industrial development": workers performed their duties at a rate and intensity that were "natural and comfortable for every man; nobody was humiliated and nobody a servant." By then, "perfect communism" had rendered "accumulating wealth" pointless, bringing a real and tangible "state of human happiness." Bacteriology and medicine played a decisive role in giving rise to and preserving this happiness; both worked toward "preventing and immunizing" people rather than curing them.

Recognition of the effectiveness of immunization was part of an overall celebration of the advances realized by biomedicine since the 1870s. There were plenty of reasons for this optimistic outlook. Roughly in the fifty years before the appearance of "Buenos Aires en el Año 2177," bacilli, viruses, and parasites associated with diseases were identified; vaccines and serums were developed; x-rays were discovered; modern chemotherapy was advanced; sulpha drugs were synthesized; the first enzyme was crystallized; and Vitamin C was isolated. In addition to these breakthroughs, there were many failures and discoveries whose advantages hadn't been fully tested and accepted, which led to a great deal of skepticism. Furthermore, there were lingering memories of the horrors of the First World War, in which science and technology had played a major role. However, for many readers of the forward-looking journalism, the future was not threatening because it was considered the inevitable consequence of material, scientific, and technological progress.[26]

Crítica's anticipatory notes reinforced trust in scientific reason as well as in science's usefulness in daily life. Believing in the power of immunization was part of this vision. If vaccines against diphtheria and tetanus had been discovered, why not believe that sooner or later there would be similar solutions for other diseases, such as tuberculosis? This optimism was born at the margins of the industrial epicenters where scientific advances were taking place: though Buenos Aires was not Paris, Berlin, or New York, its peripheral condition didn't keep *Crítica* from participating in the adventure of predicting the future and thinking that the local scientific community could be actively involved in producing effective solutions to biomedical problems. In this spirit, *Crítica* dared to predict a technologically and scientifically advanced future in Buenos Aires, not in Europe or the United States. It was in that context that, in the early twentieth century and into the late 1930s, doctors, academics, and amateur scientists with dubious credentials announced discoveries of vaccines and serums against tuberculosis in Buenos Aires. Carlos Villar in 1901, Juan Andreatti in 1927, and Jesús Pueyo in 1939 were among this group. Their discoveries turned out to be far less effective than had been claimed, as was true of many serums and vaccines produced in internationally recognized scientific European centers such as those of Behring, Ferrán, and Friedmann. *Crítica* covered in detail the search for an effective antituberculosis vaccine, often boosting the hopes of its readers by promoting new serums and vaccines but failing to adequately cover their ineffectiveness.

Crítica was perhaps the most widely read publication in Spanish during the 1920s and 1930s. It provided middle- and working-class readers with information that allowed them to imagine a better future thanks to scientific and technological advances that would affect their daily lives. It also allowed them to take part in the mythic force of modern marvels. "Buenos Aires en el Año 2177" optimistically reaffirmed the role of technology, deeming it necessary to creating and maintaining a fair and happy society in which "the proletariat [would get much more than] the crumbs from the banquet." Unlike European and American dystopias, in which technology was associated with authoritarianism, cultural misery, moral insensibility, and psychological misfortune, *Crítica*'s city wants to be perceived by the newspaper's readers as a space of social justice, equalitarianism, and happiness, a world without disease. With unbridled enthusiasm *Crítica* endorsed the technological panacea. Whereas in the Ciudad de los Hijos del Sol, Quiroule would make a cult of electricity and attack vaccines and serums that, in his view, led to racial degeneration, *Crítica* imagined a world in which vaccines rendered diseases, tuberculosis among them, a thing of the past.

Green Spaces

Starting in 1870, doctors, hygienists, politicians, city planners, and educators endorsed an agenda in which parks and public squares were deemed a valuable way to deal with the problems caused by quick urbanization and early industrialization. Picking up on European and American reformist urbanism, the pragmatism of local reformers, and the ways in which people were using parks and plazas, ideas about urban green spaces entailed rethinking the modern city in terms of its "breathing" and in terms of how the public and the private could be redefined. This agenda and its vision brought together, in different ways, a concern with living conditions; neighborhood life; the unequal distribution of services in the city's northern, western, and southern areas; efforts to control urban expansion; the real estate business; the illusion of developing bucolic rural enclaves in the metropolis; and the political will of furthering the moralization and nationalization of the urban masses. In Buenos Aires and elsewhere, these issues were also articulated in light of the impact of diseases on urban life.

Three recurrent images of green urban spaces appeared throughout the late nineteenth century and into the 1940s: green spaces as a city's lungs, green spaces as civilizing agents, and recreational green spaces. These representations were part of a regeneration program in which the metaphor of the green city was instrumental vis-à-vis the enduring goal of equipping the urban grid with more open spaces that, among the many benefits they were supposed to bring about, contributed to preventive campaigns against tuberculosis contagion.

THE GREEN CITY AND ITS URBAN LUNGS

The image of parks as urban lungs and places for physical recovery had been well defined by the last third of the nineteenth century. In 1869 an article published in *Revista Médico Quirúrgica* affirmed that "city squares ought to be large warehouses where the air is purified and then spread through the arteries we call streets, bringing life or death to the people, depending on whether the air is pure or foul." Plazas were places for "laborers, craftsmen, employees, and merchants to go during their spare time to receive the benefits of sunlight, thus enlarging their lungs, which were often sick from breathing harmful air."[27] Years before, an article in the same journal complained somewhat nostalgically that "the abundant vegetation of the past seems to have been sterilized by concrete. Not long ago our atmosphere was far richer in oxygen, which explains why a consumptive person could actually be cured while living downtown, or at least survive there for years."[28]

Depictions of the city as "a patient with asphyxia, who needs sunlight and air to revitalize its lungs" as well as images of urban green spaces as "city lungs" were consistent features from the 1870s on.[29] In 1882 Vicente Quesada highlighted the hygienic virtues of parks and squares: they provided the chance to "breathe fresh air" and "do exercise to strengthen young bodies in order to avoid paleness of children locked in their houses."[30] In 1890 a Colombian traveler praised the advantages of Buenos Aires's modest squares, where "crowds of immigrants stopped to breathe some air or get a job."[31] By the turn of the century, an article in the socialist newspaper La Vanguardia entitled "The Monopoly of Air" commented ironically on the elite's desire to limit poor people's access to the Parque de Palermo. This topic was taken up again later in defending the right of "penniless girls and shoeshine boys to a bit of oxygen."[32] In 1902 Mayor Adolfo Bullrich, in charge of the executive municipal office from 1898 to 1902, opened the Parque de los Patricios; in his speech, he stated that the creation of the park was one of the city's many efforts to "avoid diseases."[33]

The metaphor of parks as lungs and the city as a human body led to outdoor spaces being seen increasingly as "appendixes to the modern houses, many of which lacked the necessary sunlight, backyards, vegetable gardens, and corrals."[34] In the 1920s the press, city council debates, and the Proyecto Orgánico de Urbanización del Municipio (1925), an urban plan for Buenos Aires, referred to the municipal riverside beach and bathing areas as "one of the few lungs this city has." The plan recommended creating a woodsy greenbelt around Buenos Aires, "which would benefit the city's atmosphere while saving a great deal of money on hospitals and expenses for people with bronchial diseases."[35] Somewhat later Ezequiel Martínez Estrada put forth a literal representation of the metaphor coined by the city planner Eduardo Schiaffino almost twenty years earlier. As if nothing at all had changed in those two decades, he wrote in La Cabeza de Goliat that "the metropolis's lungs lie outside its body . . . the city only breathes in the periphery." No doubt Martínez Estrada found in the lack of green urban spaces another argument for his decidedly pessimistic but also very committed vision of life in Buenos Aires in the 1940s.[36]

The lung image was closely associated with individual and collective physical recovery. In 1922, when municipal summer camps for weak children worked around the clock in several city parks, there was much praise for the fact that these children now had "a rural experience for at least one month." The statement indicates how the notion of green spaces was connected to the illusion that a rural experience in the city would strengthen children's organisms.[37] And not only children's bodies, given that parks were associated with the health of the entire urban population: "The rate of tuberculosis is much higher in places without many outdoor spaces. Neighborhoods without public squares where one can breathe fresh air and take a rest from the suffocating atmosphere of unhealthy households and menacing traffic will tend to have higher rates of tuberculosis morbidity."[38]

Starting in the late nineteenth century this biological discourse on green urban spaces became associated with architecture and finance. It was said that Buenos Aires lacked sufficient avenues and parks, especially in the most densely populated areas, which "had most certainly been neglected . . . , areas where there should be a municipal effort to buy lots that would be greatly needed [for green spaces] in the future." This intervention was perceived as a way to limit "endless, mass construction," as well as to avoid a state in which "each vacant lot subject to real estate speculation will be bought at exorbitant prices when the population density demands the 'lungs' that are necessary to successfully fight the most menacing diseases."[39] Turn-of-the-century hygienic reformism insisted on the need for "urban lungs." After resignedly accepting the absence of such lungs downtown, hygienists began to work on the idea of a network of peripheral parks that would surround the city with a greenbelt and limit its growth. Starting in the 1890s, mayors of the city, especially Bullrich, sought to define the boundaries of the dense city. The parks they designed and opened—Parque Saavedra and Parque Rivadavia in the 1890s, and Parque Rancagua, Parque Patricios, and Parque Chacabuco in the 1900s—aimed to limit urban expansion. Nonetheless, at that time and during the first two decades of the twentieth century, as well urban expansion totally overran the green obstacles placed in its path. Fostered by real estate speculation, the possibility of buying lots on installment, and the growth of transportation systems, expansion advanced steadily, turning the closest *vecindarios*, very precarious settlements, into well-consolidated neighborhoods inhabited by masses of working families interested in leaving the city's most centric areas.

The city's horizontal expansion was followed by vertical expansion. The downtown area was transformed by the proliferation of many high-rise buildings and some skyscrapers. In 1940 the newspaper *La Nación* bewailed "a regime of shadows that is invading entire areas of the city; small squares are becoming antihygienic places where the benefits of green urban areas are undermined by these urban curtains."[40] Outside the downtown "the overcrowding of houses" led some to consider Buenos Aires neighborhoods as "conglomerates without empty spaces, [parts of] a city with a terrible pulmonary problem."[41] Articulated in this way, the concern was nothing new. In fact, by the end of the nineteenth century, the politician and hygienist doctor Guillermo Rawson suggested an alternative to the big central park supported by Domingo Faustino Sarmiento. Grounded on ideas of hygiene and accessibility, Rawson advocated building small squares away from the coast throughout the urban grid, which he predicted would expand westward.[42] In 1908, however, Benito Carrasco assessed Buenos Aires's growth and concluded it was pointless to think of it as a concentrated city anymore. Both inventive and realistic, Carrasco accepted the expansion of the city and sought to provide it with well-managed services and equipment. Working first in city government and later as a sort of urban critic, in the 1910s and 1920s Carrasco recommended creating new parks and transforming the existing ones into open spaces that would serve as civic centers for the expanding neighborhoods. Parque Centenario, designed to be the geographic center of the already expanded city, and Parque Avellaneda, built to serve the fast and sustained expansion toward the west, were created in those years. In addition to parks' long-standing respiratory and aesthetic functions, these two projects were also conceived in terms of social welfare. They were equipped with "large beds of flowers, games for children, sandboxes, gyms, and basketball courts."[43]

By then, it was apparent that parks and neighborhood squares had failed to limit urban growth as the mayors had wanted; they did, however, serve to create and consolidate new neighborhoods. Along with the creation of parks and public squares (indeed, sometimes in conjunction with their creation), a number of private and public initiatives took shape, including summer camps, outdoors schools, swimming pools, clubs, plants nurseries, and health care dispensaries. Such initiatives were important to neighborhood life and to forging neighborhood identities. However, at the beginning of the twentieth century and well into the 1940s, city planners claimed time and again that this type of urbanization had led to very intensive occupation of urban land, high residential density, and lack of green spaces. During the early twentieth century Carrasco repeatedly pointed out the need to establish a "system of parks and squares connected through greenways" and for this system to serve the city equitably.[44] In 1927 Schiaffino indicated that the practice of joining one house to another without leaving "a single gap to breathe in," as well as the scarcity of green spaces to refresh the city air, made it urgent to create a "central network of avenues and greenways" to connect medium-sized and large parks. In fact, he was dismissing the project set out by a municipal commission working on urban aesthetics that produced the *Proyecto Orgánico de Urbanización del Municipio* in 1925 and proposed creating fifty new small squares, each no larger than one square block. Schiaffino sarcastically called this project a great way of adding more "pulverized hygienic patches" to little or no end.[45] Somewhat later, during his visit to Argentina in the early 1930s, the German city planner Werner Hegemann, in announcing what would become a major issue in the making of the Metropolitan Area of Buenos Aires, stated that the city's growth, with its attendant massive construction of housing, had undermined the potential advantages of backyards: houses were built immediately next to each other, sometimes on very antihygienic, inadequate plots, in neighborhoods without collective equipment and basic infrastructure.[46] In 1946 the city planner Carlos Della Paolera accused the city government of neglecting the problem of urban congestion and overcrowding after having passed a building regulation in 1928 that allowed for what he considered an abusive use of urban soil. Della Paolera stated that the city government had a curious and paradoxical "notion of what green space means," a notion often shared by neighborhood mutual aid associations that, on the one hand, deemed neighborhood squares and parks great weapons against "urban suffocation" and, on the other, associated and even celebrated "neighborhood progress" in terms of building efforts on almost any vacant lot.[47] In a poll about city problems published in the magazine *Ahora*, experts underscored the need to increase the number of green spaces in the city twofold, or even by three or four; to create woods around the city; and to purchase nearby country estates that were full of trees. In all cases, the experts based their opinions on the difficulty of breathing in the city.[48] In 1940, consequently, the image of green spaces as lungs was again in vogue, as it had been in the 1870s and 1880s. This time, though, the aim was not to properly equip a modern city that its ruling elites wanted to be concentrated and self-contained, but to open green spaces throughout the entire growing urban and metropolitan grid. The issue got increasingly politicized as more and more professionals active in state-run agencies as well as civil organizations were expressing their concerns.

The language of green spaces as the city's lungs accompanied the arrival of modernity in Buenos Aires, both when the city was a kind of large village and when it was becoming a metropolis. In a way, the advocates of this discourse seemed to be striving to find in Buenos Aires the same grounds that had given rise to similar discourses in Europe, when reformists there were reacting against the unwanted consequences of the industrial revolution in Manchester and the challenges of nineteenth-century Paris. However, the grounds for this comparison were dubious, both in the late nineteenth century and in the 1930s and 1940s. In a city that was still relatively small and immediately surrounded, first, by open fields and, later, by metropolitan rings of neighborhoods and vecindarios, the tenacity of this language of green spaces was mainly connected with how relatively well-accepted and very general ideas about progress and environment in modern industrial cities were received and reinterpreted in peripheral and metropolitan Buenos Aires. It did not grow out of specific, local diagnoses and assessments of or responses to how to make breathing in Buenos Aires healthier, or at least less harmful. Tuberculosis, most often discussed in relation to the environment and overcrowding, was inevitably associated with a discourse in which green spaces were meant to ensure health, and the better the lungs in the urban grid, the better the chance of avoiding tuberculosis.

FROM THE CIVILIZING GREEN TO THE GREEN OF RECREATION

The connection between parks and the notion of green spaces as lungs—or what some called the city's respiratory tract—was tied to another image that underscored the advantages of civilization. Green spaces didn't merely rebuild and strengthen bodies; they also educated spirits in daily habits and were supposed to provide experiences that city life didn't, stimulating the ability to perceive and come into contact with new volumes, textures, sounds, and sequences. Green spaces provided oxygen, enhanced cognition, refined sensibility, and gave the illusion of a pastoral milieu that could take one by surprise and invite one to feel the sensation of the infinite, especially if the park was located near the river overlooking the Pampas in the city outskirts.

In the last third of the nineteenth century some coupled this "civilizing green" with democracy. Sarmiento was enthusiastic about creating Central Park in Buenos Aires, where the new discourse of nationality was bound to an educational project for the masses and to incipient social rights. He pointed out that "a society . . . composed of many juxtaposed societies, without cohesion or binding . . . will become a nation only by means of vast, artistic, and accessible parks: in them, and only in them, there shall be no foreigners, no natives, no plebeians." In his view, natives and Europeans, who didn't visit parks much, had to be educated in the use of "the rural atmosphere and the practice of exercise to fill their lungs with air." Rawson considered green outdoor spaces and neighborhood plazas in the urban grid a right of city dwellers, regardless of social class, stating, "We're all equals in the face of light and air, and we must provide it in abundance to everyone."[49]

However, the situation was somewhat different with the Parque de Palermo, where the Buenos Aires elite assumed that the civilizing green was theirs alone; there, they relished showing off and the social rituals of seeing and being seen, as if in a bucolic, pastoral setting. "Everybody knew everyone," wrote Adolfo Bioy Casares in *Antes del 1900* in reference to the Parque de Palermo the elite wanted for itself.[50] Notwithstanding their insularity, they were soon forced to acknowledge both urban growth and the emerging social groups. Even before the turn of the century, Parque de Palermo was attracting "people who were not part of high society." This phenomenon was called an invasion by one newspaper and, somewhat later, with the uneasiness of a surprised and resigned aristocrat, Roberto Gache described how the middle classes were taking over the park.[51] In the late 1930s Parque de Palermo had turned into a park "that everybody felt to be his own," a "neutral zone" in Buenos Aires where "lavishness and poverty go together, without trouble, like members of one large family."[52]

From the beginning, the idea of the urban green as an egalitarian milieu accompanied the gradual building of neighborhood squares in the 1910s and 1920s. Urban green spaces were bound to the democratic, civilizing visions of Sarmiento and Rawson, which led some people to think of squares and plazas as valuable resources in the state's effort to Argentinize the immigrant masses. In this context it became common for neighborhood plazas to have flagpoles, busts, and statues of national heroes as well as patriotic names celebrating the national past.[53] Along with these state-run initiatives, there were efforts by workers' and ethnic associations that found in green spaces and public squares perfect settings for picnics in which dances mixed with educational conferences and political and social activism.[54] The Catholic Church also valued plazas and parks and even attempted, sometimes successfully, sometimes not, to place big crosses in them.[55] These uses of city squares and parks were followed by others that echoed nineteenth-century ideas about the outdoors as a means of "enjoying the purest pleasures through the sheer spectacle of beauty."[56] In 1929 *Vida Comunal*, a magazine concerned with the future of Buenos Aires, pointed out that "continuous contact with well-kept gardens and the frequent contemplation of majestic trees are like melodies that move the spirit, bringing serenity and enlightenment." The article made reference to the southern neighborhood of Nueva Pompeya, and it addressed two problems. On the one hand, the apparent sordidness of that neighborhood was explained by a lack of green spaces. On the other, the urgency of establishing a large-scale park project in the southern section of the city aimed at de-

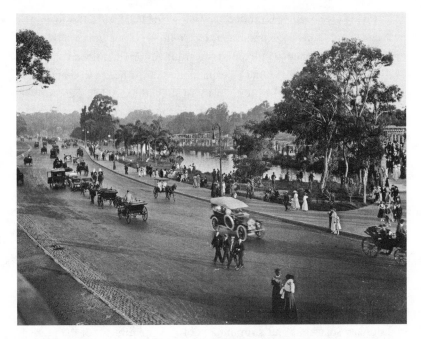

Various uses of the park by the Buenos Aires elite, ca. 1910.
(Parque Tres de Febrero, Archivo General de la Nación)

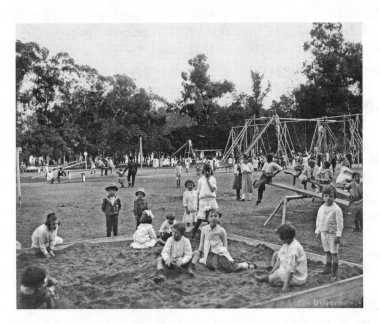

The park as open space for children's recreation, ca. 1940.
(Parque Chacabuco, Archivo General de la Nación)

mocratizing the advantages produced by Parque de Palermo in the north. The project did not materialize until the 1940s, in the face of southwestern urban expansion, with the much more modest Parque Almirante Brown.[57]

There were also more utilitarian explanations of the need for green spaces, namely, green spaces as the proper place to strengthen bodies, fight disease, practice sports, and be at leisure and rest. In the 1870s these ideas were just being formed, and a city official, for instance, thought green spaces might compensate for the negative effects of "unhealthy houses" and "the lack of space and joy." By that time Sarmiento had written, in a preview of what would be a totally naturalized feature of the park in the last third of the twentieth century, that the availability of green spaces might eventually lead medical doctors to prescribe "two or three walks around the park . . . for Buenos Aires ladies and young girls who want to lose weight."[58] Soon, doctors, hygienists, and social reformers found in parks and squares the chance to develop a recreational space ideal for exercise in order to "invigorate the physical development of youth."[59] Starting in 1890 many squares were equipped with drinking fountains, urinals, and public toilets and later with rides, playing fields, and occasionally solariums and swimming pools. As the director of the municipal department in charge of parks and plazas between 1914 and 1918, Carrasco worked to prioritize "the social functions" of green spaces in neighborhood life.[60] In the 1920s, 1930s, and 1940s all the neighborhoods wanted a plaza or a square of their own. Public squares compensated for poor living conditions that hindered incorporating the tenets of hygiene; they were instruments for rearranging local territory; and they became the setting for recreational activities of clubs, parishes, and philanthropic and ethnic associations. The shortening of the workday, and the increasing acceptance of the Saturday half-day of work and rest on Sunday, furthered the connection between parks and leisure. Not surprisingly, by the mid-1930s a city council member claimed, "Nothing can deny people access to physical exercise and recreation."[61] This new social right was swiftly embodied by the spread of sports. Ultimately, this led to squares becoming recreational spaces and sports fields. Such projects were in keeping with the discourse connecting green urban spaces to the need for children's physical education and the eugenics-influenced forging of the national race.[62] The fight against disease was also present in these discourses and agendas. A doctoral thesis of 1918 on the relationship between tuberculosis and alcoholism echoed some of these ideas, suggesting that the government should create "parks to entertain the people" and "encourage the opening of sports clubs" in order to "diminish the consumption of alcohol and tuberculosis mortality."[63]

Childhood was one of the most inspirational and powerful arguments for the recreational green and its relevance in the strengthening of individual bodies. The lack of places for leisure activities in times of expanded schooling and decreasing trends in child labor transformed the public square into an urban resource meant to facilitate the "revelation of the physical self of the child" by offering her or him close contact with "the countryside within a park."[64] These ideas were in keeping with the late nineteenth-century belief that children and children's health were the keys to shaping the nation's future. An array of discourses underscored not only the advantages of creating playgrounds and squares dedicated to exercise, sports, day summer camps, and outdoor schools, but also the transformation of what in the recent past were merely decorative squares and parks. Practically all educational agendas, no matter their ideology, from official initiatives to alternative radical projects, placed a renewed use of green spaces at the top of their list of priorities. While there might have been disagreement on the importance of enjoying learning, the notion and role of authority, the advisable physical routines, the amount of religion permissible in schools, or the role of social solidarity, everybody agreed on the importance of nature, strolls, instructive walks, and picnics in parks.[65] These agendas aimed at "replacing common, infanticidal schools that typically increased a predisposition to tuberculosis with invigorating outdoor schools . . . where in addition to teaching practical and personal hygiene, children could receive instruction outdoors, in parks and squares."[66] Informed by the American experience, starting in the 1900s doctors, city officials, architects, social workers, and educators eagerly endorsed the creation of neighborhood squares with playgrounds. The summer camps project was also linked to this effort and to the effort to provide "very poor children with weak constitutions or predisposition to tuberculosis with a scrupulous medical examination."[67] Later, in the 1920s, there were a number of projects for parks and squares with libraries and medical units for children. The plans saw these spaces as a continuation of the home: their aim was to compensate for the hardships endured by children living in "tenements and apartments lacking of space, sunlight, urban green, and hygiene."[68]

The proper use of these green spaces was regulated as they became devoted to recreation. Such regulations addressed which activities should be carried out in the parks, that is, which were the most suitable for the health and education of children. While soccer was largely discarded, exercise routines and certain group activities and games were celebrated. And although there were no explicit regulations forbidding the playing of soccer in squares, many educators discouraged it. Moreover, the people who designed the playgrounds in the city's green spaces systematically ignored soccer, and an "army of park and square guardians" was assigned to stop the pickup matches children started on the grass. By the 1920s a project presented to the City Council attempted to accelerate the transformation of decorative squares into spaces for physical exercise. It stated that "children don't go to parks in search of the space, air, and sunlight they can't find at home" because "there are no swings, trapezes, and soccer fields." According to the proposal written by the city planner and former City Council member Vicente Rotta, the aim was for "children to leave the side streets" and go instead to squares, where they could have fun and "strengthen their bodies, invigorate their team spirit, and admire our founding fathers."[69] In time, children were able to play soccer in neighborhood squares. But for quite a while the street and empty lots, urban *potreros*, were the two places where children's soccer could not be controlled by teachers, educational experts, or park guardians.

Despite widespread consensus, access to and use of green spaces weren't without conflict. By the mid-1910s the enthusiasm of an educational inspector, who celebrated how "boys and girls may now breath air and sunbathe, run, engage in rational, physical, scientific exercise, practice gym and make use of their lungs and respiratory tracts," coexisted with reports issued by the Asociación de Bibliotecas y Recreos Infantiles on the mistreatment of children in the Parque de Palermo. The report stated that "children go there to strengthen their bodies and [they're usually pulled off] the swings, and they can't even use the toilets because they're apparently reserved for the children of wealthy families."[70] According to the press, this happened only in the Parque de Palermo, not generally in the plaza neighborhoods; nevertheless, these conflicts were short-lived. If slowly, the city gradually furnished new green recreational spaces, increasing access and democratizing use. By the 1930s Parque Lezama, Parque Patricios, Parque Avellaneda, and Parque Saavedra were functioning. Municipal statistics indicated that in 1934 sixteen playing fields had been visited by more than three million children, and around seven hundred thousand children had participated in the city-organized activities in forty-four public squares.[71] The number of squares with swings and slides also increased, owing partly to the efforts of city officials and partly to requests from neighborhood associations, which, in 1929 alone, submitted forty-five requests for outdoor spaces to the City Council, sometimes offering to pay for swings and slides.[72]

In the face of shifting demands and expectations, civilizing and recreational green spaces changed over the course of seven decades. The illusory pastoral excursion that enriched the spirit without one's having to leave the city was replaced by a notion of recreation related to the use of leisure time and the strengthening of individual and collective immunity. Whereas in the late nineteenth century outdoor concerts were reserved for the ruling elite, by the 1920s a broader social sector participated in cultural and recreational events in urban green spaces. The Memoria Municipal of 1918 reported that the city government's band had given 127 concerts in ten city squares. Newspapers in the 1920s and 1930s advertised frequent movie screenings in parks as well as other forms of entertainment designed to offer a good time. Generally, the films were combined with educational shorts strongly focused on eugenic topics and seminars given by doctors on how to avoid social diseases, mainly tuberculosis, syphilis, and alcoholism. In 1942 Carrasco mentioned a state-run children's theater that functioned in the parks, "gathering kids from the poor neighborhoods" and educating them on the values of "order, discipline, and obedience."[73] All these activities and initiatives were possible in new urban green spaces with basketball courts, sandboxes, swings and slides, and, in a few cases, swimming pools and gyms.[74]

The green spaces in the modern city were also criticized for their uneven distribution in the urban grid—downtown and the older neighborhoods had the fewest green spaces—and for their sparseness. In 1935 Della Paolera showed that, in relative terms, there were more green urban spaces in 1916 than in 1932.[75] In the 1940s *Vida Comunal* stated that only 4.5 percent of the overall surface area of Buenos Aires was taken up by parks and gardens, a shocking figure when compared to London's 20 percent and the average 15 percent in American cities.[76] Rotta's book *Los espacios verdes de la ciudad de Buenos Aires* was a painstaking retrospective study and an ambitious project that sought to significantly increase the number of green spaces in the city. According to Rotta, the situation was critical: he spoke of the "sheer poverty of green spaces," the "almost absolute absence" of sports infrastructure, and the serious problems that would arise when demographic growth increased the population of the already dense areas. He also formulated an "organic plan" to correct the tendency, a plan which entailed assembling, in a "nonrational" way, small, disjointed, and exiguous green patches. Rotta claimed that there were only 3.09 square meters of green per Buenos Aires inhabitant, a figure well below the average for European and American cities; of twenty districts, two had more than 18 square meters per inhabitant, but most of the neighborhoods were well below this figure. Some lacked green spaces altogether, and others had barely 15 decimeters per inhabitant.[77]

The criticism elaborated by local experts should be read alongside others made by foreign observers, particularly those by the Swiss-French architect

Le Corbusier and articulated between 1929 and 1949. Through large architectural interventions at first, and later through ambitious urban planning, Le Corbusier planned reforms and renovations that made use of elements of the concentrated city that the urban expansion had literally swept away. Le Corbusier's plan entailed combining the projects and debates fostered by local technical and political sectors; fragments of the existent city, mostly neighborhoods with single-family homes; and the idiosyncratic tenets and urban ideology of the Modern Movement.[78] Thus, his downtown Buenos Aires would face the river; there would be areas for business, industry, leisure, and government, all of which would have gardens and parks; at the city boundaries there would be a large green ring with an array of residential towers. This was, in Le Corbusier words, a "Green City," a Buenos Aires in which "everyone will be able to breathe, see the river, walk under the trees, gaze at the waving sea of trees."[79]

The Ideal of Hygienic Housing

Between 1870 and 1940 tuberculosis was mainly discussed as a disease caused by a faulty relationship between society and the environment. Overcrowding and poor living conditions were at the core of this connection articulated by the projects, visions, regenerating imagination, and reformist discourses of professionals, academics, and politicians.

As a reaction against "poor lodgings that sicken," the ideal of the hygienic house was taking shape around changing concepts of cleanliness and the organization and improvement of domestic space. In that context fresh air and sunlight were perceived as the two most decisive resources to preventing tuberculosis contagion. Curiously enough, and despite some architectural, moral, and biomedical criticism, *conventillos* and tenements were considered for quite some time to be a kind of potentially hygienic collective housing. In 1879, for instance, a city official recommended tax exemptions for projects aiming at building "new and hygienic tenements" outside the downtown. In 1880 the municipal government proposed the construction of the Gran Casa de Inquilinato, a large, well-equipped tenement house. And in 1900 a private bank offered to finance a collective house with 270 rooms that was announced as a hygienic way to deal with the problem of housing the thousands of immigrants arriving in Buenos Aires.[80]

In spite of those initiatives, the city's growth was the result of the steady expansion of single-unit housing, not tenements or collective housing. In fact, both before and after the urban expansion no more than 20 to 25 percent of the overall population lived in tenements.[81] True, in Buenos Aires private corporations were not a major force in the expansion of the home real estate market. They did play a significant role in the construction of government buildings and large, expensive residences, as well as in the business of dividing urban land into small lots and transportation infrastructure expansion. But there is no doubt that Buenos Aires housing for middle and popular sectors was, by and large, the product of small-scale building entrepreneurs and the residents themselves. The most common habitat for popular sectors was the so-called *casa chorizo*, a house with a side courtyard, connecting rooms, and no indoor hallways. The simplest version of the house consisted of a cubicle to which could be added others with various functions, like a shed, a workshop, an extra room, a kitchen, a dining room, a room for the sick, or a room to rent. The primary way of living for the middle classes was single-family houses located outside the city downtown, structures that were built in the style of a chalet or cottage. Over the course of the twentieth century, the middle classes were also living in the first apartment buildings.

The hygienic household ideal emerged in relation to these different habitats. It was frequently linked to the notion of the hygienic neighborhood, also called the neighborhood for workers, the park neighborhood, the garden city, the peripheral neighborhood for workers and employees, the small workers' city, and the satellite city.[82] Social reformers with liberal, socialist, and social Catholic backgrounds as well as organized labor and professionals such as hygienist doctors, city planners, and educators enthusiastically endorsed the hygienic neighborhood ideal. All of them look at it as a half-urban, half-rural milieu in which the factors that had made tuberculosis into an inevitable urban calamity might disappear. Its actual impact on the city was very limited. However, at the discursive level, the ideal of the hygienic neighborhood became a recurrent topic when what was at stake was focusing on how to bring some order to urban growth and how to control the anarchic, speculative division of urban land into lots. The ideal of the hygienic neighborhood was also instrumental at the moment of imagining low-density, small, and socially homogeneous neighborhoods featuring picturesque, irregular shapes; open spaces; plenty of squares, gardens, playing fields, and solariums; and curved streets meant to break the monotonous traditional urban grid and its ninety-degree angles.

Whether part of the hygienic neighborhood or as an independent urban artifact, the idea of the hygienic house appeared occasionally and in a very cursory way in the writings of pre- and post-bacteriological revolution hygienists in the second half of the nineteenth century. An article in the *Revista Médico Quirúrgica* in 1866 spoke of the increase in the city's population, underlining that "the new homes lack the hygiene of old buildings," and the construction rush is "devastating the [urban] vegetation." According to the journal, "the atmosphere [in the city] is now poor and there is less oxygen than years before," thus increasing the recurrent threat of "tuberculosis miasmas."[83] Written in 1886, Pedro Mendez's medical school doctoral thesis, entitled "Breve Estudio sobre la Higiene de las Habitaciones," also demonstrates the growing impact of modern bacteriology on Buenos Aires. Mendez discussed, among other things, how to ensure proper ventilation, how to build appropriate windows, and how to avoid the accumulation of dust and humidity in walls, ceilings, and floors. He stressed repeatedly that "both air circulation and sunrays have a massive influence on good health."[84]

Over time the idea of the hygienic house, particularly in relation to the single-family home, became more sophisticated, if less flexible. At the beginning of the twentieth century, people would speak of houses with services (that is, kitchen, bathroom, and shower) and one or more rooms to sleep, eat, and work in, especially in the case of domiciliary work. Starting in the 1920s rooms began to have specific functions. By then, the idea of a residential, hygienic, and familial household was dominating most discourses focused on the housing of the urban population. The hygienic house was supposed to have plenty of sunlight and air, as well as a vegetable garden and a chicken coop in order to reduce food expenses and achieve some diet diversification, both instrumental for providing relief in times of hardship, unemployment, or sickness. Women's domestic chores were deemed crucial to the workings of the hygienic house, but domiciliary work, like that done by many seamstresses and laundresses, was no longer recommended.

Fresh air and the fight against dangerous dust were two crucial topics in the promise of a hygienic house in which tuberculosis was no longer a threat. Starting in the late nineteenth century, the topic of house airing was related to the advisability of having a certain "cubic space" for each habitant. Hygienists discussed it in several studies, considering the need to enforce building regulations that started as early as 1872 and continued through the 1920s and 1930s. The topic was discussed in domestic hygiene manuals as well as in specialized and popular science articles, largely in the same terms: "the need to renovate air contaminated by human breathing, combustion, and miasmas"; "altered, unhealthy air"; "the minimum amount of fresh air in the rooms according to the number of people they hold and their uses"; "good ventilation as the best antiseptic."[85] Banderoles, lace curtains, metal blinds, and double-glazed windows were some of the components extolled by a utilitarian architecture concerned with modern hygiene standards for the family house. In the 1920s and especially the 1930s there were still more studies of air renovation and movement. The "need for cubic meters"—a motto of hygienists—was gradually replaced by cries for "crossed natural ventilation," which made "stagnant air" disappear, and by a concern with room temperature control. In the framework of hygiene and prophylaxis, these shifts prioritized the search for a physical well-being increasingly connected to modern ideas of comfort.[86]

Both before and after the development of modern bacteriology, dust was a recurrent topic on the antituberculosis agenda and, indeed, a way to articulate many key domestic hygiene issues. From nineteenth-century recommendations to shorten women's skirts and keep men's faces well shaven to the celebration in the 1940s of the advantages of vacuum cleaners, the obsession with dust never waned. It influenced habits by recommending, for example, a minimal amount of furniture and decoration, straight surfaces for ease of washing, and no thick curtains or moldings. The fixation on household dust began to die down in the late forties, though that on workplace dust continued. This declining relevance was largely owing to the expanded role of laboratories in the fight against germs, the x-ray-based early detection of tuberculosis, and a greater institutionalization of protection from and struggle against contagion. In this context of an expansive and modernized public hygiene, the discourse emphasizing domestic hygiene was losing ground and ended up being relegated to a secondary role.

Throughout the first half of the twentieth century the hygienic house ideal gained specificity and new meanings. The topics of isolation and orientation, which had been highlighted by hospital architecture seeking to optimize exposure to the sun's rays for therapeutic purposes, were increasingly important to the modern building criteria regarding residential housing. In 1918 a Memoria Municipal enthusiastically presented a housing project for workers in "new park neighborhoods with chalet-style single-family homes, surrounded by gardens on three sides" and an orientation that would admit plenty of "sunlight at every hour of the day."[87] That same year La Vanguardia spoke of a "beautiful, simple small house, easy to clean, easy to straighten; . . . the sunny, hygienic house to which everyone has a right."[88] And by the early 1930s living rooms along with bedrooms were considered the epicenters of hygienic domestic life. Now, both areas were supposed to require natural light and proper, sufficient sun exposure. There was talk of special window panes that "let ultraviolet rays through, which, according to modern physiology, are very important to stimulating biological forces" and "exterior windows facing open inner doors onto corridors and halls that provide a great deal of sun during the day and a healthy, comfortable life." The hygienic house described in La Habita-

ción Popular in 1934 doesn't have "architectural pretensions" and is "devoid of superfluous adornments, moldings, pillars, and arches." Although it is "apparently austere," "anyone who really knows how to see . . . will discover a new aesthetic, the aesthetic of the house closely connected to the sun, the air, health, and life's pleasures."[89]

Years later, in an article entitled "La Casa del Futuro," the magazine *Viva Cien Años* associated the hygienic ideal of the family household with modernity. Trusting in new materials, new construction systems, and new design, the text prefigured "the house of the future," emphasizing the need for sunlight, air, and sun. The house was an alternative to the single-family home of yesteryear, a house that, regardless of its level of comfort or lavishness, was nothing but "a box with holes to get in and out that might be surrounded by some gardens." By contrast, the house of the future was supposedly in close contact with the outdoors; it had "improved bedrooms with small, independent, and outdoor lounge areas as well as a dining room directly connected to an ample garden."[90] While the magazine invited readers to "transform their houses into solar houses," architects, particularly those influenced by the Modern Movement, spoke of the need to distribute rooms according to the positions of the sun and their specific uses: rooms used during the day, like the living and dining rooms, faced the north and northwest, and bedrooms and rooms with no intensive daytime use faced the northeast and northwest.[91]

Some of the hygienic house recommendations were present to a degree in the tenements' daily life. Along with the gloomy depictions of social reformers, some of them quite extreme, other, less common images reveal that—even in tenements and conventillos—poverty, a precarious material milieu, and very modest resources didn't impede the incorporation of habits of cleanliness.

The hygienic ideal was closely associated with neighborhood households and their expectations, quite often encouraged by professional and political discourses circulating before and after the political opening of the mid-1910s. For transatlantic or domestic migrants, hygienic houses and neighborhoods were places where it was possible to reenact fragments of their previous rural lives. They were also looking for evidence of their real or imaginary participation in the adventure of social ascent. For some, single-family neighborhood houses were a ticket out of the tenement, a ticket that would eventually help them to become part of a relatively open society. For others, particularly those who arrived in Buenos Aires in periods of frantic growth—such as the years between 1904 and 1909, during which close to 250,000 immigrants arrived in Buenos Aires, many of whom ended up in new, barely occupied suburban

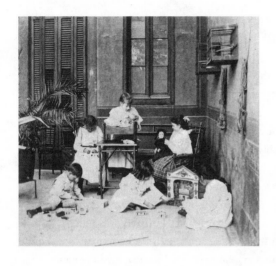

The impact of hygiene in housing for the poor: a patio in a tenement (ca. 1910), a tenement kitchen (ca. 1940), and a barrio family house (ca. 1940). (Archivo General de la Nación)

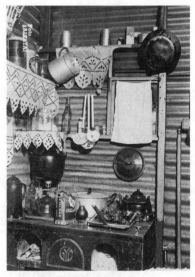

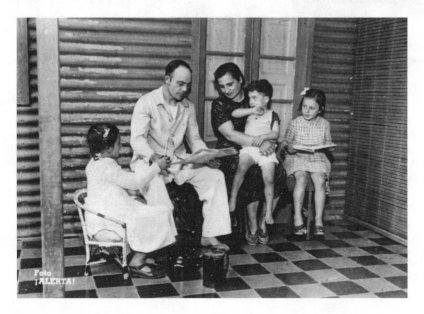

lands—stays in the tenements were short or even nonexistent. However, not everybody was equally enthusiastic about becoming homeowners and residents of single-family homes. It seems that the idea was more appealing to Italians than to Spaniards, who were less interested in leaving the city's central areas, didn't feel particularly uncomfortable being tenants, and were more inclined to gauge social ascent by other measures.

On the other hand, not all immigrants who aspired to have their own homes were able to, and many continued to rent, not in downtown tenements but in single-family houses in neighborhoods. Statistics demonstrate the phenomenon: in 1887 homeowners constituted 8 percent of Buenos Aires residents; in 1914 they were 11.7 percent; and by the mid-1940s between 17.5 percent and 24.5 percent. If these figures reveal that the city was relatively open, the less expensive tracts in the Buenos Aires metropolitan area would quite soon show its limitations: by 1947, homeowners made up 43.4 percent of the population.[92]

Whether connected to homeownership or renting, the ideal of the hygienic household was gaining ground. Regardless of ideology, practically all the groups fighting for change and social improvement embraced the idea enthusiastically. Social Catholic reformers observed the physical growth of the city, coupling it with "the inexpensive, privately owned home" and the spread of "hygiene and morality"; quite often they wanted to find in this sort of chemistry the "very key to resolving the social question."[93] Urban professionals working for the conservative republic—such as Selva and Cibils—celebrated the expansion of the urban grid, though they did discern two problems along the way. On the one hand, they pointed out that having access to sunlight and more space in the self-built and self-owned houses of the new neighborhoods entailed sacrificing access to potable water and sewage networks available in downtown tenements and to the superior hygiene standards of rental houses, two reasons that may have delayed tenants' transformation into homeowners. On the other hand, Selva and Cibils stressed that, once the market had incited the subdivision and selling of urban lands, thereby facilitating the emergence of a legion of homeowners, it was the state's responsibility and obligation to take charge of building collective infrastructure in these new outlying neighborhoods.[94] Socialist leaders encouraged the hygienic ideal yet deemed urban expansion and homeownership irrational and individualistic solutions. They promoted instead the "associated home," which was occupied by tenants, not homeowners, and in which "each house's independence [was combined with] communal life in backyards and gardens." There, shared services, including water, heating, and common playgrounds and dining rooms, would allow for great savings. They saw this type of home as an instrument for educating the immigrant masses, teaching them "hygienic, cordial, and urbane manners."[95] Anarchists celebrated the values and daily practices of home hygiene but viewed private homeownership as a "capitalist tool to control and tame workers."[96]

Somewhat later, in the mid-1930s, the Russian architect and Buenos Aires resident Wladimiro Acosta invited his readers to think of hygienic housing as a way of providing the "fresh air and sunlight crucial for health."[97] His projects attest to an intense professional experience in Buenos Aires and abroad. In Europe, Acosta had become acquainted with Ludwig Hilberseimer's architectonic rationalism and his vertical, concentrated *Grossstadt* city; with the German expressionist avant-garde seeking to restore the relationship between man and nature; with Le Corbusier's cruciform towers; and with Walter Gropius's and Martin Wagner's projects and buildings commissioned by city governments controlled by several European Social Democratic Parties. On the local scene Acosta actively participated in projects supported by the Socialist Party and carried out by the cooperative El Hogar Obrero.

Acosta's was probably the most sophisticated version of the critical urban discourse associated with the hygienic house ideal. He proposed a climate-sensitive architecture based on his "Helios system," a system intent on instilling functionality and flexibility and, mainly, facilitating house construction that optimized the reception of sunlight year-round. The Helios system is reminiscent of European rest cure mountain sanatoriums. Combining terraces, vertical hangings, covered and semicovered spaces, and filters made of various materials and placed in different positions, this sanatorium architecture strove for a regulated, systematic, controlled use of the sun according to the season, the hours of the day, and the needs of each tuberculosis patient. Acosta's Helios system is quite consistent with this agenda; with the naturism fashionable among certain groups in late 1920s and 1930s Buenos Aires; and with European architecture, which by this time suggested residential houses have rooms for sunbathing. Acosta's terrace architecture and Helios system manifested not only hygienic and aesthetic but also political concerns, in that he was convinced this kind of house represented a compensatory resource for working people living in an unhealthy atmosphere.[98]

Acosta also designed City Blocks: mammoth residential buildings situated on a rectangular base and equipped with common services, retail stores, and leisure spaces. These dwellings, too, aimed at intensifying the relationship between housing and sun. Acosta's City Blocks were cruciform at first. Later on they evolved into higher linear blocks of houses juxtaposed with lower perpendicular ones. These immense collective houses had plenty of sunlight and were a key part of a hygienic neighborhood that balanced buildings, green spaces, collective equipment, and traffic. In these neighborhoods, wrote Acosta, "nature and city ceased to be antagonistic."[99]

City Blocks were a critical response to the neighborhood house-with-a-garden, which "held a certain sentimental attraction, and" ensured "air and sunlight," and were celebrated time and again by many professional and political voices. In Acosta's view, however, the neighborhood house-with-a-garden was available only to the middle classes. The proletariat, he wrote, needs centralized services, properly available only in collective houses, in huge residential complexes.[100] Accordingly, he praised "deurbanization," hoping to bring "nature into the city, but not in the form of squares, patches of grass, gardens, trees in the streets, and flowers in baskets. [What is needed is] total, sheer nature: prairie and woods." His proposals for houses based on the Helios system and the City Blocks would be possible interventions in the real urban layout of Buenos Aires, while his "Ciudad Lineal a Escala Regional" would be a sort of urban utopian exercise. Consisting of high blocks of houses on both sides of the main road and dotted with parks, service facilities, and industries, the linear, scaled city, Acosta knew, at least in the current phase of capitalism, was a utopian project. His vision could be carried out only in a socialist system, and hence "the network of linear cities, with its light, air, and vegetation would be the end of the limited lives of beings imprisoned by the city and its monstrous overcrowding."[101]

Between 1870 and 1940 the ideal hygienic house and neighborhood varied little. Both the early twentieth-century discourses, which focused on making tenements hygienic, and the large collective buildings designed in the 1940s by avant-garde architects were facets of a project geared toward making people's lives healthier. In these discourses, the triad of fresh air, sunlight, and green spaces was crucial to the antituberculosis agenda. However, their influence on the evolution of the real city was limited and superficial. The park neighborhood, *barrios parque*, conceived by most reformists and by politicians with an array of ideological leanings, was largely irrelevant to the housing and neighborhood projects that were ultimately carried out. In Buenos Aires, only the upper classes could afford park neighborhoods, though by the late 1920s it was apparent that the initial promises of these garden enclaves in the city of the wealthy had often been distorted.[102]

As for the middle- and popular-social sectors, Buenos Aires urban history reveals that they found in the regular urban grid and the single-family home the clearest evidence of a successful integration into city life.[103] Interestingly, neighborhoods with small single-family houses and a very modest garden became a distinctive characteristic of the real city in the making. Confronting this reality, several reactive voices underlined the shortcomings of that real city, among them, its distance from the ideal of a hygienic house and neighborhood. As early as 1910 the habit of "situating a house on one of the dividing walls of the terrain, putting windows only on one side" was criticized because it limited the "available sunlight, hampered air circulation, and favored the incubation of diseases."[104] Years later, on the occasion of the "Hygienic House" competition organized in 1917 by the Comisión Nacional de Casas Baratas (which translates as "national commission on inexpensive houses"), a commentator indicated: "There are projects with plenty of cornices, columns' upper ends, and partition walls that steal air and sunlight from the rooms." Another referred to proposals that design "urban layouts following the logic of the land auctioneer selling off in monthly installments microscopic lots, disregarding the tenets of hygiene, orientation, street width, and free spaces." And a third member of the evaluating committee stated that "some proposals considered European style houses totally unfit for our climate, and others vulgar, detestable houses like those that already have infested the city neighborhoods."[105]

The situation didn't change substantially in the following decades. In the late 1920s Schiaffino criticized the habit of rich and poor alike of "erecting walls on both sides of their properties," ignoring the "incalculable advantages of hygienic living." In an urban landscape characterized by "clusters of houses that go from left to right, connected only by narrow streets where blocks finish only to begin again," Schiaffino found a decisive obstacle to both the hygienic house and park neighborhood ideal and the broader and even more ambitious goal of orienting Buenos Aires growth according to the Garden City model.[106] In 1931 Hegemann noticed that the majority of Buenos Aires neighborhoods had "conserved the most elevated of urban virtues, the private house with a garden, though this very virtue . . . has been distorted so strikingly that vicious but clean tenements are preferable to the dubious virtues of the flat house, often built in unhealthy low areas without potable water and electricity." Hegemann was also concerned with the reproduction of the same model over the emerging, much less consolidated neighborhoods of the Buenos Aires Metropolitan Area. And yet again he was not sparing in his criticism: "The chances of having a healthy house, spacious parks, woods, and appropriate roads are being irrationally destroyed."[107] In 1940 Rotta assessed the evolution of the hygienic house and neighborhood ideal and its impact on the real life of the city. He concluded that although the topic had motivated discourses and projects for more than half a century, what was actually carried out and materialized had been "marginal, timid, and exceptional."[108]

In 1955 Elda G. was strictly forbidden from consuming vinegar. Her mother was convinced that vinegar would aggravate her daughter's tuberculosis. Resignedly, Elda acceded to this prohibition, and time and again she would hear her mother asking God to move the disease from Elda's body to her own. Afraid the prayers would be heeded, Elda watched her mother closely, scrutinized how much and what she ate, whether she coughed, spit, or had fever. She observed her mother's hygiene habits, hoping she would get enough rest and go out into the fresh air of the backyard.

Elda's reactions show how—and for how long—old and new ways of dealing with tuberculosis coexisted in the mid-1950s, after the widespread use of antibiotics had transformed it, following a very slow decline over the course of the first half of the twentieth century, into a controllable disease. On the one hand, Elda's mother's belief in the harmful effects of vinegar had been around since the early nineteenth century; it was based on the image of the romantic consumptive girl who was always consuming vinegar in order to look paler. On the other, Elda's reaction shows that many tenets of the hygienic antituberculosis code—which had been spread for decades by various means, including school campaigns, the radio, newspapers, and billboards—had had an impact on society.

However, acceptance of the code was far from absolute. Much evidence suggests the limitations of the effort to model an infinite number of daily life habits. Recommendations on how, where, and when to kiss were not as observed as antituberculosis crusaders had wished. People kept spitting on the ground, despite the street signs forbidding it. Sharing straws while sipping mate remained an everyday practice. For awhile many parents ignored the calls to give their children the BCG vaccination because they didn't want to expose them to alien substances. Not many pregnant women with tuberculosis seemed to have gotten abortions, as some doctors advised. And probably most households never followed the detailed recommendations that allegedly assured hygiene.[1] But these unreformed daily habits were neither deliberate acts of ideological resistance to the hygienic code nor inevitable consequences of poverty and ignorance. To a great extent they were part of the subjective ways through which people expressed themselves and organized their routines and ordinary quotidian life.

In a context marked by the achievements of modern bacteriology and an increasing medicalization of life, habits and practices that did not conform to the recommendations of the antituberculosis code were labeled as dirty, polluted, and dangerous; these coexisted with other habits that were clearly influenced by the discourse of hygiene and consequently perceived as clean, healthy, and proper. Driven by fear of contagion, the antituberculosis code became a specific strategy to prevent disease as well as an obsessive and detailed list of daily habits and moralizing prescriptions.

Originated in the late nineteenth-century bacteriological revolution, this lay catechism of hygiene fully penetrated Buenos Aires society and culture. And although some maintained that they exceeded reasonable prevention, many understood these prescriptions as new modern necessities of urban life, both material and moral. Effecting these new hygienic practices required social marketing initiatives that took place both in the late nineteenth century, when the dominant discourse of fear and defensive hygiene was eager to combat what it saw as unrelenting dangers, and in the 1920s, when the discourse of the healthy life and positive hygiene prevailed. Thanks to the overarching fear of contagion, the code was initially disseminated throughout society, almost without significant social differentiations. Later, it turned into a public health issue that was particularly relevant to the urban poor. And it ended up, by the second quarter of the twentieth century, focusing on certain social groups, now defined by their occupation and place of residence rather than, as in the past, their lifestyles and their presumed morality. This process, like many others associated with the arrival and consolidation of a certain modernity, was bound up in consent and coercion, social imitation and learning, novelty and tradition. The new hygienic catechism was part of a culture of respectability saturated with ideas of individual improvement. In conjunction with other new values, the hygienic culture often yielded strange combinations that didn't necessarily mean the same thing to different social sectors. However, in the 1920s and 1930s and, to a greater extent, at the beginning of the first Peronist administration in the second half of the 1940s, this culture of hygiene and health became central to a set of values shared by the middle classes, the urban poor, and the increasingly politicized and unionized industrial workers. All tended to understand the culture of hygiene in terms of a new right to health care in which individual and state responsibilities were largely complementary.

Nevertheless, the tuberculosis cycle cannot be fully explained by the dissemination and acceptance of the tenets of the antituberculosis code in the first half of the twentieth century. Brimming with professional pride, some doctors and bureaucrats celebrated the building of sanatoriums, hospitals, and dispensaries as the cause of the decline in tuberculosis. Others consistently pointed out the limitations of these endeavors, emphasizing that the enduring presence of tuberculosis morbidity and mortality was owing to a lack of beds and precarious medical services. And still others called attention to medical contributions, from drug-based treatments to surgical interventions, while emphasizing that the solution lay in improving living conditions. In truth, the decline of tuberculosis had been apparent long before the medical actions at the beginning of the twentieth century. It was erratic but fast from 1870 to 1895 and then hit a plateau until 1930. Into the early 1940s the decline was steady, if minimal. In the second half of the twentieth century it fell abruptly.

In any event, the lack of reliable statistical information makes it practically impossible even to begin to assess the relative and specific impacts of educational and preventive efforts; the spread of the BCG vaccine; the new, increasingly sophisticated early diagnosis; the hospitalization of tubercular patients; modern surgery; or socioeconomic factors. Everything suggests there was no single, decisive factor; indeed, the decline in tuberculosis mortality over the course of several decades is better explained by a complex web of increasing immunity—an overall, if interrupted, tendency toward better living conditions, salaries, working conditions, and diet, as well as some medical interventions. There is no doubt, however, that by the second half of the 1940s, the decline in tuberculosis mortality accelerated as a result of the coming and relatively effective access to and fast acceptance of streptomycin. Later chemotherapies would also contribute to this process. By the end of the 1950s, tuberculosis in Buenos Aires—and, indeed, the history of tuberculosis itself as a peculiar biomedical, social, and cultural phenomenon of the last third of the nineteenth century and the first half of the twentieth—was, to a great degree, over. From then on, memories of those decades, individual and collective, began to take shape. But they did so as a very private matter, certainly not as a public issue.

In the 1960s, 1970s, and 1980s the disease was no longer an urgent public health issue riddled with despair and frustration. In the city's medical and public health circles tuberculosis was often seen as a historical phenomenon: a controlled disease currently in decline, one quite insignificant in terms of overall rates of morbidity and mortality in Buenos Aires. In this context, many artifacts produced by the tuberculosis culture were assigned recycled functions or acquired new meanings. Such is the case of the sanatoriums in the Córdoba foothills, which became union-controlled vacation hotels that offer, among other things, unusually broad galleries inherited from an architecture originally designed to serve antituberculosis rest therapies. Or the old billboards referring to a municipal ordinance prohibiting spitting on the ground that hang on the walls of coffee shops, bars, restaurants, metro stations, and movie theaters were ultimately read by passersby as a nostalgic, somewhat curious reminder of the past, not a calculated public health measure aimed at avoiding contagion.

In the 1990s this state of affairs changed considerably. Elda G. experienced once again the fears that had haunted her four decades earlier, when she was a ten-year-old girl. Tuberculosis was again wandering through Buenos Aires. This time Elda was not afraid for herself or her mother, but for her young children. Unlike her mother, she didn't forbid them to consume vinegar, but she did try to convey to them the preventative habits she had learned, namely, the antituberculosis code. Soon, however, she understood that the new tuberculosis was to a certain extent different from the old one. As in the past, the current tuberculosis cycle results from deficient immunity owing to many complex reasons, above all, poor living conditions and poverty. She also understood that the strains of the current tuberculosis cycle are resistant to antibiotics that had once been effective and accepted by the population. And adding to her fear, she learned that the HIV-AIDS epidemic is closely associated with tuberculosis.

In 2005 newspapers and epidemiological studies revealed that tuberculosis was once again becoming a public health issue in Buenos Aires.[2] Its magnitude and prevalence were and still are not as devastating as they were in earlier years; nonetheless, there is a sense of urgency in all the discourses that refer to it. While statistics show a significant increase in the number of deaths from tuberculosis connected with HIV-AIDS in the mid-1990s and the years following the economic crisis of 2001, overall tuberculosis mortality is steadily declining. The question of morbidity, however, is entirely different. In 2003 morbidity increased to 6 percent of all people infected with tuberculosis, half of whom resided in the most impoverished sections of the Buenos Aires metropolitan area. That year there were one thousand new cases of tuberculosis in the city of Buenos Aires.

The current tuberculosis cycle is not marked by the intense, persistent bio-medical uncertainties of the late nineteenth century and first half of the twen-tieth. Nowadays tuberculosis is a disease for which there are effective thera-pies. In any event, as in the past, tuberculosis has made necessary discussions and enactment of specific health policies, including allocating resources, pro-ducing early diagnosis, developing new drugs and vaccines, and providing access to treatments and follow-up programs. As in the past, antituberculosis campaigns have revealed achievements and limitations, both at the discursive level as well as in its real application. Also as in the past, its presence has once again fueled associations and metaphors, both old and new, but first of all, the fear of contagion and the facile resource of stigmatization of those who are sick, who happen to be mainly impoverished people whose immunity levels are largely a reflection of their living conditions.

As in the 1900s, so in the early years of the twenty-first century, it is appar-ent that tuberculosis is much more than a bacillus.

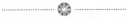
AAT	*Archivos Argentinos de Tisiología*
ABEMS	*Anales de Biotipología, Eugenesia y Medicina Social*
ACPCT	*Anales de la Cátedra de Patología y Clínica de la Tuberculosis*
ADNH	*Anales del Departamento Nacional de Higiene*
AM	*Argentina Médica*
APCCA	*Archivos de Psiquiatría, Criminología y Ciencias Afines*
ASCA	*Anales de la Sociedad Científica Argentina*
ASM	*Anales de Sanidad Militar*
ASSP	*Archivos de la Secretaría de Salud Pública de la Nación*
BC	*Brazo y Cerebro*
BDNH	*Boletín del Departamento Nacional de Higiene*
BDNT	*Boletín del Departamento Nacional del Trabajo*
BHCD	*Boletín del Honorable Concejo Deliberante de la Ciudad de Buenos Aires*
BLACA	*Boletín de la Liga Argentina contra la Tuberculosis*
BMSA	*Boletín del Museo Social Argentino*
CC	*Caras y Caretas*
CR	*Crítica*
CS	*Ciencia Social*
DSCD	*Diario de Sesiones de la Cámara de Diputados, Congreso Nacional*
DSCS	*Diario de Sesiones de la Cámara de Senadores, Congreso Nacional*
EC	*El Censor*
ED	*El Diario*
EDM	*El Día Médico*
EG	*El Gráfico*
EH	*El Hogar*
EMEC	*El Monitor de la Educación Común. Publicación de la Comisión Nacional de Educación*
EMP	*El Médico Práctico*
EN	*El Nacional*

LDC	*La Doble Cruz*
LHE	*La Higiene Escolar. Suplemento Mensual de El Monitor de la Educación Común. Publicación de la Comisión Nacional de Educación*
LLA	*La Lucha Antituberculosa*
LN	*La Nación*
LP	*La Prensa*
LPMA	*La Prensa Médica Argentina*
LPR	*La Protesta*
LR	*La Razón*
LSM	*La Semana Médica*
LV	*La Vanguardia*
LVE	*L'Avvenire. Periodico Comunista-Anarchico*
LVI	*La Voz del Interior*
MA	*Mundo Argentino*
MM	*Mundo Médico*
MMCBA	*Memoria Municipal de la Ciudad de Buenos Aires*
NT	*Nuestra Tribuna. Quincenario Femenino de Ideas, Crítica, Arte y Literatura*
PBT	*Semanario Infantil Ilustrado (Para Niños de 6 a 80 Años)*
PT	*Para Tí*
RAMA	*Revista de la Asociación Médica Argentina*
RATEP	*Revista Argentina de Tuberculosis y Enfermedades Pulmonares*
RCEMBA	*Revista del Centro de Estudiantes de Medicina de Buenos Aires*
RCMCF	*Revista del Colegio Médico de la Capital Federal*
RCPML	*Revista de Criminología, Psiquiatría y Medicina Legal*
RF	*Revista Farmacéutica*
RJA	*Revista de Jurisprudencia Argentina*
RM	*Revista Municipal*
RMQ	*Revista Médico-Quirúrgica. Órgano de los Intereses Médicos Argentinos*
RSM	*Revista de Sanidad Militar*
RT	*Revista de la Tuberculosis*
VC	*Vida Comunal*
VCA	*Viva Cien Años*
VN	*Vida Natural*
VTCD	*Versiones Taquigráficas del Concejo Deliberante de la Ciudad de Buenos Aires*

Introduction

1 Interview with Elda G., April 1996. The rest of the interviews mentioned in the text were done between May 2003 and August 2005.

2 Diego Armus, "Disease in the Historiography of Modern Latin America," in Diego Armus, ed., *Disease in the History of Modern Latin America: From Malaria to AIDS* (Durham: Duke University Press, 2003); Frank Huisman and John Harley Warner, "Medical Histories," in Frank Huisman and John Harley Warner, eds., *Locating Medical History: The Stories and Their Meanings* (Baltimore: Johns Hopkins University Press, 2004); Diego Armus and Adrián Lopez Denis, "Disease, Medicine, and Health, 1500–1950," in José Moya, ed., *The Oxford Handbook of Latin American History* (New York: Oxford University Press, 2011).

3 Charles Rosenberg, "Framing Disease: Illness, Society, and History," in Charles Rosenberg and Jeanne Golden, eds., *Framing Disease: Studies in Cultural History* (New Brunswick: Rutgers University Press, 1992), xiii.

4 Miguel Angel Scenna, *Cuando murió Buenos Aires* (Buenos Aires: Bastilla, 1974); Juan Carlos Veronelli, *Medicina, gobierno y sociedad: Evolución de las instituciones de atención de la salud en Argentina* (Buenos Aires: El Coloquio, 1975); Ernest Allen Crider, "Modernization and Human Welfare: The Asistencia Pública and Buenos Aires, 1883–1910" (Ph.D. diss., Ohio State University, 1976); Hugo Vezzeti, *La locura en la Argentina* (Buenos Aires: Folios, 1983); Diego Armus, "Enfermedad, ambiente urbano e higiene social: Rosario entre fines del siglo XIX y comienzos del XX," in Diego Armus, ed., *Sectores populares y vida urbana* (Buenos Aires: CLACSO, 1984); Alfredo Kohn Loncarica and Abel Aguero, "El contexto médico," in Héctor Biagini, ed., *El movimiento positivista argentino* (Buenos Aires: Editorial de Belgrano, 1985); Susana Belmartino et al., *Corporación médica y poder en salud: Argentina, 1920–1945* (Buenos Aires: OPS, 1988); Carlos Escudé, "Health in Buenos Aires in the Second Half of the Nineteenth Century," in C. Platt ed., *Social Welfare, 1850–1950: Australia, Argentina and Canada Compared* (London: Macmillan, 1989); Jorge Salessi, *Médicos, maleantes, maricas: Higiene, criminología y homo-*

sexualidad en la construcción de la nación Argentina (Rosario: Beatriz Viterbo, 1995); Mirta Zaida Lobato, ed., *Política, médicos y enfermedades: Lecturas de historia de la salud en la Argentina* (Buenos Aires: Biblos, 1996); Héctor Recalde, *La salud de los trabajadores en Buenos Aires (1870-1910) a través de las fuentes médicas* (Buenos Aires: Grupo Editor Universitario, 1997); Ricardo González Leandri, *Curar, persuadir, gobernar: La construcción histórica de la profesión médica en Buenos Aires, 1852-1886* (Madrid: CSIC, 1999); Diego Armus, "El descubrimiento de la enfermedad como problema social," in Mirta Lobato, ed., *Nueva historia Argentina* (Buenos Aires: Sudamericana, 2000), vol. 5; Gabriela Nouzeilles, *Ficciones somáticas: Naturalismo, nacionalismo y políticas médicas del cuerpo, Argentina 1880-1910* (Rosario: Beatriz Viterbo, 2000); Emilio de Ipola, "Estrategias de la creencia en situaciones críticas: El cáncer y la crotoxina en Buenos Aires a mediados de los años ochenta," in Diego Armus, ed., *Entre médicos y curanderos: Cultura, historia y enfermedad en la América Latina moderna* (Buenos Aires: Norma, 2003); María Silvia Di Liscia, *Saberes, terapias y prácticas médicas en Argentina, 1750-1910* (Madrid: CSIC, 2003); Adriana Alvarez, Inés Molinari, and Daniel Reynoso, eds., *Historias de enfermedades, salud y medicina en la Argentina del siglo XIX-XX* (Mar del Plata: Universidad Nacional de Mar del Plata, 2004); Kristin Ruggiero, *Modernity in the Flesh: Medicine, Law, and Society in Turn-of-the-Century Argentina* (Stanford: Stanford University Press, 2004); Marisa Miranda and Gustavo Vallejo, eds., *Darwinismo social y eugenesia en el mundo latino* (Buenos Aires: Siglo XXI, 2005); Susana Belmartino, *Atención médica en Argentina en el siglo XX: Instituciones y procesos* (Buenos Aires: Siglo XXI, 2005); Julia Rodríguez, *Civilizing Argentina: Science, Medicine and the Modern State* (Chapel Hill: University of North Carolina Press, 2006); Alejandro Kohl, *Higienismo argentino: Historia de una utopía: La salud en el imaginario colectivo de una época* (Buenos Aires: Dunken, 2006); Norma Isabel Sánchez, *La higiene y los higienistas en la Argentina (1880-1943)* (Buenos Aires: Instituto de Historia de la Medicina, 2007); Eric Carter, "'God Bless General Perón': DDT and the Endgame of Malaria Eradication in Argentina in the 1940s," *Journal of the History of Medicine and Allied Sciences*, 64, no. 1 (2009), 78–122; Adriana Alvarez and Adrián Carbonetti, eds., *Saberes y prácticas médicas en la Argentina: Un recorrido por historias de vida* (Mar del Plata: Eudem, 2008); Adrián Carbonetti and Ricardo González Leandri, eds., *Historias de salud y enfermedad en América Latina: Siglos XIX y XX* (Córdoba: Centro de Estudios Avanzados, UNC, 2008); Karina Ramacciotti, *La política sanitaria del peronismo* (Buenos Aires: Biblos, 2009); Adriana Alvarez, *Entre muerte y mosquitos: El regreso de las epidemias en la Argentina (Siglos XIX y XX)* (Buenos Aires: Biblos, 2010).

5 Isabelle Grellet and Caroline Krause, *Histoires de la tuberculose: Les fièvres de l'âme: 1800-1940* (Paris: Ramsay, 1983); Gillian Cronjé, "Tuberculosis and Mortality Decline in England and Wales, 1851-1919," in Robert Woods and John Woodward, eds., *Urban Disease and Mortality in Nineteenth Century England* (New York: St. Martin's Press, 1984); Antonio Villanueva Edo, *Historia social de la tuberculosis en*

Bizkaia (1882–1958) (Bilbao: Diputación Foral de Bizkaia, 1984); Pierre Guillaume, *Du désespoir au salut: les tuberculeux aux XIXe et XXe siècles* (Paris: Aubier, 1986); Mark Caldwell, *The Last Crusade: The War on Consumption, 1862–1954* (New York: Atheneum, 1988); Francis Barrymore Smith, *The Retreat of Tuberculosis, 1850–1950* (London: Croom Helm, 1988); Michael Teller, *The Tuberculosis Movement: A Public Health Campaign in the Progressive Era* (New York: Greenwood Press, 1988); Jorge Molero Mesa, *Historia de la tuberculosis en España, 1889–1936* (Granada: University of Granada, 1989); Randall Packard, *White Plague, Black Labor: Tuberculosis and the Political Economy of Health and Disease in South Africa* (Berkeley: University of California Press, 1989); Leonard Wilson, "The Historical Decline of Tuberculosis in Europe and America: Its Causes and Significance," *Journal of the History of Medicine and Allied Sciences* 45, no. 3 (July 1990), 366–96; A. J. Proust, ed., *History of Tuberculosis in Australia, New Zealand and Papua New Guinea* (Canberra: Brolga Press, 1991); Barbara Bates, *Bargaining for Life: A Social History of Tuberculosis, 1876–1938* (Philadelphia: University of Pennsylvania Press, 1992); Georgina Feldberg, *Disease and Class: Tuberculosis and the Shaping of the Modern North American Society* (New Brunswick: Rutgers University Press, 1995); William Johnston, *The Modern Epidemic: A History of Tuberculosis in Japan* (Cambridge: Council on East Asian Studies, Harvard University Press, 1995); Mark Harrison and Michael Worboys, "A Disease of Civilization: Tuberculosis in Britain, Africa and India," in Lara Marks and Michael Worboys, eds., *Migrants, Minorities and Health: Historical and Contemporary Studies* (London: Routledge, 1997); Antonio Pereira Loza, *La paciencia al sol: Historia social de la tuberculosis en Galicia, 1900–1950* (A Coruña: do Castro, 1999); Claudio Bertolli Filho, *História social da tuberculose e do tuberculoso: 1900–1950* (Rio de Janeiro: Editora Fiocruz, 2001); Alison Bashford, "Tuberculosis and Economy: Public Health and Labour in the Early Welfare State," *Health and History* 4 (2002), no. 2, 19–40; Emily Abel, *Tuberculosis and the Politics of Exclusion: A History of Public Health and Migration to Los Angeles* (New Brunswick: Rutgers University Press, 2007); Flurin Condrau and Michael Worboys, eds., *Tuberculosis Then and Now: Perspectives on the History of an Infectious Disease* (Montreal: McGill-Queen's University Press, 2010).

6 Diego Armus, "Salud y anarquismo: La tuberculosis en el discurso libertario argentino, 1890–1940," in Mirta Zaida Lobato, ed., *Política, médicos y enfermedades: Lecturas de historia de la salud en la Argentina* (Buenos Aires: Biblos, 1996); Adrián Carbonetti, *Enfermedad y sociedad: La tuberculosis en la ciudad de Córdoba, 1906–1947* (Córdoba: Emecor, 1998); Vera Blinn Reber, "Blood, Coughs, and Fever: Tuberculosis and the Working Class of Buenos Aires, Argentina, 1885–1915," *Social History of Medicine* 12, no. 1 (1999), 73–100; Diego Armus, "Consenso, conflicto y liderazgo en la lucha contra la tuberculosis, Buenos Aires, 1870–1950," in Juan Suriano, ed., *La cuestión social en la Argentina, 1870–1943* (Buenos Aires: La Colmena, 2000); Héctor Recalde, "La primera cruzada contra la tuberculosis. Buenos Aires, 1935," in José Panettieri, ed., *Argentina: Trabajadores entre dos guerras* (Buenos Aires: Eudeba, 2000); Vera Blin Reber, "Misery, Pain and Death:

Tuberculosis in Nineteenth Century Buenos Aires," *The Americas*, 56, no. 4 (April 2000), 497–528; Diego Armus, "Tango, Gender and Tuberculosis in Buenos Aires, 1900–1940," in Diego Armus, ed., *Disease in the History of Modern Latin America: From Malaria to AIDS*; Diego Armus, "El viaje al centro: Tísicas, costureritas y milonguitas en Buenos Aires (1910–1940)," in Diego Armus, ed., *Entre médicos y curanderos: Cultura, historia y enfermedad en la América Latina moderna*; Diego Armus, "'Queremos a vacina pueyo!!!': Incertezas biomédicas, enfermos que protestam e a Imprensa, Argentina, 1920–1940," in Gilberto Hochman and Diego Armus, eds., *Cuidar, controlar, curar: Ensaios históricos sobre saúde e doença na América Latina e Caribe* (Rio de Janeiro: Editora Fiocruz, 2004); Adrián Carbonetti, "Las entidades de beneficencia en la lucha contra la tuberculosis en la ciudad de Córdoba," in Adriana Alvarez, Irene Molinari, and Daniel Reynoso, eds., *Historias de enfermedades, salud y medicina*; Diego Armus, "Historia de enfermos tuberculosos que protestan, Argentina 1920–1940," in Diego Armus, ed., *Avatares de la medicalización en América Latina*; Sylvia Saítta, "Costureritas y artistas pobres: Algunas variaciones sobre el mito romántico de la tuberculosis en la literatura argentina," in Wolfgang Bongers and Tanja Olbrich, eds., *Literatura, cultura, enfermedad* (Buenos Aires: Paidós, 2006); Diego Armus, "Curas de reposo y destierros voluntarios: Narraciones de tuberculosos en los enclaves serranos de Córdoba," in Wolfgang Bongers and Tanja Olbrich, eds., *Literatura, cultura, enfermedad*; Amalia Pati, *Una enfermedad romántica: La tuberculosis y sus metáforas en el siglo XIX y principios del siglo XX: Un debate abierto* (Rosario; Editorial Municipal de Rosario, 2006); Elsa Rossi Raccio, *Divina Tuberculosis* (Buenos Aires: Puentes del Sur, 2008).

7 Edward Otis, *The Great White Plague* (New York: Crowell, 1909); M. Piery and J. Roshem, *Histoire de la tuberculose* (Paris: G. Doin, 1931); Charles Coury, *La tuberculose au course des âges: Grandeur et déclin d'une maladie* (Suresne: Lepetit, 1972); Frank Ryan, *The Forgotten Plague: How the Battle for Tuberculosis Was Won—and Lost* (Boston: Little, Brown, 1993).

8 René Dubos and Jean Dubos, *The White Plague: Tuberculosis, Man, and Society* (Boston: Little, Brown 1952).

9 Thomas McKeown, *The Modern Rise of Population* (London: Arnold, 1976); Thomas McKeown, *The Role of Medicine: Dream, Mirage, or Nemesis?* (Princeton: Princeton University Press, 1979); Simon Szreter, "The Importance of Social Intervention in Britain's Mortality Decline, c. 1850–1914: A Re-interpretation of the Role of Public Health," *Social History of Medicine* 1, no. 1 (1988), 1–38; Reinhard Spree, *Health and Social Class in Imperial Germany* (Oxford: Berg, 1988); Neil McFarlane, "Hospital, Housing and Tuberculosis in Glasgow, 1911–51," *Social History of Medicine* 2, no. 1 (1989), 59–85; Allan Mitchell, "An Inexact Science: The Statistics of Tuberculosis in Late Nineteenth-Century France," *Social History of Medicine* 3, no. 3 (December 1990), 387–403; Leonard Wilson, "The Historical Decline of Tuberculosis in Europe and America: Its Causes and Significance," *Journal of the History of Medicine and Allied Sciences* 45, no. 3 (July 1990), 366–96.

10 Mary Douglas, *Purity and Danger: An Analysis of the Concepts of Pollution and Taboo* (London: Routledge, 1968); Michel Foucault, *The Birth of the Clinic: An Archeology of Medical Perception* (London: Routledge, 1997 [1963]); Norbert Elias, *The History of Manners* (New York: Pantheon Books, 1982).

11 Susan Sontag, *Illness as Metaphor* (New York: Farrar, Straus and Giroux, 1978); Linda Hutcheon, *Opera: Desire, Disease, Death* (Lincoln: University of Nebraska Press, 1996); Linda Bryder, *Below the Magic Mountain: A Social History of Tuberculosis in Twentieth-Century Britain* (Oxford: Clarendon, 1988); Sheila Rothman, *Living in the Shadow of Death: Tuberculosis and the Social Experience of Illness in American History* (New York: Basic Books, 1994); David Barnes, *The Making of a Social Disease: Tuberculosis in Nineteenth-Century France* (Berkeley: University of California Press, 1995); Diego Armus, "Tango, Gender and Tuberculosis in Buenos Aires, 1900–1940," in Diego Armus, ed., *From Malaria to AIDS: Disease in the History of Modern Latin America*; Angela Porto, "Tuberculose: A pergrinação em busca da cura e de uma nova sensibilidade," in Dilene Raimundo do Nascimento and Diana Maul de Carvalho, eds., *Uma história brasileira das doenças* (Brasilia: Paralelo 15, 2004); Clark Lawlor, *Consumption and Literature: The Making of the Romantic Disease* (New York: Palgrave Macmillan, 2006).

12 Richard L. Riley, "Disease Transmission and Contagion Control," *American Review of Respiratory Diseases* 125 (1982), 16–19; Arthur M. Dannenberg Jr., "Pathogenesis of Pulmonary Tuberculosis," *American Review of Respiratory Diseases* 125 (1982), 25–27.

13 George Comstock, "Epidemiology of Tuberculosis," *American Review of Respiratory Diseases* 125 (1982), 12–14.

14 *RMQ* 11 (1875), 30; *ADNH* 2 (1936), 6–11; Juan Carlos Tassart, *El descenso de la tuberculosis en la República Argentina* (Buenos Aires, 1952), 46; *RATEP* 21, 2 (1957), 47, 49; *AAT* 25 (1949), 100–101; *RATEP* 30 (1954), fig. 8.

15 *ADNH* 2 (1936), 84.

16 *LSM*, November 10, 1927; *ADNH* 2 (1936), 82–95.

17 The historiography of public health is abundant; for example, see Gilberto Hochman, *A era do saneamento: As bases da política da saúde pública no Brasil* (São Paulo: Editora Hucitec, 1998), and the special issue of *Dynamis* 25 (2005) on health institutions in modern Latin America.

18 Examples of the literature on this topic are Marcos Cueto, ed., *Missionaries of Science: The Rockefeller Foundation and Latin America* (Bloomington: Indiana University Press, 1994); Anne-Emanuelle Birn, *Marriage of Convenience: Rockefeller International Health and Revolutionary Mexico* (Rochester: University of Rochester Press, 2006); Steven Palmer, *Launching Global Health: The Caribbean Odyssey of the Rockefeller Foundation* (Ann Arbor: University of Michigan Press, 2010).

19 For instance, Jaime Benchimol, *Dos micróbios aos mosquitos: Febre amarela e a revolução pasteuriana no Brasil* (Rio de Janeiro: Editora Fiocruz/ Editora UFRJ, 1999); Simone Petraglia Kropf, Nara Azevedo, and Luiz Otávio Ferreira, "Bio-

medical Research and Public Health in Brazil: The Case of Chagas' Disease (1909–50)," *Social History of Medicine* 16, no. 1 (April 2003), 111–29.

20 For these urban changes, see, among others, James Scobie, *Buenos Aires: Plaza to Suburb, 1870–1910* (New York: Oxford University Press, 1974); José Luis Romero and Luis Alberto Romero, eds., *Buenos Aires: Historia de cuatro siglos* (Buenos Aires: Abril, 1983); Diego Armus, ed., *Mundo urbano y cultura popular: Estudios de historia social Argentina* (Buenos Aires: Sudamericana, 1990); Richard Walter, *Politics and Urban Growth in Buenos Aires, 1910–1942* (New York: Cambridge University Press, 1993); Adrián Gorelick, *La grilla y el parque: Espacio público y cultura urbana en Buenos Aires, 1887–1936* (Buenos Aires: Universidad Nacional de Quilmes, 1998).

21 Francis Korn and Luis Alberto Romero, eds., *Buenos Aires/Entreguerras: La callada transformación, 1914–1945* (Buenos Aires: Alianza, 2006).

1. Looking for Cures

1 Clemente Alvarez, *La tuberculosis bajo el punto de vista social* (Rosario: Imprenta Federico Wentzel, 1904), 4, 21–23.

2 *AAT* 30 (1954), 146.

3 Antonio Cetrángolo, *Treinta años curando tuberculosos* (Buenos Aires: Hachette, 1945), 155.

4 Barbara Bates, *Bargaining for Life: A Social History of Tuberculosis, 1876–1938* (Philadelphia: University of Pennsylvania Press, 1992).

5 Cetrángolo, *Treinta años curando tuberculosos*, 25.

6 Accumulation of a gas, such as air, in the space between the pleurae of the lungs and the pleurae lining the chest wall (called the pleural cavity), occurring as a result of disease or injury or induced to collapse the lung in the treatment of tuberculosis and other lung diseases. A large pneumothorax is treated by inserting a syringe or a tube into the pleural cavity to aspirate air, which helps the collapsed lung to expand, cf. *American Heritage Science Dictionary* (Houghton Mifflin, 2002).

7 *MMCBA* (1880), 210–11; Samuel Gache, *Les logements ouvrières a Buenos Ayres* (Paris: G. Steinheil, 1900).

8 José Alejandro López, *Médico de pobres* (Buenos Aires: Corregidor, 1981), 32.

9 Interview, María L.

10 Angel Navarro Blasco, "La tuberculosis conyugal: Contagio y matrimonio," in Julio Noguera Toledo, ed., *Genética, eugenesia y pedagogía sexual* (Madrid: Javier Morata, 1934), 1:79.

11 Juan José Vitón, *Lo que todo tuberculoso debe saber: Anotaciones y consejos que ayudan a curar la tuberculosis y enseñan a evitarla* (Buenos Aires: El Ateneo, 1928), 29–36; Antonio Cetrángolo, *Consejos para evitar la propagación de la tuberculosis y curarse de ella* (Buenos Aires, 1930).

12 Eduardo Wilde, "Curso de higiene pública," in *Obras completas* (Buenos Aires: Talleres Peuser, 1914), 3:56.

13 *EH*, May 7, 1915.

14 D. J. G. Perez, *Medicina doméstica, o sea el arte de conservar la salud, de conocer las enfermdades, sus remedios y aplicación al alcance de todos* (Buenos Aires: Imprenta de la Revista, 1854); Pedro Chernovitz, *Diccionario de medicina popular y ciencias accesorias* (Paris: Rogen et Federico Chernovitz, 1879); *LN*, December 11, 1870; Hugo W. O'Gorman, *El médico en casa: Libro para las madres* (Buenos Aires, 1918) 2d edn.; *LV*, March 2, 1920; August 21, 1927.

15 Carlos Kozel, *Salud y curación por hierbas* (Buenos Aires, 1930).

16 *RF* 87 (1945), 357–60; *LSM*, February 13, 1941.

17 *CR*, December 22, 1940.

18 *LSM*, October 1930.

19 Arturo Montesano, *La cura natural* (Montevideo, 1911); *El Obrero Carpintero y Aserrador*, June 1924; *Acción Obrera*, October 1928.

20 César Sánchez Aizcorbe, *La salud: Tratado de higiene y medicina natural* (Buenos Aires: Kapelusz, 1919) 8, 281, 287.

21 *RF* 87 (1945), 11–26; *MM* 8 (1943), 16–17, 33–34.

22 *MM* 8 (1943), 34.

23 Alberto Borrini, *El siglo de la publicidad, 1898–1998* (Buenos Aires: Atlántida, 1998), chap. 1.

24 *CC*, January 9, 1909.

25 J. W. Sanger, "Trade Commissioner. Advertising Methods in Argentina, Uruguay, and Brazil." Department of Commerce, *Special Agents*, n. 190 (Washington: Government Printing Office, 1920), 14–16 (quoted in Fernando Rocchi, *Chimneys in the Desert*, note 67).

26 *LP*, October 28, 1883; June 10, 1901; *LR*, January 8, 1928; January 14, 1928.

27 *LP*, June 10, 1901.

28 *LV*, July 26, 1924; June 4, 1927.

29 *ADNH* 10, no. 8 (1904), 439.

30 *PT*, July 5, 1926.

31 *LR*, January 13, 1920.

32 *LR*, July 4, 1908.

33 *LR*, February 24, 1928.

34 *LR*, May 28, 1940; *LV*, July 26, 1924; June 4, 1927.

35 *LR*, May 28, 1940; May 30, 1928; July 2, 1908; *CC*, June 14, 1902.

36 *LV*, July 26, 1924; June 4, 1927.

37 *LR*, September 8, 1928.

38 *LV*, June 22, 1923.

39 *RCMCF*, April 3, 1933, 5.

40 *ED*, April 24, 1901; April 26, 1901; *LR*, September 8, 1928.

41 *Ahora* (1935).

42 *VTCD*, March–May 1921, 334.

43 *ADNH* 1, 44 (1905); *LSM*, December 31, 1925; *RCMCF*, April 3, 1933, 5; *VCA* 1 (1938) 38.

44 *El Progreso de la Boca*, December 1900; Municipalidad de la Ciudad de Buenos

Aires, Asistencia Pública, *La tuberculosis: A los niños de la Argentina* (Buenos Aires, 1927).

45 *RMQ* 21 (1866), 326; *APCCA* 4 (November–December 1905); *LSM*, March 29, 1917; *LV*, July 27, 1928; *Ahora* (1942), 750.

46 *Ahora* (1942), 750.

47 *LV*, July 27, 1928.

48 Steven Palmer, *From Popular Medicine to Medical Populism: Doctors, Healers and Public Power in Costa Rica, 1800-1940* (Durham: Duke University Press, 2003), introduction.

49 *LV*, April 5, 1925; *CC*, April 10, 1909; *LV*, March 18, 1928; *APCCA* 4 (November–December 1905); *LV*, July 27, 1928; April 5, 1925; *Ahora* (1942), 750.

50 *LN*, May 24, 1883; *LSM*, July 1905, 717; *LV*, October 27, 1924; March 18, 1928.

51 *LSM*, July 1905.

52 *La República*, November 4, 1871; *LSM*, January 7, 1926, 36.

53 *ADNH* 10, 2 (1903), 84.

54 *LR*, May 1, 1901.

55 *CC*, January 16, 1909; April 10, 1909.

56 Rogerio Holguín, *Historia del descubrimiento de medicinas vegetales para curar la tuberculosis* (Buenos Aires: Impr. San Martín, 1917), 6, 7, 113–20.

57 *LV*, October 27, 1924; *VCA* 2 (1936), 627.

58 *LSM*, July 20, 1905; December 31, 1925.

59 *AM*, July 27, 1912.

60 *Las calamidades de Buenos Aires*, April 18, 1883; *LN*, May 24, 1883.

61 *LP*, June 10, 1901; *LSM*, March 29, 1917.

62 *EP*, August 1, 1901.

63 *CR*, March 2, 1923.

64 *LV*, March 18, 1928.

65 *LSM*, May 4, 1905.

66 *APCCA* 4 (November–December 1905), 715; *LSM*, July 20, 1905, 713–17; August 2, 1934, 357–59.

67 *RMQ* 12 (1876), 335; *ADNH* 4 (1891), 206; *LSM*, March 29, 1917; *LV*, October 24, 1922; June 2, 1921; *Ahora* (1942), 750.

68 *RMQ* 12 (1876), 335; *LSM*, December 31, 1925; *CR*, March 2, 1923; *VCA* 2 (1936), 426; *Ahora* (1941), 639; Ezequiel Martínez Estrada, *La cabeza de Goliat* (Buenos Aires: Emecé, 1946).

69 *RMQ* 12 (1876), 212.

70 Ibid., 335; *ADNH* 4 (1891), 206; *LSM*, March 29, 1917; *LV*, June 2, 1921; October 19, 24, 1922; *Ahora* (1942), 750.

71 *PBT* (1909), 234.

72 *APCCA* 4 (November–December 1905), 715; *LV*, April 5, 1925, March 18, 1928; *Ahora* (1942), 750; *CR*, January 21, 1929.

73 *LP*, October 28, 1883; June 10, 1901; *VTCD* (March–May 1921), 334.

74 *EC*, September 18, 1922; *LV*, July 27, 1928.

75 *APCCA* 4 (November–December 1905), 708.

76 *Ahora* (1941), 639; *Ahora* (1942), 750; *LSM*, September 21, 1939, 680.

77 *LSM*, December 31, 1925.

78 *VTCD* (March–May 1921), 334; *LV*, July 27, 1928; *LSM*, September 21, 1939.

79 *APCCA* 4 (November–December 1905), 721; *VTCD* (March–May 1921), 334; *Ahora* (1941), 631.

80 *ADNH* (August 1909), 384.

81 César Sánchez Aizcorbe, *La salud: Tratado de higiene y medicina natural*; *El Obrero Carpintero y Aserrador*, June 1924; *NT*, September 15, 1923.

82 *RMQ* 4 (1867), 83; *Las calamidades de Buenos Aires*, April 18, 1883; *ADNH* 4 (1891), 206; *VCA* 6 (1938), 39.

83 Ricardo González Leandri, *Curar, persuadir, gobernar: La construcción histórica de la profesión médica en Buenos Aires, 1852–1886* (Madrid: CSIC, 1999), 48–55; *ADNH* 16, no. 4 (1909), 184; *LSM*, July 1934, 146.

84 *RMQ* 19 (1876), 336; *ADNH* 8 (1909), 383; Ministerio del Interior, Departamento Nacional de Higiene, *Guía oficial* (Buenos Aires, 1913), 69; *El Mundo*, July 29, 1928; *CR*, January 3, 1930.

2. Becoming a Patient

1 *LSM*, April 25, 1918.

2 *LV*, June 19, 1897; José Penna y Horacio Madero, *La administración sanitaria y la asistencia pública de la ciudad de Buenos Aires* (Buenos Aires: Kraft, 1910), 2:203, 379; Emilio Coni, *Memorias de un médico higienista* (Buenos Aires: A. Flaiban, 1923), 80, 309–12.

3 *MMCBA* (1877), 60.

4 *MMCBA* (1875), 55, 46; *RMQ* 12 (1876), 212.

5 *MMCBA* (1884), 52; *MMCBA* (1877), 53; *MMCBA* (1884), 31.

6 *LP*, January 6, 1885; *MMCBA* (1883), 25; *MMCBA* (1889), 143.

7 *MMCBA* (1878), 133.

8 *MMCBA* (1887), 507; *MMCBA* (1876), 66.

9 *MMCBA* (1884), 31.

10 *MMCBA* (1889), 148.

11 *LP*, January 13, 1904.

12 *MMCBA* (1877), 60.

13 *MMCBA* (1887), 507; *MMCBA* (1889), 364.

14 *LSM*, October 14, 1909; *MMCBA* (1893–94), 328; *MMCBA* (1897), 98; *LV*, June 24, 1899.

15 *LSM*, October 12, 1905.

16 *LSM*, October 14, 1909.

17 Penna and Madero, *La administración sanitaria*, 2:205.

18 *LSM*, December 11, 1902.

19 Penna and Madero, *La administración sanitaria*, 2:203; Municipalidad de la Ciudad de Buenos Aires, *Censo general de población, edificación, comercio e industria de la ciudad de Buenos Aires, 1909* (Buenos Aires, 1910), 2:272.

20 Penna and Madero, *La administración sanitaria*, 2:379.

21 *BDNT* 4 (1907), 191.

22 Penna and Madero, *La administración sanitaria*, 2:201.

23 *LSM*, October 14, 1909; *MMCBA* (1893–94), 328; *MMCBA* (1897), 98.

24 *MMCBA* (1912), 148; *MMCBA* (1926), 378; Coni, *Memorias de un médico higienista*, 685.

25 *MMCBA* (1918), 180.

26 *MMCBA* (1925), 420; *MMCBA* (1926), 378.

27 *MMCBA* (1926), 378.

28 *MMCBA* (1933–34), 608; *AAT* 30 (1954), 148.

29 *AAT* 5 (1928), 6.

30 *LDC* 1 (1936), 1; Liga Argentina contra la Tuberculosis, *Memoria de la cruzada antituberculosa nacional* (Buenos Aires, 1936), 2; *AAT* 5 (1928), 6.

31 *VTCD* (July–September 1933), 1561–1628; *CR*, July 3, 1933.

32 *VTCD* (December 1936), 2862; *LV*, August 3, 1926.

33 *AAT* 27 (1951), 181.

34 *MMCBA* (1910), 186; *MMCBA* (1918), 191; *MMCBA* (1935), 724; *Ahora* (1934), 622; *AAT* 15 (1939), 219.

35 *AAT* 27 (1951), 181.

36 *MMCBA* (1912), 149.

37 *MMCBA* (1935), 724; *AAT* 23 (1947), 217–18; *AAT* 27 (1951), 181.

38 Antonio Cetrángolo, *Treinta años curando tuberculosos* (Buenos Aires: Hachette, 1945), 170; *AAT* 15 (1939), 232.

39 Ibid., 212.

40 *DSCD*, September 24, 1936, 553–615.

41 *Primera conferencia nacional de asistencia social* (Buenos Aires, 1933), 1:86; *LSM*, September 1938, 573.

42 *AAT* 26 (1950), 53; *AAT* 27 (1951), 180–81.

43 *AAT* 26 (1950), 52.

44 *AAT* 15 (1939), 217.

45 Penna and Madero, *La administración sanitaria*, 2:235; *MMCBA* (1918), 188; *AAT* 27 (1951), 189; *VTCD* (1925), 2097.

46 *MMCBA* (1912), 150, *MMCBA* (1935), 725; *AAT* 15 (1939), 221–23; *AAT* 26 (1950), 55–56.

47 *MMCBA* (1912), 150; *AAT* 15 (1939), 224.

48 *MMCBA* (1909), 54.

49 *VTCD* (1921), 104–16.

50 *MMCBA* (1925), 421–22; *MMCBA* (1935), 725–26.

51 *MMCBA* (1918), 189.

52 LSM, October 19, 1905; MMCBA (1910), 184; Juan Milich, "Medicina argentina: Ligero bosquejo histórico y evolución de la higiene en la República Argentina, 1606–1910" (Ph.D. diss., Universidad de Buenos Aires, 1911), 159, 164.

53 LSM, July 30, 1925.

54 LSM, October 16, 1905; March, 29, 1938; AAT 15 (1939), 218; AAT 24 (1948), 67–72.

55 LSM, March 29, 1938; AAT 15 (1939), 214; AAT 24 (1948), 67–72; RAMA 58 (1944).

56 LSM, March 29, 1938.

57 LSM, March 21, 1935.

58 MMCBA (1926), 376.

59 AAT 25 (1939), 208.

60 LV, October 16, 1904; LSM, June 12, 1902.

61 AAT 17 (1932), 670.

62 Luis Boffi, Misión de la enfermera en la lucha antituberculosa (Buenos Aires: El Ateneo, 1939), 9.

63 AAT 7 (1931), 435.

64 LSM, April 8, 1937; August 8, 1940.

65 LSM, June 12, 1902.

66 LSM, August 5, 1920; July 30, 1925; September 5, 1935; April 8, 1937; October 8, 1940; RAMA, December 30, 1944, 1265; Eduardo Baca, Comisión Villa Crespo contra la tuberculosis (Buenos Aires, 1921); LV, April 20, 1918.

67 AAT 5 (1928), 11.

68 AAT 15 (1939), 229–61.

69 AAT 27 (1951), 193–95.

70 LDC 2, 3 (1937), 127–30.

71 LSM, March 21, 1935.

72 AAT 27 (1951), 193–95.

73 AAT 5 (1928), 17.

74 LSM, March 31, 1938.

75 Clemente Alvarez, La tuberculosis bajo el punto de vista social (Rosario: Wetzel, 1904).

76 AAT 15 (1939), 243.

77 LSM, October 12, 1905; Liga Argentina contra la Tuberculosis, Memoria de la cruzada antituberculosa nacional, 5.

78 Ahora (1941), 622.

79 LDC 28 (1941), 6.

80 LSM, March 31, 1938.

81 ATT 15 (1939), 229–61.

82 LSM, March 31, 1938.

83 LSM, July 30, 1925; March 21, 1935; AAT 5 (1928), 16–17.

84 AAT 15 (1939), 208.

85 LSM, April 8, 1937.

86 VTCD (1929), 1382.

87 *LDC* 1 (1936), 83–84.

88 Domingo Faustino Sarmiento, *Obras completas* (Buenos Aires: Luz del Día, 1951), 21:323.

89 *ADNH* 12, no. 12 (1905), 569; Alberto Martínez, *Manuel du voyageur: Baedeker de la République Argentine*, (Barcelona, 1907), 515, 518.

90 Juan José Vitón, *Lo que todo tuberculoso debe saber* (Buenos Aires: El Ateneo, 1928) 3, 7.

91 *LSM*, May 9, 1918; *LV*, February 6, 1928.

92 *CC*, January 26, 1907; *LSM*, September 6, 1917; Fenelón Matorras, "Tisis tuberculosa y neumónica: Apreciaciones propias del autor sobre la etiología, génesis, pronóstico y tratamiento en la República Argentina" (Ph.D. diss., Universidad de Buenos Aires, 1878), 110–17, 134; *LSM*, November 15, 1899; December 6, 1900; October 10, 1916; *EDM*, November 16, 1939; Francisco Súnico, *La tuberculosis en las sierras de Córdoba* (Buenos Aires: E. de Martino, 1922), 301.

93 *LLA* (1903), 531.

94 *La Semana Médica*, November 7, 1909, September 6, 1917; Cetrángolo, *Treinta años curando tuberculosos*, 174.

95 Ibid., 170, 171, 217.

96 Martínez, *Manuel du voyageur: Baedeker de la République Argentine*, 518.

97 *ADNH* 8 (1905), 390; *LDC* 2, no. 8 (1937), 2.

98 *Sanatorio Laënnec, Cosquín* (Córdoba, 1932), 6.

99 *Reflexiones*, May 1921, 20.

100 Francisco Súnico, *La tuberculosis en las sierras de Córdoba*, 259.

101 Cetrángolo, *Treinta años curando tuberculosos*, 171; *LSM*, October 16, 1919.

102 *LSM*, November 3, 1932; Cetrángolo, *Treinta años curando tuberculosos*, 176, 200.

103 *LSM*, October 19, 1905; Vitón, *Lo que todo tuberculoso debe saber*, 68.

104 *LSM*, October 19, 1905.

105 Vitón, *Lo que todo tuberculoso debe saber*, 51; Cetrángolo, *Treinta años curando tuberculosos*, 191; Antonio Cetrángolo, *Consejo a los enfermos* (Buenos Aires: 1930), 10; Pablo Barlaro, *Lecciones de patología médica: Tuberculosis* (Buenos Aires: Cadom. 1929), 2:625–26.

106 *LSM*, November 9, 1919; October 24, 1929; March 31, 1938; Cetrángolo, *Treinta años curando tuberculosos*, 38; *RAMA*, August 30, 1944.

107 *LPA* 26 (1939), 686.

108 *LV*, February 6, 1928; *LN*, December 16, 1922.

109 *LV*, January 13, 1920; August 2, 1924.

110 Ulises Petit de Murat, *El balcón hacia la muerte* (Buenos Aires: Lautaro, 1943), 68.

111 *LSM*, October 9, 1919.

112 *LSM*, November 19, 1905; *LV*, December 1, 1918; October 8, 1920.

113 Cetrángolo, *Treinta años curando tuberculosos*, 202, 27.

114 Ibid., 174.

115 *Reflexiones*, April 1922, 1.

116 Ibid., January 1922, 16.

117 Ibid., October 1921, 20.

118 Petit de Murat, *El balcón hacia la muerte*, 25.

119 *LSM*, May 11, 1899; October 16, 1919; Súnico, *La tuberculosis en las sierras de Córdoba*, 305, 428.

120 *Reflexiones*, August 1921, 18; December 1921, 2–4.

121 Petit de Murat, *El balcón hacia la muerte*; Roberto Arlt, "Ester Primavera," in *Cuentos completos* (Buenos Aires: Seix Barral, 1991); Manuel Puig, *Boquitas pintadas* (Buenos Aires: Sudamericana, 1969). The English version of the Puig book was entitled *Heartbreak Tango* [1973] and the video version *Painted Lips*.

122 Marcelo Castelli, *Cosquín: Falsedad y verdad* (Cosquín, Córdoba, 1954), 341, 360–62, 431.

123 Ibid., 431, 218.

124 Ibid., 214, 374, 439.

125 Ibid., 14.

126 Ibid., 360–62, 431.

127 *Ahora* (1941), 578; Carlos Desmaras, *Tiempo libre de los trabajadores: Vacaciones y centros de descanso* (Buenos Aires, 1942).

3. Unruly and Well-Adjusted Patients

1 Juan José Vitón, *Lo que todo tuberculoso debe saber: Anotaciones y consejos que ayudan a curar la tuberculosis y enseñan a evitarla* (Buenos Aires: El Ateneo, 1928), 83–87.

2 Ulises Petit de Murat, *El balcón hacia la muerte* (Buenos Aires: Lautaro, 1943), 57.

3 Antonio Cetrángolo, *Treinta años curando tuberculosos* (Buenos Aires: Hachette, 1945), 194.

4 Diego Armus, "Historias de Enfermos Tuberculosos que Protestan: Argentina, 1920–1940," in Diego Armus, ed., *Avatares de la medicalización en América Latina, 1870–1970* (Buenos Aires: Lugar Editorial, 2005), 65–74.

5 Cetrángolo, *Treinta años curando tuberculosos*, 188; *LV*, October 20, 1923; *CR*, October 28, 1940; November 29, 1940; July 2, 1941; *Ahora* (1941), 560.

6 *LV*, February 16, 1920; *LVI*, December 30, 1919; *La Montaña*, May 20, 1930; June 30, 1934.

7 *LV*, March 13, 1912; December 29, 1919; January 4, 1920; *La Montaña*, June 30, 1934.

8 *LV*, March 9, 1924.

9 *LV*, April 6, 1920; February 12, 1922; October 22, 1922; October 29, 1922; December 12, 1922; *LSM*, November 3, 1932; *LVI*, February 25, 1930; *La Montaña*, September 25, 1937.

10 *LV*, January 31, 1922; April 7, 1922; April 11, 1922; August 15, 1922; *RCEMBA*, October 23, 1922.

11 *LV*, October 23, 1922; Francisco Súnico, *La tuberculosis en las sierras de Córdoba* (Buenos Aires: de Martino, 1922); *LV*, January 8, 1920; January 13, 1920; Cetrángolo, *Treinta años curando tuberculosos*, 189–92.

12 Cetrángolo, *Treinta años curando tuberculosos*, 192; Marcelo Castelli, *Cosquín: Falsedad y verdad* (Cosquín, Córdoba, 1954), 32.

13 *LV I*, March 10, 1920; *LV*, October 6, 1922.

14 *LM*, November 24, 1932.

15 *LVI*, February 5, 1920; *La Montaña*, May 20, 1930.

16 *LV*, June 19, 1897; June 9, 1918; June 16, 1918; *LVI*, March 28, 1920.

17 *Idea Hospitalaria*, July 6, 1922; *LV*, June 17, 1918; August 11, 1918.

18 *LV*, January 16, 1920; *LVI*, March 25, 1920.

19 *LV*, January 16, 1920; February 17, 1923; July 26, 1924. On Spaniards, Galicians, and tuberculosis, see chapter 7.

20 *LV*, January 13, 1920.

21 *LV*, February 7, 1922; December 28, 1919; October 23, 1922; April 12, 1920; *LSM*, October 9, 1919; *LN*, October 27, 1922; *LVI*, October 28, 1922.

22 *Los Principios*, November 12, 1941.

23 Comisión Nacional de Investigaciones, *Libro negro de la segunda tiranía* (Buenos Aires, 1958), 43–44.

24 *Ahora* (1941), 560, 578, 591, 624, 645, 719; *LV*, August 28, 1914; June 17, 1918; June 23, 1918; August 11, 1918; January 13, 1920.

25 *LV*, October 6, 1922.

26 Cetrángolo, *Treinta años curando tuberculosos*, 47.

27 *LV*, January 14, 1920.

28 *La Montaña*, November 24, 1932.

29 *LV*, July 26, 1924; June 28, 1924; October 24, 1924; February 3, 1925.

30 *La Montaña*, May 20, 1930.

31 *LSM*, November 3, 1932; *LDC* 2, 8 (1937), 3.

32 *La Montaña*, September 25, 1937.

33 *Reflexiones*, June 1921.

34 Cetrángolo, *Treinta años curando tuberculosos*, 55; *LSM*, November 3, 1932; *LV*, February 7, 1922; July 18, 1924; Petit de Murat, *El balcón hacia la muerte*, 253.

35 *LV*, February 19, 1923.

36 Petit de Murat, *El balcón hacia la muerte*, 22, 78, 82, 114, 118, 190; Cetrángolo, *Treinta años curando tuberculosos*, 195; *LSM*, July 30, 1925; *VCA* 11, no. 4 (1940), 273.

37 *La Montaña*, May 20, 1930.

38 Ibid., December 1, 1932.

39 Ibid., December 15, 1932.

40 Gregorio Berman, *La explotación de los tuberculosos* (Buenos Aires: Editorial Claridad, 1941), chaps. 11, 12.

41 Castelli, *Cosquín: Falsedad y verdad*, 319, 320, 352, 391, 452. For a more detailed discussion on sanitoriums, see chapter 2.

42 *LSM*, June 5, 1941, 315–24.

43 Augusto Bunge, *La tuberculosis vencida: Su cura y extinción por la vacuna Friedmann* (Buenos Aires: La Facultad, 1934); *LSM*, July 12, 1934, 130–36; August 9, 1934,

428–31; August 30, 1934, 663; September 27, 1934, 993–94; October 18, 1934, 1197–204; *Revista de Medicina Legal y Jurisprudencia Médica* 2 (1936), 87–108.

44 *LN*, April 22, 1901.

45 *El País*, April 26, 1901; April 29, 1901.

46 *ED*, April 25, 1901; *LP*, April 29, 1901; *CC*, May 4, 1901.

47 *ED*, May 15, 1901; *LN*, April 22, 1901; *El País*, July 6, 1901.

48 *El País*, April 30, 1901.

49 Ibid., May 1, 1901.

50 *ED*, May 12, 1091.

51 *LSM*, July 18, 1901, 425–30.

52 *El País*, July 6, 1901.

53 Enrique de Cires, *La proteinoterapia es argentina: El Dr. Carlos L. Villar, su vida y su obra*, (Buenos Aires: El Ateneo, 1936); *LSM*, June 5, 1933; March 1, 1934; *EDM* 4, 42 (1934).

54 *VCA* 11 (1941), 208.

55 *Ahora* (1941), 560, 591, 624, 645, 719.

56 Jesús Pueyo, *La burocracia de la medicina contra los tuberculosos: Síntesis documentada y antecedentes reales de mi vacuna antituberculosa: Yo acuso* (Buenos Aires: Editorial Científica, 1942).

57 *VCA* 15 (1941), 364.

58 *Ahora* (1941), 645, 560.

59 Ibid., 578.

60 *LDC* 2, 10 (1938), 22.

61 *VCA* 11 (1941), 213, 254; *VCA* 15 (1941), 393.

62 *CR*, October 21, 1940; January 3, 1941; *Ahora* (1941), 14; Pueyo, *La Burocracia de la Medicina*, 23–28, 73–103; *VCA* 9 (1941), 254.

63 *VCA* 9 (1941), 254.

64 *CR*, November 8, 1940.

65 Ibid., December 4, 1940.

66 *Ahora* (1941), 578.

67 Ibid.

68 Ibid.

69 Ibid., 580.

70 Ibid., 591.

71 *DSCD*, July 29, 1941; August 12, 1941; August 19, 1941; August 26, 1941.

72 *Ahora* (1941), 642.

73 Ibid., 651.

74 *CR*, October 14, 1941; November 2, 1941; November 17, 1941; December 25, 1941; January 12, 1942.

75 *Ahora* (1941), 578.

76 Ibid. (1942), 719.

77 Ibid. (1941), 578.

78 Juan José Vitón, *Lo que todo tuberculoso debe saber*, 83.

79 *El Obrero Panadero*, October 16, 1894; October 9, 1897; April 5, 1900; August 1, 1911; March 1913; April 1913; August 1913; February 1921; May 1926; January 1928; March 1936.

80 *AAT* 23 (1947), 216; *LPMA* 24 (1938), 87–88; *LPMA* 28 (1941), 880–90.

4. *The Fight against Tuberculosis*

1 José Antonio Wilde, *Compendio de higiene pública y privada al alcance de todos* (Buenos Aires: Jacobo Peuser, 1868); Intendencia Municipal de la Capital, *Instrucciones contra la propagación de la tuberculosis* (Buenos Aires, 1894); *ADNH* 16, no. 12 (1909); Municipalidad de Buenos Aires, *Los peligros de las moscas: Medios eficaces para destruirlas* (Buenos Aires, 1914); Municipalidad de Buenos Aires, *Disposiciones generales para evitar la propagación de enfermedades epidémicas* (Buenos Aires, 1916); Municipalidad de la Ciudad de Buenos Aires, *Preceptos de higiene y economía alimenticias* (Buenos Aires, 1924); Pedro Escudero, *El contagio tuberculoso por el consumo de leche en la ciudad de Buenos Aires* (Buenos Aires, 1936); Cátedra de Higiene Médica y Preventiva, *Educación sanitaria popular y propaganda higiénica* (La Plata: Universidad Nacional de La Plata, Facultad de Ciencias Médicas, 1942).

2 Roque Izzo and Florencio Escardó, *Una campaña de propaganda sanitaria* (Buenos Aires: Centro de Investigaciones Tisiológicas, 1940), 16, 25.

3 *RT* (1901), 184; *LLA* (1902), 200–201; *LSM*, April 10, 1902.

4 *LSM*, May 29, 1902; May 22, 1919; Eduardo Hansen, "Profilaxia de la tuberculosis" (Ph.D. diss., Universidad de Buenos Aires, 1918).

5 *LDC*, October 15, 1936, 8–9.

6 Wilde, *Compendio de higiene pública y privada*, 24.

7 Congreso Nacional, *Leyes Sancionadas*, (1899), 2:930; *DSCD*, June 19, 1912, 277; July 17, 1912, 543.

8 Ibid., June 26, 1899; September 6, 1899; June 8, 1908.

9 Ibid., July 26, 1906, 392–93.

10 Emilio Tenti Fanfani, *Estado y pobreza: Estrategias típicas de intervención* (Buenos Aires: CEAL, 1989), 71.

11 Tulio Halperín Donghi, *Vida y muerte de la república verdadera (1910–1930)* (Buenos Aires: Ariel, 1999), 153–64.

12 *DSCD*, July 28, 1915; September 2, 1918; March 2–3, 1921; October 21, 1924; June 24, 1925; August 10, 1927.

13 Ibid., May 20, 1918; June 6, 1918; July 29, 1918; September 2, 1918; June 9, 1920; June 10, 1920; March 2–11, 1921; June 3, 1921; June 8, 1921; July 30, 1921; August 1, 1924; August 21, 1924; September 30, 1924; May 15, 1925; September 17, 1925; September 3, 1926; September 28, 1926; August 10, 1927; September 7, 1927; September 23, 1927; June 13, 1919; September 13, 1929.

14 *LSM*, June 17, 1920; November 19, 1925; *ADNH* 34 (1930), 12; Liga Argentina contra la Tuberculosis, *Memoria de la cruzada antituberculosa nacional* (Buenos Aires, 1936), 103–5.

15 *LSM*, June 17, 1919; *LV*, May 10, 1925; Liga Argentina contra la Tuberculosis, *Memoria de la cruzada antituberculosa nacional*, 61–68, 79; *AAT* 3 (1937), 279; *MMCBA*, *Año 1933–1934*, 715–33.

16 Susana Belmartino et al., *Fundamentos históricos de la construcción de relaciones de poder en el sector salud: Argentina 1940–1960* (Buenos Aires: OPS, 1991), chap. 4; Peter Ross, "Policy Formation and Implementation of Social Welfare in Peronist Argentina, 1943–1955" (Ph.D. diss., University of New South Wales, Sydney, 1988), chap. 2.

17 Tenti Fanfani, *Estado y pobreza*, 75.

18 Liga Argentina contra la Tuberculosis, *Memoria de la cruzada*, 139–42.

19 Secretaría de Salud Pública de la Nación, *Plan analítico de salud pública* (Buenos Aires, 1947), 2:1086.

20 Belmartino et al., *Fundamentos históricos de la construcción*, 363–64.

21 *MMCBA*, *Año 1883*, 24–36.

22 *MMCBA*, *Año 1918*, 1818–1819; *MMCBA*, *Año 1925*, 418–22; *MMCBA*, *Año 1933–1934*, 602–42; *MMCBA*, *Año 1935*, 715–34; *MMCBA*, *Año 1936*, 2:545–85; *AAT* 15, no. 2 (1939), 204–61.

23 Harold Wilensky, "The Professionalization of Everyone?," *American Journal of Sociology* 70, no. 2 (September 1964), 137–58.

24 *RAMA* 47 (1933); *ACPCT* (1942–50).

25 *LSM*, August 28, 1941, 548; September 4, 1941, 608.

26 Ibid., December 12, 1940, 1380.

27 *DSCD*, August 13, 1924.

28 *LN*, October 22, 1941.

29 Liga Argentina contra la Tuberculosis, *Memoria de la cruzada*, 12.

30 Emilio Coni, *Memorias de un médico higienista* (Buenos Aires: Flaiban, 1918), 518–20, 592–93; *LSM*, July 12, 1917.

31 *LV*, November 11, 1925; Liga Argentina contra la Tuberculosis, *Memoria de la cruzada*, 3.

32 Liga Argentina contra la Tuberculosis, *Memoria de la cruzada*, 16.

33 *Reflexiones*, November 1921, 5.

34 Ibid., 117–18.

35 Liga Argentina contra la Tuberculosis, *Memoria de la cruzada*, 110–18, 156–60.

36 Héctor Recalde, "La primera cruzada contra la tuberculosis. Buenos Aires, 1935," in José Panettieri, ed., *Argentina: Trabajadores entre dos guerras* (Buenos Aires: Eudeba, 2000), 80.

37 Liga Argentina contra la Tuberculosis, *Memoria de la cruzada*, 29–31, 143–44.

38 Izzo and Escardó, *Una campaña de propaganda sanitaria*, 25.

5. The Obsession with Contagion

1 *LDC* 2, 17 (1938), 2.

2 *RMQ* 5 (1868), 199.

3 Emilio de Arana, *La medicina y el proletariado* (Rosario: Tipografía El Comercio, 1899).

4 *MMCBA, Año 1912*, 150.

5 *LSM*, November 10, 1926.

6 *La Habitación Popular*, March 1935, 4.

7 *Revista Grafa* (1943–44); *CGT* (1942–44).

8 *AAT* 23, nos. 3–4 (1947), 169.

9 *LDC* 1, 1 (1936), 9.

10 Ibid., 11.

11 Ibid., 13.

12 *VCA* 9, 6 (1940), 363–64.

13 Intendencia Municipal de la Capital, Dirección General de la Administración y Asistencia Pública, *Instrucciones contra la propagación de la tuberculosis* (Buenos Aires: Lotería Nacional, 1894), 3–4.

14 *LDC* 1, 1 (1936), 12–13, 16.

15 *CC*, June 8, 1907; *LV*, October 23, 1928.

16 *La República*, July 25, 1871.

17 *LHE* (1901–5); Francisco Súnico, *Nociones de higiene escolar* (Buenos Aires: Taller Tipográfico de la Penitenciaría Nacional, 1902).

18 *EMEC*, February 1922, 100–101.

19 Ibid., July 31, 1924, 47.

20 Municipalidad de la Ciudad de Buenos Aires, Asistencia Pública, *La tuberculosis: A los niños de la Argentina* (Buenos Aires: Imprenta Mazzucco, 1927).

21 María Arcelli, *Ciencias domésticas: Apuntes de higiene de la habitación* (Buenos Aires: Moly, 1936), 44–45.

22 *DSCD*, July 30, 1921.

23 Ibid., May 5, 1933.

24 *EMEC*, February 1922, 101.

25 Silvina Gvirtz, "Higiene, moral y ciencia: Las funciones del tema 'cuerpo humano' en la escuela (Argentina 1920–1940)," in Adrián Ascolani, ed., *La educación en la Argentina: Estudios de historia* (Rosario: Ediciones del Arca, 1999), 185–96.

26 *AAT* 23, nos. 3–4 (1947); *ABEMS* 4, no. 6 (1933).

27 J. G. Pérez, *Nueva medicina doméstica, o sea el arte de conservar la salud, de conocer las enfermedades, sus remedios y aplicación al alcance de todos* (Buenos Aires: Imprenta de la Revista, 1854).

28 Nancy Tomes, "Spreading the Germ Theory: Sanitary Science and Home Economics, 1880–1930," in Sarah Stage and Virginia Vincent, eds., *Rethinking Home Economics: Women and the History of a Profession* (Ithaca: Cornell University Press, 1997).

29 Intendencia Municipal de la Capital, Dirección General de la Administración y Asistencia Pública, *Instrucciones contra la propagación de la tuberculosis* (Buenos Aires: Lotería Nacional, 1894), 3.

30 *AAT* 17, no. 2 (1941), 238.

31 *ASM* 3 (1901), 738; *LSM*, October 24, 1918, 510.

32 Antonio Cetrángolo, *Consejos para evitar la propagación de la tuberculosis* (Buenos Aires, 1930), 16.

33 *ADNH* 19, no. 3 (1912), 1007.

34 Nicolás Lozano, "Contribución al estudio de la etiología y profilaxis de la tuberculosis desde el punto de vista sociológico," in *Proceedings of the Second Pan American Scientific Congress*, Washington, December 1915, Washington, 1917, 435.

35 Norbert Elias, *The History of Manners* (New York: Pantheon, 1978), 156–60.

36 *LSM*, March 14, 1905.

37 Roque Izzo and Florencio Escardó, *Una campaña de propaganda sanitaria* (Buenos Aires: Centro de Investigaciones Tisiológicas, 1940), 47.

38 Cetrángolo, *Consejos para evitar la tuberculosis*, 18, 20, 23.

39 Lozano, "Contribución al estudio de la etiología y profilaxis de la tuberculosis desde el punto de vista sociológico," in *Proceedings Second Pan American Scientific Congress*, 427, 428.

40 *El Progreso de la Boca*, January 17, 1904; *LV*, December 24, 1919; *EMEC*, April 1927, 101; *LDC* 1, no. 1 (1936), 18; *VCA* 3, no. 7 (1937), 473.

41 Marcelo Castelli, *Cosquín: Falsedad y verdad* (Cosquín, Córdoba, 1954), 353, 439.

42 *LDC* 1, no. 2 (1936).

43 José Antonio Wilde, *Compendio de higiene pública y privada* (Buenos Aires: Casa Peuser, 1884 [1868]); Pilar Pascual de San Juan, *Guía de la mujer o lecciones de economía doméstica* (Buenos Aires, 1880); Municipalidad de la Capital, *Instrucciones generales para el vecindario sobre higiene pública y privada* (Buenos Aires: Kraft, 1891); Gregorio Aráoz Alfaro, *El libro de las madres: Pequeño tratado práctico de higiene del niño* (Buenos Aires: Etchepareborda, 1899); Municipalidad de Buenos Aires, Administración y Asistencia Pública, *Disposiciones generales para evitar la propagación de enfermedades epidémicas* (Buenos Aires: Kraft, 1916); Aurora S. Del Castaño, *El vademécum del hogar: Tratado práctico de economía doméstica y labores* (Buenos Aires: Imprenta Tragant, 1906 [1903]); *LV*, May 20, 1912; Angel Bassi, *Gobierno, administración e higiene del hogar* (Buenos Aires: Cabaut Editores, 1914); *ASM* 6 (1917); Luis Barrantes Molina, *Para mi hogar: Síntesis de economía y sociabilidad domésticas* (Buenos Aires, 1923); *LDC* 2, no. 11 (1938); María Arcelli, *Ciencias domésticas: Apuntes de higiene de la habitación* (Buenos Aires, 1936); Luis Boffi, *La misión de la enfermera en la lucha antituberculosa* (Buenos Aires, 1939); Roque Izzo and Florencio Escardó, *Una campaña de propaganda sanitaria.*

44 Bassi, *Gobierno, administración e higiene del hogar*, 83.

45 Gregorio Aráoz Alfaro, "Errores perjudiciales y nociones nuevas en materia de tuberculosis," *Reflexiones*, March 1922, 3.

46 Izzo and Escardó, *Una campaña de propaganda sanitaria*, 110.

47 Richard L. Riley, "Disease Transmission and Contagion Control," *American Review of Respiratory Disease* 125 (1982), 16–19.

48 Pascual de San Juan, *Guía de la mujer o lecciones de economía doméstica*, 38; Del Castaño, *El vademécum del hogar*, 8; Barrantes Molina, *Para mi hogar*, 18–19.

49 Pascual de San Juan, *Guía de la mujer o lecciones de economía doméstica*, 61.

50 Del Castaño, *El vademécum del hogar*, 4.

51 Bassi, *Gobierno, administración e higiene del hogar*, 14.

52 Barrantes Molina, *Para mi hogar*, 23, 21.

53 Juan P. Riera, "Influencia de las costumbres en las enfermedades" (Ph.D. diss., Universidad de Buenos Aires, 1878), 39; Municipalidad de la Ciudad de Buenos Aires, *Digesto de ordenanzas* (Buenos Aires, 1884); *LSM*, October 15, 1903; *LV*, June 9, 1906.

54 Manuel Augusto Montes de Oca, "Ensayo sobre las efermedades de Buenos Aires" (Ph.D. diss., Universidad de Buenos Aires, 1854), 38, 39.

55 Arturo Balbastro, "La mujer argentina: Estudio médico social" (Ph.D. diss., Universidad de Buenos Aires, 1892), 78–82.

56 Elvira Rawson de Dellepiane, "Apuntes sobre higiene de la mujer" (Ph.D. diss., Universidad de Buenos Aires, 1892), 18, 24, 42, 46.

57 *AM*, February 2, 1914, 127.

58 García Romero, "Psicología, terreno y ambiente en la tuberculosis pulmonar," in Enrique Noguera and Luis Huerta, *Genética, eugenesia y pedagogía sexual* (Madrid: Javier Morata, 1934), 54.

59 Ibid., 53; Riera, "Influencia de las costumbres en las enfermedades," 24.

60 Barrantes Molina, *Para mi hogar: Síntesis de economía y sociabilidad domésticas*, 181.

61 Bassi, *Gobierno, administración e higiene del hogar*, 53.

62 *VCA*, August 1941, 616–17, 621; *VN* 3, no. 30 (1938), 27.

63 *EG*, February 10, 1923.

64 Ibid., December 13, 1919; June 13, 1925.

65 *Revista Fray Mocho* 103 (1914).

66 *CC*, May 28, 1910; *Vida Porteña* 37 (1914); *EG*, April 17, 1920; *PBT* 44 (1905); *Revista Fray Mocho* 103 (1914).

67 *PBT* 237 (1909).

68 *PBT* 47 (1905); *PBT* 237 (1909).

69 *LR*, August 8, 1945.

70 *Chicas*, January 27, 1949.

71 Montes de Oca, "Ensayo sobre las enfermedades," 39.

72 José Antonio Wilde, *Compendio de higiene pública y privada al alcance de todos* (Buenos Aires, Imprenta Bernheim, 1868), 65.

73 Bassi, *Gobierno, administración e higiene del hogar*, 371.

74 Barrantes Molina, *Para mi hogar*, chap. XII.

75 *PT*, January 20, 1925.

76 David Kunzle, *Fashion and Fetishism: A Social History of the Corset, Tight-lacing and Other Forms of Body Sculpture in the West* (Totowa, N.J.: Rowman and Little-field, 1982), 18, 42; Leigh Summers, *Bound to Please: A History of the Victoria Corset* (New York: Berg, 2001), 213.

77 Eugenio Ramírez, "La tuberculosis debe ser un impedimento para la celebración del matrimonio" (Ph.D. diss., Universidad de Buenos Aires, 1880), 40; APCCA 8 (1909), 264; Angel Navarro Blasco, "La tuberculosis conyugal: Contagio y matrimonio," in Enrique Noguera and Luis Huerta, *Genética, eugenesia y pedagogía*, 2:70; LSM, December 5, 1940.

78 Antonio Cetrángolo, *Treinta años curando tuberculosos* (Buenos Aires: Hachette, 1945), 101.

79 Navarro Blasco, "La tuberculosis conyugal: Contagio y matrimonio," 71.

80 LV, December 16, 1899.

81 Izzo and Escardó, *Una campaña de propaganda sanitaria*, 99.

82 EMEC, July 1906, 10.

83 LDC 2, no. 17–18 (1938), 6; Antonio Cetrángolo, *La tuberculosis: Consejos*, 11.

84 Carlos Fonso Gandolfo and Hector Norrie, "Cómo vive el tuberculoso indigente," in *Segunda conferencia nacional de profilaxis antituberculosa* (Rosario, 1919), 318.

85 LDC 2, no. 17–18 (1938), 6.

86 Florencio Sánchez, "Los derechos de la salud," in *El teatro de Florencio Sánchez* (Buenos Aires: Tor, 1917), 19.

87 Alejandro Albarracín, "Consideraciones sobre la tisis pulmonar" (Ph.D. diss., Universidad de Buenos Aires, 1875), 83.

88 Lozano, "Contribución al estudio de la etiología y profilaxis de la tuberculosis," 433.

89 Navarro Blasco, "La tuberculosis conyugal," 71; NT, September 15, 1923.

90 Ibid., 70; *Ideas*, March 3, 1929; LSM, March 25, 1919.

91 VCA, February 1937, 308.

92 Cetrángolo, *La tuberculosis: Consejos a los enfermos*, 14; Navarro Blasco, "La tuberculosis conyugal," 81.

93 Lozano, "Contribución al estudio de la etiología y profilaxis," 433.

94 Carlos Bernaldo de Quirós, *Eugenesia jurídica y social: Derecho eugenésico argentino* (Buenos Aires: Ideas, 1943), 44–45.

95 Ramirez, "La tuberculosis debe ser un impedimento," 41–43.

96 Juan Carlos Loz, *La familia en el código civil argentino* (Córdoba, 1935), 343–44; LSM, March 17, 1910, 420; Jorge Frías, *El matrimonio: Sus impedimentos y nulidades, derecho comparado* (Buenos Aires, 1941), 155–61.

97 Paulina Luisi, *Por una mejor descendencia* (Buenos Aires, 1919), 25–26.

98 LV, November 22, 1916; November 15, 1916; January 5, 1917.

99 LSM, October 6, 1912, 471.

100 VCA November 1936, 133–34.

101 José Lascano and Gumersido Sayago, "Tuberculosis y embarazo," *II congreso argentino de obstetricia y ginecología* (Buenos Aires: Caporaleti, 1934), 57.

102 Juan Lazarte, *La socialización de la medicina: Estructurando una nueva sanidad* (Buenos Aires: Imán, 1934), 70; *La revolución sexual de nuestro tiempo* (Buenos Aires, 1932).

103 *LP*, October 12, 1915; January 11, 1907; January 16, 1907; January 12, 1909; October 12, 1915; September 28, 1925; *ER*, January 1, 1907; *El Obrero Ebanista*, May 1920; *Ideas*, August 1921; *Acción Obrera*, March 1926; *Brazo y Cerebro*, January 5, 1926.

104 *El Obrero Ebanista*, May 1929; *Brazo y Cerebro*, January 5, 1926.

105 Luis Jimenez de Asúa, "La esterilización y la castración de anormales y delincuentes," *Revista La Ley*, February 12, 1941; Bernaldo de Quirós, *Eugenesia jurídica y social*, 108.

106 *LV*, January 5, 1917; Carlos Bernaldo de Quirós, *La esterilización* (Buenos Aires, 1934); Manuel Luis Pérez, *Esterilización* (Buenos Aires, 1940).

107 Hugo Vezzetti, *Aventuras de Freud en el país de los argentinos: De José Ingenieros a Enrique Pichón Riviere* (Buenos Aires: Paidós, 1996), chap. 2.

108 T. H. Van de Velde, *Fertilidad e infertilidad en el matrimonio* (Buenos Aires: Claridad, 1940), 225, 429.

109 Ricardo Schwarcz, "Embarazo, parto y aborto artificial en la mujer tuberculosa," *IATRIA: Revista del consorcio de médicos católicos*, October 1939.

110 Juan P. Munzinger, "Algunas consideraciones sobre tuberculosis y embarazo" (Ph.D. diss., Universidad de Buenos Aires, 1920).

111 *LSM*, July 10, 1919; October 2, 1919; Alejandro Bunge, *Una nueva Argentina* (Buenos Aires: Kraft, 1940), 48–49.

112 *BMSA* 19, no. 103–5 (1931), 94.

113 Eduardo Wilde, *Curso de higiene pública: Lecciones en el colegio nacional de Buenos Aires* (Buenos Aires: Mayo, 1878).

114 *LSM*, May 25, 1919.

115 *LV*, December 15, 1916.

116 *BMSA* 28, no. 221–22 (1940), 376.

117 Cetrángolo, *La tuberculosis: Consejos a los enfermos*, 14.

118 Bernaldo de Quirós, *Eugenesia jurídica y social* 2:14, 15.

119 *VCA* 3, no. 2 (1936), 133–34; Hugo Vezzetti, "Viva cien años: Algunas consideraciones sobre familia y matrimonio en Argentina," in *Punto de Vista: Revista de Cultura*, August 1986, 9.

120 *LSM*, December 5, 1901.

121 *ABEMS* 3, 36 (1935).

122 Enrique Díaz de Guijarro, *El impedimento matrimonial de la enfermedad: Matrimonio y eugenesia* (Buenos Aires: Kraft, 1944), 330–31.

123 Alfredo Palacios, *La justicia social* (Buenos Aires: Claridad, 1954 [1922]), 323; Nancy Stepan, *"The Hour of Eugenics": Race, Gender and Nation in Latin America* (Ithaca: Cornell University Press, 1991), 118–19.

124 Bernaldo de Quirós, *Eugenesia jurídica y social*, 213; *ABEMS* 1 (1933), 14–16.

125 Carlos Bernaldo de Quirós, *Problemas demográficos argentinos* (Buenos Aires: Kraft, 1942), 99.

126 *ABEMS* 2, no. 30–31 (1934).

127 Palacios, *La justicia social*, 323.

128 *DSCD* 9 (1946), 16.

129 Antonio Cetrángolo, "El instinto de conservación frente a la tuberculosis," *Reflexiones*, July 1921, 2–3.

130 *APCCA* 8 (1909), 267; *AAT* 32, no. 1–2 (1947), 189.

131 *La República*, July 25, 1871; Eduardo Wilde, "El hipo" (Ph.D. diss., Universidad de Buenos Aires, 1870), 7–8.

132 *PBT* 2, no. 26 (1905), 62.

133 Súnico, *La tuberculosis en las sierras de Córdoba*, 385, 253; Telémaco Susini, "Prólogo," in Súnico, *La tuberculosis en las sierras de Córdoba*, xiv.

134 Súnico, *La tuberculosis en las sierras de Córdoba*, 253; *LSM*, June 13, 1918; *LDC* 1, no. 1 (1936); *LDC* 2, no. 7 (1937).

135 *LV*, March 25, 1917; November 18, 1920.

136 *PBT* 3, no. 85 (1906), 87.

137 *LR*, February 10, 1921.

138 *El Rebelde*, June 22, 1901; *LPR*, July 27, 1901.

139 *Ciencia Social* 2 (1900).

140 *El Obrero en Madera*, October 1906.

141 *Acción Obrera*, June 1927; October 1928.

142 *Ideas*, April 30, 1936.

143 *LPR*, October 5, 1901; *El Rebelde*, September 29, 1901; *Acción Obrera*, May 1928.

144 *El Obrero en Dulce* 7 (1921).

145 *Acción Obrera*, May 1928.

146 *Ideas*, July 1923.

147 *Acción Obrera*, October 1928; *LPR*, October 24, 1903; *El Azote*, October 1911; *El Rebelde*, September 29, 1901; *NT*, September 15, 1923.

148 Súnico, *La tuberculosis en las sierras de Córdoba*, v, vii, xii, xiii, 654, 659, 663.

149 *LSM*, March 31, 1938; *AAT* 17, no. 2 (1941), 230; *VCA* 6, no. 10 (1939), 636; *LDC* 2, no. 10 (1938); Navarro Blasco, "La tuberculosis conyugal," 81.

150 *VCA* 3, no. 2 (1936), 162; *LDC*, October 10, 1936, 10.

151 Secretaría de Salud Pública de la Nación, *Plan analítico de salud pública* (Buenos Aires, 1947), 2:1067.

6. A Disease of Excesses

1 Nicolás Lozano, "Contribución al estudio de la etiología y profilaxis de la tuberculosis desde el punto de vista sociológico," in *Proceedings of the Second Pan American Scientific Congress*, Washington, 1917, 431.

2 *La Educación: Periódico Quincenal*, September 14, 1886, 336.

3 Luis Boffi, *Misión de la enfermera en la lucha antituberculosa* (Buenos Aires: El Ateneo, 1939), 15; Luis Oscar Romero, *Es contagiosa la tuberculosis?* (Buenos Aires: Claridad, 1924), 24.

4 *LSM*, October 11, 1900, 526; Susan Sontag, *Illness and Its Metaphors* (New York: Farrar, Straus and Giroux, 1978), 46.

5 *VCA* 11 (1936), 154, 125.

6 Antonio Cetrángolo, *Treinta años curando tuberculosos* (Buenos Aires: Hachette, 1945), 169; *ABEMS* 1, no. 4 (1933), 9, 8.

7 *VCA* 11 (1936), 125.

8 Hugo Vezzetti, *Aventuras de Freud en el país de los argentinos: De José Ingenieros a Enrique Pichon Riviere* (Buenos Aires: Paidós, 1996), 49, 112–14.

9 Dora Barrancos, "Anarquismo y Sexualidad," in Diego Armus, ed., *Mundo urbano y cultura popular: Estudios de historia social Argentina* (Buenos Aires: Sudamericana, 1990), 17–37.

10 *LSM*, August 5, 1926, 345.

11 Julio Noguera Toledo, "El instinto sexual del tuberculoso," in Enrique Noguera and Luis Huerta, *Genética, eugenesia y pedagogía sexual* (Madrid: Javier Morata, 1964), 2:59, 62.

12 Eugenio Ramírez, "La tuberculosis debe ser un impedimento para la celebración del matrimonio" (Ph.D. diss., Universidad de Buenos Aires, 1880), 41.

13 Angel Navarro Blasco, "La tuberculosis conyugal: Contagio y matrimonio," in Enrique Noguera and Luis Huerta, *Genética, eugenesia y pedagogía sexual*, 79.

14 Eugenio Perez, "Opúsculo sobre la Tisis pulmonar" (Ph.D. diss., Universidad de Buenos Aires, 1843), 37; Juan P. Riera, "Influencia de las costumbres en las enfermedades" (Ph.D. diss., Universidad de Buenos Aires, 1878), 22; *El Despertar Gallego* 1 (1906); *Ideas* 11 (1927); *LSM*, October 11, 1900, 529.

15 Vezzetti, *Aventuras de Freud en el país de los argentinos*, 119, 78.

16 Noguera Toledo, "El instinto sexual del tuberculoso," 62.

17 *Reflexiones*, October 1921, 11.

18 Jean Baptiste Baumes, *De la pthisie pulmonaire* (1783); P. Ch. A. Louis, *Recherches anatomico-pathologiques et therapéutiques sur la pthisie* (1843); G. Daremberg, *Les différents formes cliniques et sociales de la tuberculose* (1905), quoted in Pierre Guillaume, *Du desespoir au salut: Les tuberculeux aux XIX et XX siecles* (Paris: Aubier, 1986), 73, 161.

19 Ramírez, "La tuberculosis debe ser un impedimento," 41.

20 *APCCA* 8 (1909), 264.

21 Navarro Blasco, "La tuberculosis conyugal," 70; *LSM*, December 5, 1940.

22 *LSM*, January 18, 1934; *VTCD* 1 (1921), 96, 104–16; José García Romero, "Psicología, terreno y ambiente en tuberculosis pulmonar," in Noguera and Huerta, *Genética, eugenesia y pedagogía sexual*, 2:42.

23 Pablo Barlaro, *Lecciones de patología médica* (Buenos Aires: CADOM, 1929), 2:632.

24 Antonio Cetrángolo, *La tuberculosis: Consejos para evitar la propagación de la tuberculosis y curarse de ella* (Buenos Aires: Sociedad Luz, 1930), 8.

25 Ulises Petit de Murat, *El balcón hacia la muerte* (Buenos Aires: Lautaro, 1943), 146.

26 *ADNH* 37 (1936), 54.

27 *LSM*, August 5, 1926; June 13, 1940; *LV*, September 17, 1904; Gumersindo Sayago

and Francisco Torres, "Encuesta epidemiológica de las bailarinas en Córdoba," in vol. 2 of *V Congreso Panamericano de la Tuberculosis, 1940* (Buenos Aires: 1941).

28 *Ideas*, March 3, 1929.

29 Navarro Blasco, "La tuberculosis conyugal," 70.

30 LSM, August 5, 1926; Cetrángolo, *La tuberculosis: Consejos a los enfermos*, 14.

31 VTCD 1 (1921), 106.

32 ABEMS (1933), 8; Antonio Cetrángolo, *Treinta años curando tuberculosos*, 163–64; LSM, August 5, 1936, 352; EDM, January 4, 1943; AAT 30, no. 3–4 (1954).

33 Noguera Toledo, "El instinto sexual del tuberculoso," 58, 63.

34 *La Voz de la Mujer*, January 31, 1896; *El Rebelde*, January 6, 1901.

35 Petit de Murat, *El balcón hacia la muerte*, 147.

36 García Romero, "Psicología, terreno y ambiente en tuberculosis pulmonar," 42.

37 Navarro Blasco, "La tuberculosis conyugal," 79.

38 Manuel Puig, *Boquitas pintadas* (Buenos Aires: Sudamericana, 1969), 64.

39 APCCA 6 (1907), 710.

40 Francisco Súnico, *La tuberculosis en las sierras de Córdoba* (Buenos Aires: de Martino, 1922), 217, 219; APCCA 6 (1907), 710, 715–19.

41 *El Obrero Panadero*, May 1913.

42 Carlos Lanús, "El alcoholismo" (Ph.D. diss., Universidad de Buenos Aires, 1876); Juan P. Riera, "Influencia de las costumbres en las enfermedades" (Ph.D. diss., Universidad de Buenos Aires, 1878); Avelino Sandoval, "El alcohol tomado como alimento de ahorro o antidesnutrimiento de los pobres y trabajadores" (Ph.D. diss., Universidad de Buenos Aires, 1878); Jacobo García, "Estudio sobre el alcohol y el alcoholismo" (Ph.D. diss., Universidad de Buenos Aires, 1881); Manuel de la Cárcova, "Alcoholismo" (Ph.D. diss., Universidad de Buenos Aires, 1882).

43 Benjamin Canard, "La embriaguez" (Ph.D. diss., Universidad de Buenos Aires, 1872); LSM, June 25, 1913, 1471; September 11, 1919, 307; Luis Poviña, "Contribución al estudio del alcoholismo en la República Argentina" (Ph.D. diss., Universidad de Buenos Aires, 1896), 27.

44 Poviña, "Contribución al estudio del alcoholismo," 18–20, 34.

45 LV, January 1, 1917; VN 7, no. 90 (1944), 12; VCA 19 (1945), 351–54.

46 Lanús, "El alcoholismo," 61.

47 LSM, October 11, 1900, 528.

48 Esteban Lucotti, "Alcoholismo y tuberculosis" (Ph.D. diss., Universidad de Buenos Aires, 1918), 75.

49 BLAT 7, 1 (1907); Luis Boffi, *Alcoholismo y tuberculosis* (Buenos Aires, 1939), 5.

50 Eduardo Menéndez, "'Saber médico' y 'saber popular': El modelo hegemónico y su función ideológica en el proceso de alcoholización," *Estudios Sociológicos* 3, 8 (1985), 292–94.

51 LV, February 10, 1916.

52 Lozano, "Contribución al estudio de la etiología y profilaxis de la tuberculosis," 431.

53 Boffi, *Alcoholismo y tuberculosis*, 6; LSM, June 19, 1913, 1468; DSCD, August 20, 1912.

54 *LSM*, December 5, 1901, 774; Eduardo Rojas, "El sweating system: Su importancia en Buenos Aires" (Ph.D. diss., Universidad de Buenos Aires, 1913), chap. 3; Clemente Alvarez, "Plan general de profilaxis antituberculosa en la república," in *Actas y trabajos* (Córdoba, 1917), 59.

55 Sandoval, "El alcohol tomado como alimento de ahorro," 9, 40–43.

56 Poviña, "Contribución al estudio," 50.

57 *LSM*, October 10, 1912.

58 *LPR*, October 24, 1903; Juan B. Obarrio, *Efectos del alcoholismo en la infancia* (Buenos Aires, 1926), 3.

59 Alberto Martinez, *Manuel du voyageur: Baedeker de la République Argentine* (Barcelona: López Robert, 1907), 515–18.

60 *RSM* 16 (1917), 616.

61 *ABEMS* 8, no. 94 (1940), 15.

62 *ADNH* 11, no. 8 (1904), 438; *LP*, October 26, 1883; *El Progreso de la Boca*, December 1900; *MA*, May 1917; *LV*, July 12, 1925.

63 *ADNH* 37, no. 2 (1936), 35.

64 *El Obrero Panadero*, September 9, 1900; *BDNT*, March 31, 1910, 73; *El Obrero en Madera*, September 1911; Floreal Ferrara, *El alcoholismo en América Latina* (Buenos Aires: Palestra, 1961), 120.

65 *LSM*, December 11, 1902, 1012.

66 Ferrara, *El alcoholismo en América Latina*, 198.

67 Joseph Gusfield, "Passage to Play: Rituals of Drinking Time in American Society," in Mary Douglas, ed., *Constructive Drinking: Perspectives on Drink from Anthropology* (Cambridge, 1987), 79–83.

68 *LSM*, November 27, 1901; *LV*, February 10, 1916; *Anuario Socialista, 1928* (Buenos Aires: La Vanguardia, 1929), 226.

69 Libros de Notas de la Policía, 37, January 6, 1884, quoted in Sandra Gayol, "Ebrios y divertidos: La estrategia del alcohol en Buenos Aires, 1860–1900," *Siglo XIX*, 13 (1993), 78; *BDNT*, March 31, 1910, 73.

70 Augusto Bunge, *El alcoholismo* (Buenos Aires, 1912), 30, 7.

71 *LPR*, July 20, 1901; August 11, 1904; January 9, 1906; February 9, 1906; December 3, 1907.

72 Sociedad Luz, *Guerra al alcohol: Antología antialcohólica* (Buenos Aires: Sociedad Luz, 1926).

73 *El Rebelde*, July 7, 1900.

74 *ADNH* 16, no. 7 (1909), 324.

75 *LSM*, July 16, 1942, 147–49.

76 Ibid., November 16, 1938, 1138–39; February 14, 1940, 278–85.

77 Estela Ferreiros and Martha Morey, *Enfermedades del trabajador* (Buenos Aires: Hammurabi, 1985), 67–68; Departamento Nacional del Trabajo, *Boletín Informativo*, May 1934, 3920; *LPMA* 24, no. 1 (1938), 87–88; *AAT* 23, no. 3–4 (1947), 216.

78 *DSCD*, September 19, 1941.

79 *LPMA* 28, no. 17 (1941), 880–90; *LPMA* 36, no. 39 (1949), 1972–76; *AAT* 24, no. 1–2 (1948), 74–77; *Revista de Jurisprudencia Argentina* 1 (1949), 565.

80 *El Obrero Panadero,* October 10, 1894; *El Obrero Textil,* June 1912; *Acción Obrera,* October 1928; *El Obrero Textil,* April 1941.

81 Daniel James, *Doña María: History, Memory and Political Identity in Argentina* (Durham: Duke University Press, 2004), 246.

82 José Ingenieros, *La jornada de trabajo* (Buenos Aires: Librería Obrera, 1899), 15–16.

83 *DSDC,* June 8, 1908.

84 Augusto Bunge, *Las conquistas de la higiene social: Informe presentado al excelentísimo gobierno nacional* (Buenos Aires: Imprenta Coni, 1910), 1:12, 79, 188, 133, 190.

85 Francisco Súnico, *La tuberculosis en las sierras de Córdoba* (Buenos Aires: de Martino, 1922), 654.

86 Carlos Caminos, "Prólogo a la primera edición de 1923," in Alfredo Palacios, *La fatiga y sus proyecciones sociales: Investigaciones de laboratorio en los talleres del estado* (Buenos Aires: La Vanguardia, 1935), 14–15.

87 Palacios, *La fatiga y sus proyecciones sociales,* 307, 324, 325.

88 *El Rebelde,* June 22, 1901; *LPR,* July 27, 1901.

89 Ernesto Demarco, "Trabajo y tuberculosis," in *Primer congreso argentino de medicina del trabajo* (Buenos Aires, 1948), 2:149–52.

90 *EMP* 4 (1948), 35.

91 *ADNH* 33 (1927), 210.

92 Alain Cottereau, "La tuberculose: Maladie urbaine ou maladie de l'usure au travail? Critique d'une epidémiologie officielle: le cas de Paris," *Sociologie du Travail* 20, no. 2 (1978), 193–207; Karl Figlio, "Chlorosis and Chronic Disease in Nineteenth-Century Britain: The Social Construction of Somatic Illness in a Capitalist Society," *Social History* 3, no. 2 (1978), 167–98; Paul Weindling, ed., *The Social History of Occupational Health* (London, 1985); Diego Armus, "Enfermedad, ambiente urbano e higiene social: Rosario entre fines del siglo XIX y comienzos del XX," in Diego Armus, ed., *Sectores populares y vida urbana* (Buenos Aires: CLACSO, 1984).

93 *LSM,* May 16, 1918.

94 *RATEP* 21 (1957), 95.

95 *LPM,* January 5, 1938, 87–88; April 23, 1941, 880–90; October 1, 1949, 1972–76; *AAT* (1947), 212–19; *AAT* (1948), 74–77; *BDNT,* May 1934, 3920.

96 Mirta Zaida Lobato, *Historia de las trabajadoras en la Argentina, 1869–1960* (Buenos Aires: Edhasa, 2007), chap 1.

97 Ricardo Etcheberry, "La ley Argentina sobre reglamentación del trabajo en las mujeres y niños" (Ph.D. diss., Universidad de Buenos Aires, 1918).

98 Rojas "El Sweating System"; Bunge, *Las conquistas de la higiene social,* 132, 144; *BDNT* 30 (1915), 80–82, 85–87, 106.

99 Rojas, "El Sweating System," chap. 5; *BDNT* 30 (1915), 106.

100 *ADNH* 11 (1904), 438.

101 *La Nación: Edición aniversario de la independiencia* (Buenos Aires: La Nación, 1916), 59; *BNDT* 30 (1915), 84.

102 *LSM*, May 16, 1918.

103 *LN*, July 12, 1904; *El País*, January 22, 1900; *BDNH*, June 1910, 621, 622.

104 *BMSA* 7, no. 75–84 (1918).

105 *BMSA* 6, no. 71–72 (1917), 683.

106 *MA*, September 17, 1919.

107 *BMSA* 2, no. 15–16 (1913), 65.

108 *MMCBA, Año 1918*, 191; *VTCD*, July–September 1933, 1888; *MMCBA, Año 1935*, 724.

109 *LSM*, January 10, 1918; *ADNH* 33 (1927), 210.

110 *LV*, April 9, 1924.

111 *ADNH* 15, 5 (1909), 191.

112 *AAT* (April–June 1947), 215–17.

113 *MMCBA, Año 1908*, 190; *MMCBA, Año 1933–1934*, 1935, 723.

114 *BDNT* 24 (1913), 558.

115 Bunge, *Las conquistas de la higiene social*, 195; *LSM*, July 16, 1942; *LDC* 2, no. 17–18 (1938), 6; *RATEP* 21, no. 2 (1957), 100.

116 *LSM*, October 9, 1902; Liga Argentina contra la Tuberculosis, *Memoria de la cruzada antituberculosa naciona* (Buenos Aires: Liga Argentina contra la Tuberculosis, 1936), 207.

117 *ADNH* 32 (1926), 100–103.

118 *El Obrero Panadero*, October 16, 1894; *LV*, November 13, 1908.

119 *ADNH* 11, no. 10 (1904), 444–45; *El Obrero Panadero*, August 1913.

120 *El Obrero Panadero*, August 1913.

121 *ADNH* 11, no. 10 (1904), 444–45.

122 *El Obrero Panadero*, January 1928.

123 Ibid., March 1913.

124 *BDNT* 24 (1913), 555, 558; *LSM*, May 16, 1918.

125 Bunge, *Las conquistas de la higiene social*, 195; *LPMA* 36, no. 40 (1949), 2195; *LV*, December 18, 1913; February 13, 1921.

126 *Idea Hospitalaria* 1, no. 6 (July 1922).

127 *AAT* 28, no. 1–2 (1952), 28.

128 Bunge, *Las conquistas de la Higiene social*, 128, 193; *RATEP* 21, no. 2 (1957), 96.

129 *ADNH* 16, no. 9 (1909), 451; Walter Pagel et al., *Pulmonary Tuberculosis: Bacteriology, Pathology, Diagnosis, Management, Epidemiology, and Prevention* (Oxford, Oxford University Press, 1964), 66.

130 *ADNH* 16, no. 9 (1909), 451; *RATEP* 21, no. 2 (1957), 96–97; *Ahora* (1941), 640.

131 *BDNT* 24 (1913), 554.

132 Bunge, *Las conquistas de la higiene social*, 128; *El Obrero Gráfico*, June 16, 1908; September 1913; *Acción Obrera*, November 17, 1914.

133 Adrián Patroni, *Los trabajadores en la Argentina* (Buenos Aires, 1898), 136–37.

134 *BDNT* 24 (1913), 554.

135 Ibid., 557; Bunge, *Las conquistas de la higiene social*, 124.

136 *ADNH* 11, no. 10 (904), 436.

137 *BDNT* 24 (1913), 558.

138 *ADNH* 16, no. 9 (1909), 450.

139 *LV*, February 2, 1916.

140 *RMQ* 3 (1866), 51–52.

141 Ciudad de Buenos Aires, *Censo general de población, edificación, comercio e industria de la ciudad de Buenos Aires, 1887* (Buenos Aires: 1889), 193.

142 Samuel Gache, *Les logements ouvrières a Buenos Ayres* (Paris: G. Steinheil, 1900), 64, 75; José Penna and Horacio Madero, *La administración sanitaria y asistencia pública de la ciudad de Buenos Aires* (Buenos Aires, 1910), vol. 1, chap. 6; *RMQ* 3 (1866), 37; *LSM*, October 10, 1900; Francisco Súnico, *La tuberculosis en las sierras de Córdoba* (Buenos Aires: de Martino, 1922), 136; *LDC* 1, no. 1 (1936), 17; *LLA* 6 (1906), 92; *Infancia y Juventud*, July 1943, 138.

143 Guillermo Rawson, *Escritos y discursos* (Buenos Aires: Compañía Sudamericana de Billetes, 1891), 1:108.

144 Ibid., 83, 88.

145 Eduardo Wilde, "Curso de higiene pública," in *Obras completas* (Buenos Aires, 1914), 3:30; Rawson, *Escritos y discursos*, 1:108; Gache, *Les logements ouvrières a Buenos Ayres*, 94.

146 Rawson, *Escritos y discursos*, 1:47.

147 Wilde, "Curso de higiene pública," 30.

148 *MMCBA*, *Año 1879* (Buenos Aires: Martín Biedma, 1880), 27–29.

149 Rawson, *Escritos y discursos*, 1:115.

150 Gache, *Les logements ouvrières a Buenos Ayres*, 55.

151 *BDNT* 3 (1907), 480.

152 *LV*, February 26, 1918.

153 *BMSA*, May 1920, 188–89; *Ideas*, August 1921.

154 *Anuario Socialista* (Buenos Aires: La Vanguardia, 1942), 97.

155 Municipalidad de Buenos Aires, *Anuario estadístico de la ciudad de Buenos Aires* (Buenos Aires: Dirección General de Estadística Municipal, 1892), 139.

156 Gache, *Les logements ouvrières a Buenos Ayres*, 64, 75.

157 Oficina Demográfica Nacional, *Boletín demográfico argentino* (Buenos Aires: Ministerio del Interior, 1900).

158 Municipalidad de la Ciudad de Buenos Aires, *Censo general de la ciudad de Buenos Aires de 1904* (Buenos Aires, 1906), 29, 31, 123.

159 *LSM*, October 11, 1900; December 5, 1901.

160 Ibid., December 5, 1901; *ADNH* 9, no. 3 (1901), 123.

161 *LSM*, March 3, 1918.

162 *ADNH* 37, no. 2 (1936), 66–67; *Infancia y Juventud*, July 1934, 138; *Vida Comunal*, January 3, 1932.

163 *LV*, October 30, 1928.

164 *ADNH* 37, no. 2 (1936), 69.

165 José María Balbi Robecco, "Tuberculosis y hacinamiento: Estudio sobre 98 familias," in *RAMA* 60 (1946), 583; "Vivienda y tuberculosis," in *Revista de Medicina y Ciencias Afines*, September 1945; Raúl Vacarezza, "Tuberculosis y vivienda: Estudio sobre 250 grupos familiares," in *ACPCT* 3 (1941).

7. Immigration, Race, and Tuberculosis

1 *ADNH* 43 (1936), 70–71, 85; Generoso Schiavone, "Indice de tuberculinización según el carácter étnico de nuestra población," in *V congreso panamericano de la tuberculosis, Córdoba, 1940* (Córdoba, 1940), 2:593.

2 Domingo Salvarezza, "Tisis pulmonar" (Ph.D. diss., Universidad de Buenos Aires, 1866), 11–12; D. J. G. Pérez, *Medicina doméstica, o sea el arte de conservar la salud, de conocer las enfermedades, sus remedios y aplicación, al alcance de todos* (Buenos Aires: Imprenta de la Revista, 1854), 226.

3 Abel Domíngues, "Tratamiento climatérico de la tuberculosis pulmonar en la República Argentina" (Ph.D. diss., Universidad de Buenos Aires, 1895), 41; Marcelo Viñas, "La herencia en la tuberculosis" (Ph.D. diss., Universidad de Buenos Aires, 1896); Leticia Acosta, "La defensa de la infancia contra la tuberculosis" (Ph.D. diss., Universidad de Buenos Aires, 1918); Leónidas Silva, "Conceptos modernos sobre tuberculosis pulmonar" (Ph.D. diss., Universidad de Buenos Aires, 1919); Juan Munzinger, "Algunas consideraciones sobre tuberculosis y embarazo" (Ph.D. diss., Universidad de Buenos Aires, 1920); Pedro Bottinelli, "Tuberculosis y embarazo" (Ph.D. diss., Universidad de Buenos Aires, 1921).

4 Antonio Cetrángolo, *Treinta años curando tuberculosos* (Buenos Aires: Hachette, 1945), 113.

5 Oscar Terán, *Vida intelectual en el Buenos Aires fin-de-siglo (1880–1910), Derivas de la "cultura científica"* (Buenos Aires: Fondo de Cultura Económica, 2000).

6 Tzvetan Todorov, *Nosotros y los otros: Reflexión sobre la diversidad humana* (Mexico City: Siglo XXI, 1991), 117–18.

7 Juan Bautista Alberdi, *Bases y puntos de partida para la organización política de la República Argentina* (Buenos Aires: Plus Ultra, 1984), 237.

8 Agustín Alvarez, *Ensayo de piscología política (1894)* (Buenos Aires: La Cultura Argentina, 1918), 219.

9 Lucas Ayarragaray, *Cuestiones y problemas argentinos contemporáneos*, 3d edn. (Buenos Aires: Talleres Ross, 1937) 2:228, 451; *Boletín del Museo Social Argentino*, nos. 227–28 (1941).

10 Maria Silvia Di Liscia, *Saberes, terapias y prácticas médicas en Argentina (1750–1910)* (Madrid: CSIC, 2002), 70–76; *BMSA*, 225–26 (1941), 107.

11 Juan Alsina, *La inmigración en el primer siglo de la independencia* (Buenos Aires: Edición de Felipe Alsina, 1910), 204–25.

12 Carlos Bernaldo de Quirós, *Eugenesia jurídica y social (Derecho eugenésico argentino)* (Buenos Aires: Editorial Ideas, 1943), 142.

13 *LN*, August 18, 1894.

14 Juan B. Justo, *Discursos y escritos políticos* (Buenos Aires: 1933).

15 *LN*, June 29, 1894.

16 José María Ramos Mejía, *Las multitudes argentinas* (Buenos Aires: Secretaría de Cultura de la Nación, 1994 [1889]), 164.

17 Carlos Octavio Bunge, *Nuestra América: Ensayo de psicología social* (Buenos Aires: Abeledo Editor, 1905 [1903]), 160, 143; Terán, *Vida intelectual en el Buenos Aires fin-de-siglo*, 202.

18 Jose Ingenieros, *Sociología Argentina* (Buenos Aires: Elmer Editor, 1957 [1915]), 327.

19 Ricardo Rojas, *Eurindia*, 2d edn., *Obras completas* (Buenos Aires: Juan Roldán, 1924), 5:134.

20 *BMSA* (1919) 8, 27, 85–90.

21 *ABEMS* 46 (1935).

22 Ayarragaray, *Cuestiones y problemas argentinos*, 55, 59, 454–56.

23 *BMSA* (1941), 227–28, 157.

24 Nancy Leys Stepan, *The Hour of Eugenics: Race, Gender and Nation in Latin America* (Ithaca: Cornell University Press, 1991).

25 Rodolfo Pasqualini, *Medicina interna* (Buenos Aires: Intermédica, 1964), 299.

26 Maurice Lefford, "Immunology of Mycobacterium tuberculosis," in Andre Nahmias and Richard O'Reilly, eds., *Immunology of Human Infection* (New York, 1981), 1:349, cited in F. B. Smith, *The Retreat of Tuberculosis 1850-1950* (London: Croom Helm, 1988), 40.

27 Alsina, "Breves consideraciones sobre la higiene del inmigrante" (Ph.D. diss., Universidad de Buenos Aires, 1899).

28 *BMSA* 8, no. 85–90 (1919), 8–90.

29 Fernando Devoto, *Historia de la inmigración en la Argentina* (Buenos Aires: Sudamericana, 2003), 358.

30 Alsina, "Breves consideraciones sobre la higiene del inmigrante," 44; *LSM*, January 10, 1918.

31 *LSM*, August 5, 1926.

32 Ibid., no. 2, October 14, 1909; no. 3, February 28, 1918.

33 Ayarragaray, *Cuestiones y problemas argentinos contemporáneos*, 60.

34 *ADNH* 33 (1927), 210.

35 *MMCBA 1894* (Buenos Aires: Lotería Nacional, 1894), 275.

36 Manuel Gil y Casares, "La herencia y el contagio de la tuberculosis pulmonar y la lepra en Galicia," *Congreso español internacional de la tuberculosis* (Santiago: Tipografía el Eco, 1912), 13; "La profilaxis de la tuberculosis desde los puntos de vista del contagio y de la herencia," *I congreso de la lucha antituberculosa en Galicia* (Santiago: Tipografía el Eco, 1925).

37 E. Hervada García, *La lucha antituberculosa en Galicia* (La Coruña: Tipografía El Noroeste, 1923), 45.

38 Antonio Pereira Loza, *La paciencia al sol: Historia social de la tuberculosis en Galicia, 1900-1950* (A Coruña: do Castro, 1999), 34.

39 Gil y Casares, "La herencia y el contagio de la tuberculosis," 10, 13.

40 *Galicia Clínica*, January 15, 1930, 2, cited in Pereira Loza, *La paciencia al sol*, 35.

41 *Galicia Clínica*, September 15, 1933, 373, 374; April 15, 1935, 2.

42 X. L. García, ed., *Castelao, Otero Pedrayo, Villar Ponte, Suárez Picallo: Discursos parlamentarios (1931–1933)* (Sada: do Castro, 1978), 95–110. Cited in Xosé Nuñez Seixas, "Emigración y exilio antifascista en Alfonso R. Castelao: de la Pampa solitaria a la Galicia ideal" (mimeo, 2005).

43 Ramón Baltar Domínguez, *Castelao ante la medicina, la enfermedad y la muerte* (Santiago: Editorial de los Bibliófilos Gallegos, 1979); María Victoria Carballo-Calero Ramos, *Os castelaos de ourense* (La Coruña: Editorial Atlántico, 1985).

44 Xosé Nuñez Seixas, "Colón y Farabutti: discursos hegemónicos de la elite gallega de Buenos Aires (1880–1930)," in Xosé Nuñez Seixas, ed., *La Galicia austral: La inmigración gallega en la Argentina* (Buenos Aires: Biblos, 2001), 240, 219–20.

45 José R. De Uriarte, ed., *Los baskos en la nación Argentina* (Buenos Aires: La Baskonia, 1916), 394.

46 Ibid., 446, 442, 447.

47 *BMSA* 8, nos. 85–90 (1919), 78, 83.

48 José Moya, *Cousins and Strangers: Spanish Immigrants in Buenos Aires, 1850–1930* (Berkeley: University of California Press, 1998), 253, 229.

49 Antonio Villanueva Edo, *Historia social de la tuberculosis en Bizkaia (1882–1958)* (Bilbao: Diputación Foral de Bizkaia, 1984), chap. 2.

50 *LSM*, February 28 (1918); March 7 (1918).

51 Municipalidad de Buenos Aires, *Memoria de la intendencia municipal de Buenos Aires, presentada al honorable concejo deliberante, año 1909* (Buenos Aires: Guillermo Kraft, 1910), 59.

52 Alan Kraut, *Silent Travelers: Germs, Genes and the "Immigrant Menace"* (New York, 1994), chap. 3.

53 *LN*, August 26, 1881.

54 Daniel Lvovich, *Nacionalismo y antisemitismo en la Argentina* (Buenos Aires: Javier Vergara, 2003), 100–104.

55 Jorge Salessi, *Médicos, maleantes y maricas: Higiene, criminolgía y homosexualidad en la construcción de la nación Argentina (Buenos Aires 1871–1914)* (Rosario: Beatriz Viterbo Editora, 1995), 248.

56 *El Pueblo*, January 28, 1913.

57 *BMSA* 8, no. 85–90 (1919).

58 Ibid., 7.

59 Ayarragaray, *Cuestiones y problemas argentinos contemporáneos*, 237–38, 451.

60 *Crisol*, April 2, 1933, 1.

61 Haim Avni, *Argentina y la historia de la inmigración judía, 1810–1950* (Jerusalem: Magnes/AMIA, 1983).

62 Ibid.

63 José Sanarelli's work is discussed in Elías Singer, "La tuberculosis en el pueblo judío" (Ph.D. diss., Universidad de Buenos Aires, 1936), 40.

64 Singer, "La tuberculosis en el pueblo judío," 44–45, 48–49.

65 Federico Barbará, *Manual de la lengua pampa* (Buenos Aires: La Cultura Argentina, 1990), 140, cited in Di Liscia, *Saberes, terapias y prácticas médicas en Argentina*, 134.

66 Octavio Bunge, *Nuestra América: Ensayo de psicología social* (Buenos Aires: Valerio Abeledo, 1905), 167.

67 Ibid., 156.

68 The reference to Gache in Carlos Urien and Ezio Colombo, *La República Argentina en 1910* (Buenos Aires: Maucci Hermanos, 1910), 1:131.

69 RMQ (1886), 154, 279–81, cited in Di Liscia, *Saberes, terapias y prácticas médicas en Argentina*, 125, 127. See also chap. 1.

70 LSM, October 14, 1909; March 7, 1918; February 28, 1918; ADNH 32 (1927), 33.

71 Antonio Cetrángolo, *Treinta años curando tuberculosos* (Buenos Aires: Hachette, 1945), 115–19; "Herencia y Contagio," *Quinto congreso panamericano de la tuberculosis* (Buenos Aires: 1940), 243–57.

72 Raúl Entraigas, *El mancebo de la tierra: Ceferino Namuncurá* (Buenos Aires: Instituto Salesiano, 1974), 45, 146.

73 LSM, October 4, 1909, Februray 28, 1918.

74 ASM 1, no. 4 (1899), 224–27.

75 ADNH 43 (1936), 73.

76 Manuel Vidaurreta, *Vacunación antituberculosa: La BCG en nuestros soldados* (Buenos Aires: Pergamino, 1937), 3–4.

8. A Female Disease

1   AAT 30 (1954), 8.

2   Eugenio Cambaceres, *En la sangre* (Buenos Aires: Imprenta de Sud América, 1887), 117.

3   Florencio Sánchez, "Los derechos de la salud," in *El teatro de Florencio Sánchez* (Buenos Aires: Tor, 1917), 24.

4   Horacio Quiroga, *Cuentos completos* (Montevideo: Ediciones de la Plata, 1978), 151.

5   Nicolás Olivari, *La musa de la mala pata* (Buenos Aires: Deucalión, 1956).

6   Elías Castelnuovo, "Lázaro," in *Malditos* (Buenos Aires: Claridad, 1924), 98, 104, 117.

7   Enrique González Tuñón, *Camas desde un peso* (Buenos Aires: Ameghino, 1998 [1932]), 83, 94.

8   Roberto Arlt, "Ester primavera," in *Ester primavera y otros cuentos* (Montevideo: Signos, 1993 [1928]); Ulises Petit de Murat, *El balcón hacia la muerte* (Buenos Aires: Lautaro, 1943); Manuel Puig, *Boquitas pintadas* (Buenos Aires: Sudamericana, 1969).

9   Juana Manuela Gorriti, "Peregrinaciones de una alma triste," in *Obras completas* (Salta: Fundación del Banco del Noroeste: 1992 [1876]).

10 Lea Fletcher, "Patriarchy, Medicine, and Women Writers in Nineteenth-Century

Argentina," in Bruce Clarke and Wendell Alock, eds., *The Body and the Text* (Austin: Texas Tech University Press, 1990); Cristina Iglesia, ed., *El ajuar de la patria: Ensayos críticos sobre Juana Manuela Gorriti* (Buenos Aires: Feminaria, 1993); Francesca Denegri, *El abanico y la cigarrera: La primera generación de mujeres ilustradas en el Perú* (Lima: Flora Tristán/IEP, 1996).

11 Gorriti, "Peregrinaciones de una alma triste," 192.

12 Ibid., 75–86.

13 D. J. G. Pérez, *Medicina doméstica, o sea el arte de conservar la salud, conocer las enfermedades, sus remedios y aplicación al alcance de todos* (Buenos Aires: Imprenta de la Revista, 1854), 49, 197; Lucas Ayarragaray, *Pasiones: Estudios médico-sociales* (Buenos Aires: Jacobo Peuser, 1893), 289–90.

14 Pérez, *Medicina doméstica*, 226.

15 Susan Sontag, *Illness as Metaphor* (New York: Farrar, Strauss and Giroux, 1978).

16 *PBT* 2, no. 31 (1905), 26.

17 *PT*, December 15, 1931.

18 *VCA* 4, no. 6 (1937), 426.

19 Janet Oppenheim, *"Shattered Nerves": Doctors, Patients, and Depression in Victorian England* (New York: Oxford University Press, 1991), 86.

20 *LN*, December 2, 1898; *LR*, July 2, 1908; September 8, 1908.

21 *LR*, September 11, 1928.

22 Arturo Ameghino and Alejandro Raimondi, "Confusión mental por shock emotivo en un tuberculoso," *RCPML* 11 (1924), 257–392; Arturo Ameghino and Alejandro Raimondi, "Otro caso de confusión mental postemotiva en un tuberculoso," *RCPML* 11 (1924), 513–17; Arturo Ameghino, "Alrededor de la etiología tuberculosa en los enfermos mentales," *RCPML* 12 (1925), 204–13; Ramón Melgar, *Tuberculosis y psicopatías* (Buenos Aires: Imprenta Gasterine, 1937).

23 León Charosky and Antonio Dalto, "La psicopatología de los tuberculosos," *LPMA*, January 24, 1934, 186–200; *LSM*, May 18, 1930.

24 Gregorio Bermann, *La explotación de los tuberculosos* (Buenos Aires: Claridad, 1941), 176, 177.

25 Ibid., 186, 181–83.

26 Jorge Luis Borges, "Evaristo Carriego," in *Obras completas* (Buenos Aires: Emecé, 1974 [1930]), 1:142.

27 All references to Carriego's poetry are from Evaristo Carriego, *Poesías completas* (Buenos Aires: Eudeba, 1968 [1926]).

28 José Ingenieros, *La jornada de trabajo* (Buenos Aires: Librería Obrera, 1899).

29 Elvira Rawson de Dellepiane, "Apuntes sobre higiene en la mujer" (Ph.D. diss., Universidad de Buenos Aires, 1892), 27.

30 Augusto Bunge, *Las conquistas de la higiene social: Informe presentado al excelentísimo gobierno nacional* (Buenos Aires: Imprenta Coni, 1910), 1:12, 79, 188, 133, 190.

31 For tango lyrics, Eduardo Romano, ed., *Las letras de tango: Antología cronológica* (Rosario: Ross, 1989).

32 Josué Quesada, "La costurerita que dio aquel mal paso," and Julio Fingerit, "La hija del taller," in *La novela semanal, 1917–1926* (Buenos Aires: Página 12/UNQ, 1999); Alvaro Yunque, "Pasa una obrera," *Reflexiones*, January 1922; Roberto Arlt, *Aguafuertes porteñas* (Buenos Aires: Losada, 1998 [1928–42]); Mariela Méndez, Graciela Queirolo, and Alicia Salomone, eds., *Nosotras . . . y la piel: Selección de ensayos de Alfonsina Storni* (Buenos Aires: Alfaguara, 1998).

33 María del Carmen Feijóo, "Las mujeres trabajadoras porteñas a comienzos de siglo," in Diego Armus, ed., *Mundo urbano y cultura popular: Estudios de historia social Argentina* (Buenos Aires: Sudamericana, 1990), 286–300. For more on working women and tuberculosis, see chapter 6.

34 Gabriela L. de Coni, *Proyecto de ley de protección del trabajo de la mujer y del niño en las fábricas* (Buenos Aires: Liga Argentina contra la Tuberculosis, 1902); Eduardo Rojas, "El sweating system: Su importancia en Buenos Aires" (Ph.D. diss., Universidad de Buenos Aires, 1913); BDNT 30 (1915); Ricardo Etcheberry, "La ley argentina sobre reglamentación del trabajo en las mujeres y niños" (Ph.D. diss., Universidad de Buenos Aires, 1918).

35 *LSM*, May 16, 1918.

36 Borges, *Obras completas*, 1:127.

37 Ismael Moya, *El arte de los payadores* (Buenos Aires: Berutti, 1959).

38 Andrés Cepeda, "Marta la tísica," in *La guitarra de los payadores* (Buenos Aires, n/d) and "La tísica," in Víctor Cavallaro Cadeillac, ed., *Glorias del terruño: Selección gauchesca nativista y lírica de poesía popular y alta poesía* (Montevideo: Cumbre, n/d).

39 Enrique González Tuñón, *Tangos* (Buenos Aires: Gleizer, 1926), 125, 8.

40 Beatriz Seibel, *Historia del teatro argentino, desde los rituales hasta 1930* (Buenos Aires: Corregidor, 2002), part 4.

41 Blas Matamoro, *La ciudad del tango* (Buenos Aires: Galerna, 1969), 47–72.

42 Harold Segel, *Turn-of-the-Century Cabaret: Paris, Barcelona, Berlin, Munich, Vienna, Cracow, Moscow, St. Petersburg, Zurich* (New York: Columbia University Press, 1987), Introduction.

43 Tania, *Discepolín y yo* (Buenos Aires: La Bastilla, 1973), 28–29.

44 Ibíd., 28–33.

45 Blas Matamoro, *La ciudad del tango*, 121–24; Donna Guy, *Sex and Danger in Buenos Aires: Prostitution, Family and Nation in Argentina* (Lincoln: Nebraska University Press, 1990), 144.

46 Jorge Miguel Couselo, *El Negro Ferreyra: Un cine por instinto* (Buenos Aires: Freeland, 1969), 131–45.

47 González Tuñón, *Tangos*, 125, 8.

48 Eduardo Archetti, "Masculinity in the Poetics of Argentinian Tango," in Eduardo Archetti, ed., *Exploring the Written: Anthropology and the Multiplicity of Writing* (Oslo: Scandinavian University Press, 1994), 110.

49 Catalina Wainerman and Rebeca Barck de Raijman, *Sexismo en los libros de lectura de la escuela primaria* (Buenos Aires: IDES, 1987), chap. 2; Beatriz Sarlo, *El*

imperio de los sentimientos (Buenos Aires: Catálogos, 1986); Marcela Nari, "La educación de la mujer: O acerca de cómo cocinar y cambiar a su bebé de manera científica," in Mora, *Revista del Instituto Interdisciplinario de Estudios de Género* 1 (1995).

50 Gabriela Nouzielles, "An Imaginary Plague in Turn-of-the-Century Buenos Aires: Hysteria, Discipline, and Languages of the Body," in Diego Armus, ed., *From Malaria to AIDS: Disease in the History of Modern Latin America* (Durham: Duke University Press, 2003).

51 Julio Fingerit, "La hija del taller," in *La novela semanal, 1917–1926*.

52 Olivari, "La costurerita que dio aquel mal paso," in Olivari, *La musa de la mala pata*.

53 *Crítica*, October 4, 1925.

54 Storni, "La costurerita a domicilio," in *Nosotras . . . y la piel*; Tania Diz, "Deshilvanar los vestidos: Mujeres solteras en la literatura argentina" (mimeo, 2000).

9. Forging the Healthy Body

1 *Revista Médica de Rosario* 27 (1937), 56.

2 Domingo Faustino Sarmiento, *Obras completas* (Buenos Aires: Luz del Día, 1951), 22:268–69.

3 *ASM* 15 (1916), 517.

4 *VCA* 12, no. 8 (1942), 572; *Infancia y Juventud*, January–May 1944; *VCA* 12, no. 10 (1944), 440–49.

5 *VCA* 5, no. 1 (1940), 26; *VCA* 11, no. 9 (1941), 617–18.

6 *LV*, August 23, 1925; November 11, 1923.

7 Próspero Alemandri, *Moral y deporte* (Buenos Aires: Librería del Colegio, 1937), 8–19; Gregorio Marañón, *Sexo, moral y deporte* (Buenos Aires: Claridad, 1926), 20; *VCA* 9, 1 (1940), 52.

8 *VC*, January 1, 1929; *Club Grafa: Revista Oficial* (1943), 31–32; *Anuario Socialista* (1937).

9 *Ideas*, January 1923; *LV*, May 1, 1921.

10 *Ideas*, October 1923; *LV*, January 8, 1922.

11 Julio Frydenberg, "Prácticas y valores en el proceso de popularización del fútbol, Buenos Aires 1900–1910," *Entrepasados: Revista de Historia* 6, no. 12 (1997), 10.

12 Próspero Alemandri, *Cincuentenario del club Gimnasia y Esgrima de Buenos Aires, 1880–1930* (Buenos Aires, 1931), 167; *VC*, January 1, 1929.

13 *VCA* 4, no. 8 (1938), 541; *LV*, August 23, 1925.

14 *Acción Obrera*, September 1927; April 1930; *El Obrero del Mueble*, November 1924; *LV*, August 30, 1926; *La Internacional*, July 9, 1926.

15 Justino Ramos Mexía, "Higiene y educación física de la mujer" (Ph.D. diss., Universidad de Buenos Aires, 1898), 41; *LV*, October 15, 1898; Domingo Faustino Sarmiento, *Obras completas*, vol. 41; *El Nacional*, October, 2, 1892.

16 Arturo Balbastro, "La mujer argentina: Estudio médico-social" (Ph.D. diss., Universidad de Buenos Aires, 1892), 8.

17 Ramos Mexía, "Higiene y educación física de la mujer," 26.

18 César Sánchez Aizcorbe, *La salud: Tratado de higiene y medicina natural* (Buenos Aires: Kapelusz, 1919), 459, 464.

19 *LV*, January 7, 1925; October 10; Edmundo de Amicis, *Amor y gimnástica* (Buenos Aires: Kapelusz, 1946).

20 Alemandri, *Moral y deporte*, 33.

21 *VCA* 4, no. 1 (1937), 31, 35.

22 *Club Grafa: Revista Oficial* (1943), 31–32.

23 Ruth Schwarz de Morgenroth, *Gimnasia para la mujer* (Buenos Aires: Librería de la Salud, 1938).

24 Elvira Rawson de Dellepiane, "Apuntes sobre higiene en la mujer" (Ph.D. diss., Universidad de Buenos Aires, 1892), 9.

25 *VCA* 4, no. 1 (1938), 20–23.

26 *VCA* 11, no. 9 (1941), 617–20.

27 Enrique Romero Brest, "Concepto de la educación física," in *Primera conferencia nacional de asistencia social* (Buenos Aires, 1936), 3:328.

28 Eugenio Pérez, "Opúsculo sobre la tisis pulmonar" (Ph.D. diss., Universidad de Buenos Aires, 1843), 67.

29 *LDC* 1, no. 1 (1936), 12–14.

30 Emilio Coni, *Progrès de l'hygiene dans la république argentine* (Paris: Baillière, 1887), 4. Gregorio Aráoz Alfaro, *Libro de las madres: Pequeño tratado práctico de higiene del niño con indicaciones sobre el embarazo, parto y tratamiento de los accidentes* (Buenos Aires: Librería Científica, 1899).

31 Emilio Coni, *Higiene social, asistencia y previsión social: Buenos Aires caritativo y previsor* (Buenos Aires: Imprenta Spinelli, 1918), chaps. 8–10, 14.

32 María José Billorou, "'Esta sociedad ha llegado en un momento oportuno: Nació aunando pensamiento y ejecución': La creación de la sociedad de puericultura de Buenos Aires," in Adriana Alvarez, Irene Molinari, and Daniel Reynoso, eds., *Historias de enfermedades, salud y medicina en la Argentina del siglo XIX y XX* (Mar del Plata: Universidad Nacional de Mar del Plata, 2004), 189–297.

33 Victoria Mazzeo, *La mortalidad infantil en la ciudad de Buenos Aires, 1856-1986* (Buenos Aires: CEAL, 1993), 29–31.

34 Alfredo Casaubón, "Prólogo," in Félix Liceaga, *La crianza del niño* (Buenos Aires: Cabaut, 1930), 7.

35 *LSM*, February 13, 1940, 387–93.

36 *ADNH* (1927–33), 175.

37 *LSM*, January 16, 1919; *LPMA*, June 20, 1915.

38 Pedro Guerrero, *Tuberculosis común: Estudios de vulgarización sobre medicina social e higiene de la tuberculosis* (Buenos Aires: Talleres Lorenzo, 1928), 141–42.

39 *LSM*, November 9, 1933, 1449.

40 Coni, *Higiene social, asistencia y previsión social*, 195; LSM, May 20, 1920, 698.

41 *Revista de Estadística Municipal* (1931), 69.

42 LPMA, April 1, 1936, 849.

43 Ibid., 849–52.

44 Sandra Carli, "El campo de la niñez: Entre el discurso de la minoridad y el discurso de la educación nueva," in Adriana Puiggrós, ed., *Escuela, democracia y orden, 1916–1943* (Buenos Aires: Galerna 1992), 101.

45 LHE, September 5, 1906, 56.

46 VCA 9, no. 6 (1940), 353.

47 EMEC, July–September 1917, 96.

48 Ibid., June 1905, 644.

49 Enrique Romero Brest, *Elementos de gimnástica fisiológica* (Buenos Aires: Librería del Colegio, 1939), 25, 54, 236–37.

50 Angela Aisenstein, "Historia de la educación física en Argentina: Una mirada retrospectiva de la escolarización del cuerpo," *Revista Educación y Pedagogía*, May–August 2003, 3–4.

51 EMEC (1888), 861; EMEC (1891), 1215.

52 Ibid., July 1893, 411; November 1893, 413; July 1901, 45.

53 Ibid., September 1894, 1067, 1082.

54 Ibid., June 1905.

55 Ibid., June 1905; July–September 1917; LSM, May 27, 1909.

56 LSM, May 22, 1909, 719–26.

57 Enrique Romero Brest, *El sentido espiritual de la educación física: Evolución de una escuela argentina: El Instituto Nacional de Educación Física* (Buenos Aires: Librería del Colegio, 1938), 222.

58 Ibid., 205.

59 Aisenstein, "Historia de la educación física en Argentina," 9.

60 Tulio Halperín Donghi, *Vida y muerte de la república verdadera, 1910–1930* (Buenos Aires: Ariel, 1999), 153.

61 EMEC, March 15, 1890; Sarmiento, *Obras completas*, 22:268; Carlos Octavio Bunge, *La educación contemporánea* (Madrid: Espasa-Calpe, 1903), 353.

62 Sánchez Aizcorbe, *La salud: Tratado de higiene y medicina natural*, 77, 78.

63 VCA, December 15, 1937, 385.

64 EMEC 615 (1924), 96; Romero Brest, *Pedagogía de la educación física*, 98; *El sentido espiritual de la educación física*, 72.

65 Romero Brest, "Concepto de la educación física," 328.

66 LHE, October 1906, 68.

67 Romero Brest, *El sentido espiritual de la educación física*, 72.

68 DSCD, August 18, 1915, 733–36.

69 VTCD, April–June (1925), 88–89.

70 VCA, August 7, 1940, 552.

71 "Discurso del General Perón ante participantes de los campeonatos Evita,"

March 18, 1952, quoted in Cristina Acevedo; "La preconscripción," in Héctor Cucuzza ed., *Estudios de historia de la educación durante el primer peronismo, 1943–1955* (Buenos Aires: Universidad Nacional de Luján, 1997), 191; Angel Gamboa, "Contribución a la protección social de la infancia: Centros de recreación infantil," in *Archivos de la Secretaría de Salud Pública de la Nación*, vol. 5, February 1949.

72 Acevedo, "La preconscripción," 198.

73 *Primera conferencia nacional de asistencia social* (Buenos Aires, 1934), vol. 3, part 2, 122.

74 Coni, *Higiene social, asistencia y previsión social*, chap. 9.

75 *Revista del Consejo Nacional de Mujeres*, November 1925, 49; EMEC, April–June (1930).

76 EMEC 781 (1938).

77 Genaro Sisto, *Segundo congreso médico latino-americano: Establecimientos preventivos infantiles, necesidad de su creación en la República Argentina y urgencia para la ciudad de Buenos Aires* (Buenos Aires: Kraus, 1904); Hamilton Cassinelli, "Contribución al estudio de los niños débiles y retardados en edad escolar" (Ph.D. diss., Universidad de Buenos Aires, 1912), LSM, May 28, 1933.

78 Sisto, *Segundo congreso médico latino-americano*, 18; Coni, *Higiene social*, 192.

79 EMEC 781 (1938).

80 Ibid., January–March 1911, 51.

81 Cassinelli, "Contribución al estudio de los niños débiles"; EMEC, April–June 1930.

82 Sisto, *Establecimientos preventivos infantiles*, 17.

83 EMEC, January–March 1921, 148; January–March 1924, 39–42.

84 Cassinelli, "Contribución al estudio de los niños débiles"; EMEC, January–March (1911), 148–53; May–June 1921, 65–83; *Memoria del Hospital Tornú, 1927* (Buenos Aires, 1928), 8–12.

85 EMEC, January–March (1910), 1036–37.

86 Coni, *Higiene social*, 195.

87 MMCBA, *Año 1925* (Buenos Aires: Peuser, 1926), 375.

88 EMEC, April–June 1913; January–March 1914; July–September 1914, 136; EH, November 1935, 1.

89 Vicente Rotta, *Los espacios verdes de la ciudad de Buenos Aires* (Buenos Aires: Concejo Deliberante, 1940), 62, 42, 41.

90 EMEC, January–May 1924.

91 Ibid., January–March 1911, 51; Coni, *Higiene social*, 195.

92 Municipalidad de Buenos Aires, *Memoria del departamento ejecutivo Dr. Mariano de Vedia y Mitre, intendente municipal: Año 1933–1934* (Buenos Aires: Municipalidad de la Ciudad de Buenos Aires, 1935), 495.

93 MMCBA, *Año 1935*, 575.

10. Tuberculosis and Regeneration

1 René Dubos, "Medical Utopias," *Daedalus* (1959) Summer, 413; Diego Armus, "La ciudad higiénica entre Europa y Latinoamérica," in Antonio Lafuente, ed., *Mundialización de la ciencia y cultura nacional* (Madrid: Doce Calles, 1993), 589.

2 Aquiles Sioen, *Buenos Aires en el año 2080: Historia verosímil* (Buenos Aires: Igon Hermanos, 1879), 62.

3 Jules Verne, *Le cinq cents millions de la begum* (Paris: J. Hetzel, 1879); Benjamin Richardson, *Hygeia, A City of Health* (London: Macmillan. 1876).

4 Sioen, *Buenos Aires en el año 2080*, 62, 101.

5 Ibid., 105.

6 Alberto de Paula, "Una modificación del diseño urbano porteño proyectada en 1875," in *Anales del Instituto de Arte Americano e Investigaciones Estéticas "Mario J. Buschiazzo"* 19 (1966), 72–74.

7 Juan de Cominges, *Obras escogidas* (Buenos Aires, 1892), 345, 346.

8 Felix Weinberg, *Dos utopías argentinas de principios de siglo* (Buenos Aires: Hyspamerica, 1986), 63–65.

9 Pierre Quiroule, *La ciudad anarquista americana, obra de construcción revolucionaria* (Buenos Aires: La Protesta, 1914), 248.

10 Ana María Rigotti, *Dos utopías argentinas en el debate sobre el habitat obrero de principios de siglo* (Rosario: Cuadernos de Curdiur, 1986), 17.

11 Quiroule, *La ciudad anarquista americana*, 74, 159, 161.

12 Ibid., 244, 245, 68, 87–88, 98–100.

13 Ibid., 99.

14 Ibid., 99, 133, 101, 126, 142, 129.

15 Ibid., 102, 75, 72, 76.

16 Paul Scheerbart, *Glassarchitecture* (New York: Preager, 1972 [1914]), 35; Quiroule, *La ciudad anarquista americana*, 72, 76.

17 Emilio Coni, "La ciudad argentina ideal o del porvenir," in *LSM*, April 3, 1919.

18 Benjamín Richardson, "Hygeia, la ciudad de la salud," in *RMQ* 12 (1876), 113, 117, 142, 166, 186; Emilio Coni, *Progrès de l'hygiène dans la République Argentine* (Paris: Bailliere, 1887).

19 Emilio Coni, *Memorias de un médico higienista: Contribución a la historia de la higiene pública y social* (Buenos Aires: A. Flaiban, 1918).

20 Coni, "La ciudad argentina ideal o del porvenir," 466.

21 Manuel Gálvez, *Historia de arrabal* (Buenos Aires: Agencia General de Librería y Publicaciones, 1922); Enrique González Tuñón, "Parque Patricios," in *CC*, December 12, 1925; Domingo Selva, "La habitación higiénica para el obrero," in *Revista Municipal*, December 19, 1904; Benito Carrasco, "La ciudad del porvenir," in *CC*, February 1908; Francisco R. Cibils, "La descentralización urbana de la ciudad de Buenos Aires," in *BDNT*, March 31, 1911.

22 Coni, "La ciudad argentina ideal o del porvenir," 466.

23 Diego Armus, "La ciudad higiénica entre Europa y Latinoamérica," in Antonio Lafuente, ed., *Mundialización de la ciencia y cultura nacional*, 594.

24 Lewis Munford, *The Story of Utopias, Ideal Commonwealths and Social Myths* (New York: Knopf, 1922); F. E. Manuel and F. P. Manuel, *Utopian Thought in the Western World* (Cambridge: Belknap, 1979).

25 *CR*, October 23, 1927.

26 Beatriz Sarlo, *La imaginación técnica: Sueños modernos de la cultura argentina* (Buenos Aires: Nueva Visión, 1993), chap. 3.

27 *RMQ* 6 (1869), 350.

28 *RMQ* 3 (1866), 51–52.

29 *MMCBA, Año 1873*, 6.

30 Vicente Quesada, *Memorias de un viejo: Escenas de costumbres de la República Argentina* (Buenos Aires: Peuser, 1888), 64–65.

31 Antonio Samper, "La República Argentina vista por un colombiano," in Julio Cortázar et al., eds., *Buenos Aires: De la fundación a la angustia* (Buenos Aires: De la Flor, 1968), 63.

32 *LV*, May 19, 1894; December 7, 1901; December 21, 1901.

33 *ED*, September 11, 1902.

34 *MMCBA, Año 1896*, 56.

35 *LV*, April 25, 1926; *VTCD*, January–May 1923, 195; Intendencia Municipal, Comisión de Estética Edilicia, *Proyecto orgánico para la urbanización del municipio: El plano regulador y de reforma de la Capital Federal* (Buenos Aires: Peuser, 1925), 395.

36 Ezequiel Martínez Estrada, *La cabeza de Goliat* (Buenos Aires: Emecé, 1946), 135; Eduardo Schiaffino, *Urbanización de Buenos Aires* (Buenos Aires: Gleizer, 1927), 48.

37 *LV*, December 12, 1922.

38 *VC*, September 1, 1929.

39 *MMCBA, Año 1897*, 34; *MMCBA, Año 1908*, 27.

40 *LN*, April 10, 1940.

41 *LN*, January 20, 1936.

42 Guillermo Rawson, *Escritos y discursos* (Buenos Aires: Compañía Sudamericana de Billetes, 1891), 123.

43 Benito Carrasco, "Evolución de los espacios verdes," *BHCD* 33–34 (1942), 497.

44 Ibid., 496.

45 Schiaffino, *Urbanización de Buenos Aires*, 50.

46 Jorge Tartarini, "La visita de Werner Hegemann a la Argentina en 1931," in *DANA* 37/38 (Buenos Aires, 1995).

47 Carlos Della Paolera, *Buenos Aires y sus problemas urbanos* (Buenos Aires: Oikos, 1946), 39, 48, 49.

48 *Ahora*, April 7, 1942.

49 Rawson, *Escritos y discursos*, 123.

50 Adolfo Bioy, *Antes del 900* (Buenos Aires: Guías de Estudio Ediciones, 1958), 264.

51 Diego Armus, "La idea del verde en la ciudad moderna: Buenos Aires 1870–1940," in *Entrepasados: Revista de Historia* 10 (1996), 9–22; Roberto Gache, *Glosario de la farsa urbana* (Buenos Aires: Cooperativa Editorial, 1919), 67.

52 Martínez Estrada, *La cabeza de Goliat*, 135.

53 Manuel Zuloaga, *Nuestra raza: Condición del extranjero en la Argentina* (Buenos Aires: Ferrari, 1931), 168.

54 *LV*, January 15, 1898; January 4, 1913; April 26, 1913; July 24, 1913; January 29, 1918.

55 *VTCD*, September–November 1936, 1727.

56 Cominges, *Obras escogidas*, 342.

57 *VC*, September 1, 1929.

58 Cominges, *Obras escogidas*, 345–46; Doming Faustino Sarmiento, *Obras completas* (Buenos Aires: Luz del Día, 1956), 41:355, 195.

59 *APCCA*, May–June 1904, 347; *LV*, January 25, 1908.

60 Carrasco, "Evolución de los espacios verdes," 498.

61 *VTCD*, September–November 1934, 2163.

62 Ibid., 2868; Rotta, *Los espacios verdes de la ciudad de Buenos Aires*, 41.

63 Esteban Lucotti, "Alcoholismo y tuberculosis" (Ph.D. diss., Universidad de Buenos Aires, 1918).

64 *BMSA* 20 (1913), 241.

65 *EMEC*, January 31, 1891; November 30, 1901; December 31, 1902; *LHE* 5, 6, 7 (1905); *L'Avvenire, Periódico Comunista-Anarchico*, January 13, 1908; *LSM*, May 27, 1909; *El Azote*, October 22, 1911; *Boletín de Educación Racionalista*, May 1915; *Acción Obrera*, December, 1925; *LV*, June 28, 1926; *BMSA*, September–October 1934, 147–48.

66 Francisco Súnico, *La tuberculosis en las sierras de Córdoba* (Buenos Aires: E. de Martino, 1922), 371; Carlos Octavio Bunge, *La educación contemporánea* (Madrid, 1903), 354; *BMSA*, September October 1934, 266–67.

67 *LHE*, October 1906, 68.

68 *LV*, July 30, 1922; *VTCD*, August–December 1924, 125; January–May 1929, 1445.

69 *VTCD*, April–June 1925, 88–89.

70 *EMEC*, April–June 1916, 151; *LV*, December 7, 1914.

71 *MMCBA*, Año 1935, 561, 564.

72 *VTCD*, July–September 1933, 1998.

73 Carrasco, "Evolución de los espacios verdes," 498.

74 Intendencia Municipal, Comisión de Estética Edilicia, *Proyecto orgánico para la urbanización del municipio*, 395; *MMCBA*, Año 1916, 333; *LV*, January 4, 1913; January 16, 1922; November 15, 1923; *BMSA*, July–August 1939, 214; *Acción Obrera* 9 (1926).

75 Della Paolera, *Urbanización de Buenos Aires*, 48.

76 *VC*, November 1, 1942.

77 Rotta, *Los espacios verdes de la ciudad de Buenos Aires*, 41, 52, 53.

78 Pablo Pschepiurca and Francisco Liernur, "Precisiones sobre los proyectos de Le Corbusier en la Argentina, 1929–1949," *Summa* 243 (1987), 44–45, 48–49.

79 Quoted in Sonia Berjman, *Plazas y parques de Buenos Aires: La obra de los paisajistas franceses* (Buenos Aires: Fondo de Cultura Económica, 1998), 270–71.

80 MMCBA, *Año 1882*, 1, 221; ASCA 26 (1886), 133–44; Samuel Gache, *Les logements ouvrières a Buenos Ayres* (Paris: G. Steinheil, 1900), 100.

81 Diego Armus, "Un balance tentativo y dos interrogantes sobre la vivienda popular entre fines del siglo XIX y comienzos del XX," in *La vivienda en Buenos Aires* (Buenos Aires: Instituto de Historia de la Ciudad de Buenos Aires, 1985).

82 DSCD, July 20, 1910; June 11, 1913; May 29, 1914; LV, May 9, 1915; MMCBA, *Año 1918*, 561–65; Intendencia Municipal, Comisión de Estética Edilicia, *Proyecto orgánico para la urbanización del municipio*, 13–18; VC, October 1, 1931, 18; Vicente Rotta, *Los fenómenos regresivos del urbanismo porteño* (Buenos Aires: Amigos de la Ciudad, 1931), 49; BMSA, July–August 1945, 232–38.

83 RMQ 3 (1866), 51–52.

84 Pedro Méndez, "Breve estudio sobre la higiene de las habitaciones" (Ph.D. diss., Universidad de Buenos Aires, 1886), 106.

85 José Antonio Wilde, *Compendio de higiene pública y privada al alcance de todos* (Buenos Aires: Jacobo Peuser, 1884), 19; Angel Bassi, *Gobierno, administración e higiene del hogar: Curso de ciencia doméstica* (Buenos Aires: Cabaut, 1914), 85; Luis Barrantes Molina, *Para mi hogar: Síntesis de economía y sociabilidad domésticas* (Buenos Aires, 1923), 160.

86 *Diccionario de arquitectura, habitat y urbanismo, edición preliminar* (Buenos Aires: SAC/FADU, 1992), 408.

87 MMCBA, *Año 1918*, 565.

88 LV, March 14, 1918.

89 *La Habitación Popular* 3 (1934), 121–31.

90 VCA October 6, 1943, 72–77.

91 Ibid., February 2, 1946, 208–9; *Diccionario de arquitectura, habitat y urbanismo*, 313.

92 Horacio Torres, "Evolución de los procesos de estructuración espacial urbana: El caso de Buenos Aires," *Desarrollo Económico: Revista de Ciencias Sociales* (July–September 1975), 281–306; Anahí Ballent, *Las huellas de la política: Vivienda, ciudad, peronismo en Buenos Aires, 1943–1955* (Buenos Aires: UNQ/Prometeo, 2006), chap. 1.

93 DSCD, May 29, 1914.

94 Domingo Selva, "La habitación higiénica para el obrero," in *Revista Municipal*, December 19, 1904; Cibilis, "La descentralización urbana de la ciudad de Buenos Aires," BDNT, March 31, 1911.

95 LV, October 26, 1918.

96 *El Obrero en Madera*, January 1914; *Acción Obrera*, December 20, 1913.

97 Wladimiro Acosta, *Vivienda y ciudad, Problemas de la arquitectura contemporánea* (Buenos Aires: Aresti, 1936).

98 Francisco Liernur, "Wladimiro Acosta y el expresionismo alemán," in *Wladimiro Acosta, 1900–1967* (Buenos Aires: FADU, 1987), 25–26.

99 Acosta, *Vivienda y ciudad*, 109, 10, 11, 138–60.

100 *VCA*, November 2, 1939, 130–33.

101 Wladimiro Acosta, "Bosquejo de la ciudad del futuro," in *Segundo ciclo de conferencias sobre temas argentinos* (La Plata, 1938), 33–34; Acosta, *Vivienda y ciudad*, 13, 170, 172.

102 Schiaffino, *Urbanización de Buenos Aires*, 57, 59.

103 Adrián Gorelik, *La grilla y el parque: Espacio público y cultura urbana en Buenos Aires, 1887–1936* (Buenos Aires: Universidad de Quilmes, 1998), 290.

104 *LV*, December 24, 1910.

105 Ibid., May 20, 1917.

106 Schiaffino, *Urbanización de Buenos Aires*, 57, 56.

107 Hegemann, "La vivienda barata en Buenos Aires y otras ciudades del mundo," 289; *Als Stadtebauer in Sudamerika*, 148, quoted in Gorelik, *La grilla y el parque*, 349, 350.

108 Rotta, *Los espacios verdes de la ciudad de Buenos Aires*, 123.

Epilogue

1 Antonio Cetrángolo, *Treinta años curando tuberculosos* (Buenos Aires: Hachette, 1945), 163; *La Habitación Popular*, March 5, 1935.

2 Instituto Nacional de Enfermedades Respiratorias Dr. Emilio Coni, "Mortalidad por tuberculosis: República Argentina, 2003," PRO.TB. DOC.TEC. 06/2005; *La Nación*, April 12, 2005.

This very selective bibliography includes neither all the materials consulted during the research process nor all those sources that appear as full citations in the notes to each chapter. Several long historiographical notes appear in the introduction, referencing disease, medicine, and public health in Argentina and Latin America; the history of tuberculosis worldwide; and the history of Buenos Aires. All of the sources cited therein have informed my narrative and analysis to varying degrees.

Official Documents

Censos municipales (1887, 1904, 1936).

Censos nacionales (1895, 1909).

Concejo Deliberante de la ciudad de Buenos Aires, Versiones taquigráficas del Honorable Concejo Deliberante (1920–1941).

Congreso de la Nación, Cámara de Diputados, Diario de Sesiones (1873–1955).

Congreso de la Nación, Cámara de Senadores, Diario de Sesiones (1873–1955).

Intendencia Municipal. Comisión de Estética Edilicia, *Proyecto orgánico para la urbanización del municipio. El plano regulador y de reforma de la Capital Federal*, Buenos Aires: Peuser, 1925.

Intendencia Municipal de la Capital, Dirección General de la Administración y Asistencia Pública, *Instrucciones contra la propagación de la tuberculosis*. Buenos Aires: Lotería Nacional, 1894.

Municipalidad de la Ciudad de Buenos Aires, Memorias municipales (1883–1935).

Secretaria de Salud Pública de la Nación. *Plan analítico de salud pública*. Buenos Aires, 1947.

Periodicals

Acción Obrera

Ahora

Anales de Biotipología, Eugenesia y Medicina Social

Anales de la Cátedra de Patología y Clínica de la Tuberculosis
Anales del Departamento Nacional de Higiene
Archivos Argentinos de Tisiología
Archivos de la Secretaría de Salud Pública de la Nación
L'Avvenire. Periódico Comunista-Anarchico
Boletín de la Liga Argentina contra la Tuberculosis
Boletín del Departamento Nacional de Higiene
Boletín del Departamento Nacional del Trabajo
Boletín del Museo Social Argentino
Brazo y Cerebro
Caras y Caretas
Crítica
El Día Médico
La Doble Cruz
El Gráfico
La Habitación Popular
La Higiene Escolar
El Hogar
Iatria. Revista del Consorcio de Médicos Católicos
Idea Hospitalaria
La Lucha Antituberculosa
El Médico Práctico
El Monitor de la Educación Común
Mundo Argentino
La Nación
El Nacional
La Novela Semanal
El Obrero del Mueble
El Obrero Gráfico
El Obrero Panadero
El Obrero Textil
Para Tí
PBT: Semanario Infantil Ilustrado (Para niños de 6 a 80 años)
La Prensa
La Prensa Médica Argentina
La Protesta
La Razón
El Rebelde
Revista Argentina de Tuberculosis y Enfermedades Pulmonares
Revista de Jurisprudencia Argentina
Revista de la Asociación Médica Argentina
Revista de la Tuberculosis
Revista de Sanidad Militar

Revista Farmacéutica
Revista Médico Quirúrgica. Órgano de los Intereses Médicos Argentinos
La Semana Médica
La Vanguardia
Vida Comunal
Vida Natural
Vida Porteña
Viva Cien Años
La Voz de la Mujer

Other

Acosta, Leticia. 1918. "La defensa de la infancia contra la tuberculosis." Ph.D. diss., Facultad de Ciencias Médicas, Universidad de Buenos Aires.

Acosta, Wladimiro. 1938. "Bosquejo de la ciudad del futuro." *Segundo ciclo de conferencias sobre temas argentinos*, La Plata.

Aisenstein, Ángela. 2003. "Historia de la educación física en Argentina: Una mirada retrospectiva de la escolarización del cuerpo." *Revista de Educación y Pedagogía* 15, no. 36.

Alemandri, Próspero. 1937. *Moral y deporte*. Buenos Aires: Claridad.

Alsina, Juan. 1899. "Breves consideraciones sobre la higiene del inmigrante." Ph.D. diss., Facultad de Ciencias Médicas, Universidad de Buenos Aires.

Álvarez, Clemente. 1904. *La tuberculosis bajo el punto de vista social*. Rosario: Imprenta Federico Wetzel.

Aráoz Alfaro, Gregorio. 1899. *Libro de las madres: Pequeño tratado práctico de higiene del niño con indicaciones sobre el embarazo, parto y tratamiento de los accidentes.* Buenos Aires: Librería Científica.

Arcelli, María. 1936. *Ciencias Domésticas: Apuntes de higiene de la habitación.* Buenos Aires: Moly.

Archetti, Eduardo, ed. 1994. *Exploring the Written: Anthropology and the Multiplicity of Writing.* Oslo: Scandinavian University Press.

Arlt, Roberto. 1993 [1928]. *Ester Primavera y otros cuentos.* Montevideo: Signos.

Armus, Diego. 1996a. "La idea del verde en la ciudad moderna: Buenos Aires 1870–1940." *Entrepasados: Revista de Historia* 10.

———. 1996b. "Salud y anarquismo: La tuberculosis en el discurso libertario Argentino, 1890–1940." In *Política, Médicos y Enfermedades: Lecturas de Historia de la Salud en la Argentina*, ed. Mirta Zaida Lobato. Buenos Aires: Biblos.

———. 2000a. "Consenso, conflicto y liderazgo en la lucha contra la tuberculosis: Buenos Aires, 1870–1950." *La cuestión social en la Argentina, 1870–1943*, ed. Juan Suriano. Buenos Aires: La Colmena.

———. 2000b. "El descubrimiento de la enfermedad como problema social." *Nueva Historia Argentina*, vol. 5, ed. Mirta Lobato. Buenos Aires: Sudamericana.

———. 2003. "Tango, Gender, and Tuberculosis in Buenos Aires, 1900–1940." In *Dis-

ease in the History of Modern Latin America: From Malaria to AIDS, ed. Diego Armus. Durham: Duke University Press.

—. 2004. "'Queremos a vacina Pueyo!!!': Incertezas biomédicas, enfermos que protestam e a imprensa, Argentina, 1920–1940." *Cuidar, controlar, curar: Ensaios históricos sobre saúde e doença na América Latina e Caribe*, ed. Gilberto Hochman and Diego Armus. Rio de Janeiro: Editora Fiocruz.

—. 2007. *La ciudad impura: Salud, tuberculosis y cultura en Biuenos Aires, 1870–1950*. Buenos Aires: Edhasa.

Avni, Haim. 1983. *Argentina y la historia de inmigración judía (1810–150)*. Jerusalem: Editorial Universitaria Magnes/AMIA.

Ayarragaray, Lucas. 1937 [1926]. *Cuestiones y problemas argentinos contemporáneos*. Buenos Aires: Talleres Rosso.

Ballent, Anahí. 2005. *Las huellas de la política: Vivienda, ciudad, peronismo en Buenos Aires, 1943–1955*. Buenos Aires: Universidad Nacional de Quilmes/Prometeo.

Baltar Domínguez, Ramón. 1979. *Castelao ante la medicina, la enfermedad y la muerte*. Santiago: Editorial de los Bibliófilos Gallegos.

Barlaro, Pablo. 1929. *Lecciones de patología médica*. Buenos Aires: Cadom.

Barnes, David. 1995. *The Making of a Social Disease: Tuberculosis in Nineteenth-Century France*. Berkeley: University of California Press.

Barrantes Molina, Luis. 1923. *Para mi hogar: Síntesis de economía y sociabilidad domésticas*. Buenos Aires: n. p.

Bashford, Alison.2002. "Tuberculosis and Economy: Public Health and Labour in the Early Welfare State," *Health and History* 4, no. 2: 19–40.

Bassi, Ángel. 1914. *Gobierno, administración e higiene del hogar: Curso de ciencia doméstica*. Buenos Aires: Cabaut Editores.

Bates, Barbara. 1992. *Bargaining for Life: A Social History of Tuberculosis, 1876–1938*. Philadelphia: University of Pennsylvania Press.

Belmartino, Susana. 2005. *Atención médica en Argentina en el siglo XX: Instituciones y procesos*. Buenos Aires: Siglo XXI.

Bermann, Gregorio. 1941. *La explotación de los tuberculosos*. Buenos Aires: Claridad.

Bernaldo de Quirós, Carlos. 1943. *Eugenesia jurídica y social (derecho eugenésico argentino)*. Buenos Aires: Ideas.

Bertoni, Lilia Ana. 2001. *Patriotas, cosmopolitas y nacionalistas: La construcción de la nacionalidad argentina a fines del siglo XIX*. Buenos Aires: FCE.

Bioy, Adolfo. 1958. *Antes del 900*. Buenos Aires: Guías de Estudios Ediciones.

Boffi, Luis. 1939. *Misión de la enfermera en la lucha antituberculosa*. Buenos Aires: El Ateneo.

Borges, Jorge Luis. 1974. "Evaristo Carriego." *Obras completas*, vol. 1. Buenos Aires: Emecé.

Borrini, Alberto. 1998. *El siglo de la publicidad, 1898–1998: Historias de la publicidad gráfica argentina*. Buenos Aires: Atlántida.

Bottinelli, Pedro. 1921. "Tuberculosis y embarazo." Ph.D. diss., Facultad de Ciencias Médicas, Universidad de Buenos Aires.

Bryder, Linda. 1988. *Below the Magic Mountain: A Social History of Tuberculosis in Twentieth-Century Britain*. Oxford: Clarendon.

Bunge, Alejandro. 1940. *Una nueva Argentina*. Buenos Aires: Kraft.

Bunge, Augusto. 1910. *Las conquistas de la higiene social (Informe presentado al excelentísimo Gobierno Nacional)*. Buenos Aires: Imprenta Coni.

———. 1912. *El alcoholismo*. Buenos Aires: La Vanguardia.

Bunge, Carlos Octavio. 1903. *La educación contemporánea*. Madrid: Daniel Jorro.

———. 1905 [1903]. *Nuestra América: Ensayo de psicología social*. Buenos Aires: Valerio Abeledo.

Cambaceres, Eugenio. 1887. *En la sangre*. Buenos Aires: Imprenta de Sud América.

Candioti, Marcial. 1920. *Bibliografía doctoral de la Universidad de Buenos Aires y catálogo cronológico de las tesis en su primer centenario: 1821-1920*. Buenos Aires: Talleres Gráficos del Ministerio de Agricultura.

Carli, Sandra. 1992. "El campo de la niñez: Entre el discurso de la minoridad y el discurso de la Educación Nueva." *Escuela democracia y orden (1916-1943)*, ed. Adriana Puiggrós. Buenos Aires: Galerna.

Carriego, Evaristo. 1968 [1926]. *Poesías completas*. Buenos Aires: Eudeba.

Castelli, Marcelo. 1954. *Cosquín: falsedad y verdad*. Cosquín: n.p.

Castelnuovo, Elías. 1924. *Malditos*. Buenos Aires: Claridad.

Cetrángolo, Antonio. 1945. *Treinta años curando tuberculosos*. Buenos Aires: Hachette.

Comstock, George. 1982. "Epidemiology of Tuberculosis." *American Review of Respiratory Diseases* 125: 12–14.

Coni, Emilio. 1887. *Progrès de l'hygiène dans la République Argentine*. Paris: Bailliere.

———. 1918a. *Higiene social: Buenos Aires caritativo y previsor*. Buenos Aires: Spinelli.

———. 1918b. *Memorias de un médico higienista*. Buenos Aires: A. Flaiban.

Couselo, Jorge Miguel. 1969. *El negro Ferreyra: Un cine por instinto*. Buenos Aires: Freeland.

Cronjé, Gillian. 1984. "Tuberculosis and Mortality Decline in England and Wales, 1851–1919." *Urban Disease and Mortality in Nineteenth-Century England*, ed. Robert Woods and John Woodward. New York: St. Martin's Press.

Cucuzza, Héctor, ed. 1997. *Estudios de historia de la educación durante el primer peronismo, 1943-1955*. Buenos Aires: Universidad Nacional de Luján.

De Amicis, Edmundo. 1946. *Amor y gimnástica*. Buenos Aires: Kapelusz.

De Arana, Emilio. 1899. *La medicina y el proletariado*. Rosario: Tipografía El Comercio.

De Cires, Enrique. 1936. *La proteinoterapia es argentina: El Dr. Villar, su vida y su obra*. Buenos Aires: El Ateneo.

De Cominges, Juan. 1892. *Obras escogidas*. Buenos Aires: J. A. Alsina.

De Ipola, Emilio. 2003. "Estrategias de la creencia en situaciones críticas: El Cáncer y la crotoxina en Buenos Aires a mediados de los años ochenta." *Entre médicos y curanderos: Cultura, historia y enfermedad en la América Latina moderna*, ed. Diego Armus. Buenos Aires: Norma.

Del Castaño, Aurora. 1906 [1903]. *El vademécum del hogar: Tratado práctico de economía doméstica y labores*. Buenos Aires: Imprenta Tragant.

Della Paolera, Carlos. 1977 [1946]. *Buenos Aires y sus problemas urbanos*. Buenos Aires: Editorial Oikos.

Devoto, Fernando. 2003. *Historia de la inmigración en la Argentina*. Buenos Aires: Sudamericana.

Díaz de Guijarro, Enrique. 1944. *El impedimento matrimonial de la enfermedad: Matrimonio y eugenesia*. Buenos Aires: Kraft.

Diccionario de arquitectura, hábitat y urbanismo (ed. preliminar). Buenos Aires: Sociedad Central de Arquitectos y FADU-UBA. 1992.

Domínguez, Abel. 1895. "Tratamiento climatérico de la tuberculosis pulmonar en la República Argentina." Ph.D. diss., Facultad de Ciencias Médicas, Universidad de Buenos Aires.

Douglas, Mary. 1968. *Purity and Danger: An Analysis of the Concepts of Pollution and Taboo*. London: Routledge.

Dubos, René, and Jean Dubos. 1952. *The White Plague: Tuberculosis, Man, and Society*. Boston: Little, Brown.

Elias, Norbert. 1978. *The History of Manners*. New York: Pantheon.

Entraigas, Raúl. 1974. *El mancebo de la tierra: Ceferino Namuncurá*. Buenos Aires: Instituto Salesiano.

Escudé, Carlos. 1989. "Health in Buenos Aires in the Second Half of the Nineteenth Century." *Social Welfare, 1850–1950: Australia, Argentina and Canada Compared*, ed. C. Platt. London: Macmillan.

Feijóo, María del Carmen. 1990. "Las mujeres trabajadoras porteñas a comienzos de siglo." *Mundo urbano y cultura popular: Estudios de historia social argentina*, ed. Diego Armus. Buenos Aires: Sudamericana.

Ferreiros, Estela, and Martha Morey. 1985. *Enfermedades del trabajador*. Buenos Aires: Hammurabi.

Figlio, Karl. 1978. "Chlorosis and Chronic Disease in Nineteenth-Century Britain: The Social Construction of Somatic Illness in a Capitalist Society." *Social History* 3, no. 2.

Fletcher, Lea. 1990. "Patriarchy, Medicine, and Women Writers in Nineteenth-Century Argentina." *The Body and the Text*, ed. Bruce Clarke and Wendell Aycock. Lubbock: Texas Tech University Press.

Fonso Gandolfo, Carlos. 1919. "Cómo vive el tuberculoso indigente." *Segunda conferencia nacional de profilaxis antituberculosa*. Rosario: Talleres de la Biblioteca Argentina.

Foucault, Michel. 1997 [1963]. *The Birth of the Clinic: An Archeology of Medical Perception*. London: Routledge.

Frydenberg, Julio. 1997. "Prácticas y valores en el proceso de popularización del fútbol: Buenos Aires 1900–1910." *Entrepasados: Revista de Historia*, no. 12.

Gache, Roberto. 1920. *Glosario de la farsa urbana*. Buenos Aires: Cooperativa Editorial.

Gache, Samuel. 1900. *Les logements ouvrières á Buenos Ayres*. Paris: G. Steinheil.

Gil y Casares, Manuel. 1912. "La herencia y el contagio de la tuberculosis pulmonar y la lepra en Galicia." *Congreso español internacional de la tuberculosis.* Santiago: Tipografía el Eco.

González Leandri, Ricardo. 1999. *Las profesiones: Entre la vocación y el interés corporativo. Fundamentos para su estudio histórico.* Madrid: Catriel.

González Tuñón, Enrique. 1998 [1932]. *Camas desde un peso.* Buenos Aires: Ameghino.

Gorelik, Adrián. 1998. *La grilla y el parque: Espacio público y cultura urbana en Buenos Aires, 1887-1936.* Bernal: Universidad Nacional de Quilmes.

Gorriti, Juana Manuela. 1992 [1876]. "Peregrinaciones de un alma triste." *Obras completas,* vol. 1. Salta: Fundación del Banco del Noroeste.

Guerrero, Pedro. 1928. *Tuberculosis común: Estudios de vulgarización sobre medicina social e higiene de la tuberculosis.* Buenos Aires: Talleres Lorenzo.

Guillaume, Pierre. 1986. *Du désespoir au salut: les tuberculeux aux XIXe et XXe Siècles.* Paris: Aubier.

Halperín Donghi, Tulio. 1999. *Vida y muerte de la república verdadera (1910-1930).* Buenos Aires: Ariel.

Hervada García, E. 1923. *La lucha antituberculosa en Galicia.* La Coruña: Tipografía El Noroeste.

Holguín, Rogerio. 1917. *Historia del descubrimiento de medicinas vegetales para curar la tuberculosis.* Buenos Aires: Impr. San Martín.

Huisman, Frank, and John Harley Warner, eds. 2004. *Locating Medical History: The Stories and Their Meanings.* Baltimore: Johns Hopkins University Press.

Hutcheon, Linda. 1996. *Opera: Desire, Disease, Death.* Lincoln: University of Nebraska Press.

Iglesia, Cristina, ed. 1993. *El ajuar de la patria: Ensayos críticos sobre Juana Manuela Gorriti.* Buenos Aires: Feminaria.

Ingenieros, José. 1899. *La jornada de trabajo.* Buenos Aires: Librería Obrera.

———. 1957 [1915]. *Sociología argentina.* Buenos Aires: Elmer Editor.

Izzo, Roque, and Florencio Escardó. 1940. *Una campaña de propaganda sanitaria.* Buenos Aires: Centro de Investigaciones Tisiológicas.

Johnston, William. 1995. *The Modern Epidemic: A History of Tuberculosis in Japan.* Cambridge: Council on East Asian Studies, Harvard University Press.

Korn, Francis, and Luis Alberto Romero, eds. 2006. *Buenos Aires / Entreguerras: La callada transformación, 1914-1945.* Buenos Aires: Alianza.

Kozel, Carlos. 1930. *Salud y curación por hierbas.* Buenos Aires: n.p.

Kraut, Alan. 1994. *Silent Travelers: Germs, Genes, and the "Immigrant Menace."* New York: Basic Books.

Kunzle, David. 1982. *Fashion and Fetishism: A Social History of the Corset, Tight-lacing, and Other Forms of Body Sculpture in the West.* Totowa, N.J.: Rowman and Littlefield.

Laperriere de Coni, Gabriela. *Proyecto de ley de protección del trabajo de la mujer y del niño en las fábricas.* Buenos Aires: Liga Argentina contra la Tuberculosis, 1902.

Liernur, Jorge Francisco. n.d. "Wladimiro Acosta y el expresionismo alemán." AA.VV., *Wladimiro Acosta, 1900-1967.* Buenos Aires: FADU–UBA.

Lozano, Nicolás. 1917. "Contribución al estudio de la etiología y profilaxis de la tuberculosis desde el punto de vista sociológico." *Proceedings of the Second Pan-American
Scientific Congress, Washington, D.C., December 1915.* Washington.

Luisi, Paulina. 1919. *Por una mejor descendencia.* Buenos Aires: La Vanguardia.

Lvovich, Daniel. 2003. *Nacionalismo y antisemitismo en la Argentina.* Buenos Aires:
Javier Vergara.

Manuel, Frank E., and Fritzie P. Manuel. 1979. *Utopian Thought in the Western World.*
Cambridge: Belknap.

Marañón, Gregorio. 1926. *Sexo, moral y deporte.* Buenos Aires: Claridad.

Martínez, Alberto. 1907. *Manuel du voyageur: Baedeker de la république argentine.* Barcelona: López Robert.

Matamoro, Blas. 1969. *La ciudad del tango.* Buenos Aires: Galerna.

Mazzeo, Victoria. 1993. *La mortalidad infantil en la ciudad de Buenos Aires, 1856–1986.*
Buenos Aires: CEAL.

McFarlane, Neil. 1989. "Hospital, Housing, and Tuberculosis in Glasgow, 1911–51," *Social History of Medicine,* 2, no. 1, 59–85.

McKeown, Thomas. 1976. *The Modern Rise of Population.* London: Arnold.

———. 1979. *The Role of Medicine: Dream, Mirage, or Nemesis?* Princeton: Princeton
University Press.

Melgar, Ramón. 1937. *Tuberculosis y psicopatías.* Buenos Aires: Imprenta Gasterine.

Menéndez, Eduardo. 1985. "'Saber médico' y 'saber popular': El modelo hegemónico
y su función ideológica en el proceso de alcoholización." *Estudios Sociológicos* 3,
no. 8.

Mitchell, Allan. 1990. "An Inexact Science: The Statistics of Tuberculosis in Late
Nineteenth-Century France." *Social History of Medicine* 3, no. 3 (July), 387–403.

Moya, Ismael. 1959. *El arte de los payadores.* Buenos Aires: Berutti.

Moya, José. 1998. *Cousins and Strangers: Spanish Immigrants in Buenos Aires, 1850–1930.*
Berkeley: University of California Press.

Mumford, Lewis. 1922. *The Story of Utopias, Ideal Commonwealths and Social Myths.*
New York: Boni and Liveright.

Munzinger, Juan. 1920. "Algunas consideraciones sobre tubercuslosis y embarazo:
Ph.D. diss., Facultad de Ciencias Médicas, Universidad de Buenos Aires.

Nari, Marcela. 1995. "La educación de la mujer (o acerca de cómo cocinar y cambiar a
su bebé de manera científica)." *Mora: Revista del Área Interdisciplinaria de Estudios de la Mujer* No. 1.

Newman, Kathleen. 1990. "The Modernization of Femininity: Argentina, 1916–1926,"
in *Women, Culture, and Politics in Latin America.* Berkeley: University of California Press.

Noguera, Enrique, and Luis Huerta. 1934. *Genética, eugenesia y pedagogía sexual.*
Madrid: Javier Morata.

Nouzeilles, Gabriela. 2000. *Ficciones somáticas: Naturalismo, nacionalismo y políticas
del cuerpo, Argentina 1880–1910.* Rosario: Beatriz Viterbo.

Nuñez Seixas, Xosé, ed. 2001. *La Galicia austral: La inmigración gallega en la Argentina*. Buenos Aires: Biblos.

Olivari, Nicolás. 1956 [1926]. *La musa de la mala pata*. Buenos Aires: Deucalión.

Palacios, Alfredo. 1935 [1923]. *La fatiga y sus proyecciones sociales. Investigaciones de laboratorio en los talleres del estado*. Buenos Aires: La Vanguardia.

———. 1954 [1922]. *La justicia social*. Buenos Aires: Editorial Claridad.

Penna, José, and Horacio Madero. 1910. *La administración sanitaria y asistencia pública de la ciudad de Buenos Aires*. Buenos Aires: Kraft.

Pereira Loza, Antonio. 1999. *La paciencia al sol: Historia social de la tuberculosis en Galicia, 1900–1950*. Coruña: Edicios do Castro.

Petit de Murat, Ulises. 1943. *El balcón hacia la muerte*. Buenos Aires: Lautaro.

Pueyo, Jesús. 1942. *La burocracia de la medicina contra los tuberculosos: Síntesis documentada y antecedentes reales de mi vacuna antituberculosa (Yo Acuso)*. Buenos Aires: Editorial Científica.

Puig, Manuel. 1969. *Boquitas pintadas*. Buenos Aires: Sudamericana.

Quiroga, Horacio. 1978. *Cuentos completos*. Montevideo: Ediciones de la Plata.

Quiroule, Pierre. 1914. *La ciudad anarquista americana: Obra de construcción revolucionaria*. Buenos Aires: La Protesta.

Rawson, Guillermo. 1891. *Escritos y discursos*. Buenos Aires: Compañía Sudamericana de Billetes.

Recalde, Héctor. 2000. "La primera cruzada contra la tuberculosis: Buenos Aires, 1935." *Argentina: Trabajadores entre dos guerras*, ed. José Panettieri. Buenos Aires: Eudeba.

Rigotti, Ana María. 1986. "Dos utopías argentinas en el debate sobre el hábitat obrero de principios de siglo." *Cuadernos del CURDIUR*. Rosario.

Romano, Eduardo. 1989. *Las letras de tango: Antología cronológica*. Rosario: Ross.

Romero, José Luis, and Luis Alberto Romero, eds. 1983. *Buenos Aires: Historia de cuatro siglos*. Buenos Aires: Editorial Abril.

Romero, Luis Oscar. 1924. *¿Es contagiosa la tuberculosis?* Buenos Aires: Claridad.

Romero Brest, Enrique. 1911. *Pedagogía de la educación física*. Buenos Aires: Cabaut.

———. 1938. *El sentido espiritual de la educación física: Evolución de una escuela argentina: El Instituto Nacional de Educación Física*. Buenos Aires: Librería del Colegio.

Rosenberg, Charles, and Jeanne Golden, eds. 1992. *Framing Disease: Studies in Cultural History*. New Brunswick: Rutgers University Press.

Rothman, Sheila. 1994. *Living in the Shadow of Death: Tuberculosis and the Social Experience of Illness in American History*. New York: Basic Books.

Rotta, Vicente. 1940. *Los espacios verdes de la ciudad de Buenos Aires*. Buenos Aires: Imprenta La Argentina.

Saítta, Sylvia. 2006. "Costureritas y artistas pobres: Algunas variaciones sobre el mito romántico de la tuberculosis en la literatura argentina." *Literatura, cultura, enfermedad*, ed. Wolfgang Bongers and Tanja Olbrich. Buenos Aires: Paidós.

Sánchez, Florencio. 1917. *El teatro de Florencio Sánchez*. Buenos Aires: Tor.

Sánchez Aizcorbe, César. 1919. *La salud: Tratado de higiene y medicina natural*. Buenos Aires: Kapelusz.

Sarlo, Beatriz. 1993. *La imaginación técnica: Sueños modernos de la cultura argentina*. Buenos Aires: Nueva Visión.

Sarmiento, Domingo Faustino. 1951. *Obras completas*. Buenos Aires: Luz del Día.

Schiaffino, Eduardo. 1927. *Urbanización de Buenos Aires*. Buenos Aires.

Schwarz de Morgenroth, Ruth. 1938. *Gimnasia para la mujer*. Buenos Aires: Librería de la Salud.

Scobie, James. 1974. *Buenos Aires: Plaza to Suburb, 1870–1910*. New York: Oxford University Press.

Segel, Harold. 1987. *Turn-of-the-Century Cabaret: Paris, Barcelona, Berlin, Munich, Vienna, Cracow, Moscow, St. Petersburg, Zurich*. New York: Columbia University Press.

Seibel, Beatriz. 2002. *Historia del teatro argentino: Desde los rituales hasta 1930*. Buenos Aires: Corregidor.

Singer, Elías. 1936. "La tuberculosis en el pueblo judío." Ph.D. diss., Facultad de Ciencias Médicas, Universidad de Buenos Aires.

Sioen, Aquiles. 1879. *Buenos Aires en el año 2080: Historia verosímil*. Buenos Aires: Igon Hermanos.

Sisto, Genaro. 1904. *Establecimientos preventivos infantiles: Necesidad de su creación en la República Argentina y urgencia para la ciudad de Buenos Aires*. Buenos Aires: L. E. Kraus.

Sontag, Susan. 1978. *Illness as Metaphor*. New York: Farrar, Straus and Giroux.

Steinberg, Oscar, and Oscar Traversa. 1997. *Estilo de época y comunicación mediática*. Buenos Aires: Atuel.

Stepan, Nancy. 1991. *The Hour of Eugenics: Race, Gender, and Nation in Latin America*. Ithaca: Cornell University Press.

Súnico, Francisco. 1902. *Nociones de higiene escolar*. Buenos Aires: Taller Tipográfico de la Penitenciaría Nacional.

———. 1922. *La tuberculosis en las sierras de Córdoba*. Buenos Aires: E. de Martino.

Szreter, Simon. 1988. "The Importance of Social Intervention in Britain's Mortality Decline, c. 1850–1914: A Reinterpretation of the Role of Public Health." *Social History of Medicine* 1, no. 1, 1–38.

Tania. 1973. *Discepolín y yo: Memorias transcriptas por Jorge Miguel Couselo*. Buenos Aires: La Bastilla.

Tartarini, Jorge. 1995. "La visita de Werner Hegemann a la Argentina en 1931." *Revista documentos de arquitectura nacional y americana (DANA)* Nos. 37–38.

Tassart, Juan Carlos. 1952. *El descenso de la tuberculosis en la República Argentina*. Buenos Aires: Ministerio de Salud Pública de la Nación.

Terán, Oscar. 2000. *Vida intelectual en el Buenos Aires fin-de-siglo (1880–1910): Derivas de la "cultura científica."* Buenos Aires: FCE.

Todorov, Tzvetan. 1991. *Nosotros y los otros: Reflexión sobre la diversidad humana*. Mexico City: Siglo XXI.

Tomes, Nancy. 1977. "Spreading the Germ Theory: Sanitary Science and Home Economics, 1880–1930." *Rethinking Home Economics: Women and the History of a Profession*, ed. Sarah Stage and Virginia Vincent. Ithaca: Cornell University Press.

Uriarte, José R., ed. 1916. *Los baskos en la nación argentina*. Buenos Aires: La Baskonia.

Urien, Carlos, and Ezio Colombo. 1910. *La República Argentina en 1910*. Buenos Aires: Maucci Hermanos.

Van de Velde, T. H. 1940. *Fertilidad e infertilidad en el matrimonio*. Buenos Aires: Claridad.

Vezzetti, Hugo. 1996. *Aventuras de Freud en el país de los argentinos: De José Ingenieros a Enrique Pichon Rivière*. Buenos Aires: Paidós.

Villanueva Edo, Antonio. 1984. *Historia social de la tuberculosis en Bizkaia (1882–1958)*. Bilbao: Diputación Foral de Bizkaia.

Viñas, Marcelo. 1896. "La herencia en la tuberculosis." Ph.D. diss., Facultad de Ciencias Médicas, Universidad de Buenos Aires.

Vitón, Juan José. 1928. *Lo que todo tuberculoso debe saber*. Buenos Aires: El Ateneo.

Walter, Richard. 1993. *Politics and Urban Growth in Buenos Aires, 1910–1942*. New York: Cambridge University Press.

Weinberg, Félix. 1986. *Dos utopías argentinas de principios de siglo*. Buenos Aires: Hyspamérica.

Wilde, Eduardo. 1917. *Obras completas*. Buenos Aires: Talleres Peuser.

Wilde, José Antonio. 1868. *Compendio de higiene pública y privada al alcance de todos*. Buenos Aires: Imprenta Bernheim.

Wilson, Leonard. 1990. "The Historical Decline of Tuberculosis in Europe and America: Its Causes and Significance." *Journal of the History of Medicine and Allied Sciences* 45, no. 3 (July): 366–96.

Zimmerman, Eduardo. 1998. *Los liberales reformistas*. Buenos Aires: Universidad de San Andrés and Sudamericana.

Zuloaga, Manuel. 1931. *Nuestra raza: Condición del extranjero en la Argentina: Contribución al estudio de la ciudadanía de los extranjeros*. Buenos Aires: Ferrari Hnos.

fear: antituberculosis messages and, 70, 115–16, 139, 151–52, 183–85; of contagion, 15, 145–46, 174, 183, 282, 346; of hospitals, 52; of tuberculosis, 1, 15, 24, 183–85, 186–88

forgery, of medicines, 33

Gache, Samuel, 61, 216, 246

Galicians, 92, 233–40

gender relations, 254, 272–73, 275, 280, 283

General Roca's Indians, 244–50

germ theory, 151

green spaces, 309–11, 322–33

government: children's health and, 298–302; health care and, 14, 51, 98, 117; as labor arbitrator, 121; physical education and, 289, 293; public health role of, 119–26; tuberculosis treatments regulated by, 105–7, 119, 123–27, 129

gymnastics, 277–79, 281, 289–96

healers: as alternatives to institutionalized medicine, 38, 45–47; consultations with, 24, 47; herbalists as, 14, 24, 38; hybrid, 39–40, 47; institutionalized medicine in dialogue with, 42–43, 44; marketing strategies of, 39–41; naturalists as, 43–44, 47; regulation of, 44, 48; self-cure encouraged by, 43; stereotypes of, 38

health cards, 182

health care: access to, 125; government's impact on, 119; as social issue, 119, 135

health care network, 120–25; expansion of, 126–27, 283

health care professionals, 50

health visitors, 61–63, 283

Helios system, 341

heredity, 222, 232–36, 247, 253, 282

higienistas, 119, 120

historiography: of disease, 3–6; of tuberculosis, 6–8, 9–13

home care, 14, 24, 25–27, 84; advocates of, 28–29; hybrid healers and, 39; family's role in, 27, 49, 50; home medicine manuals, 27; hygienic code used in, 26; medicalization's impact on, 27

home hygiene, 157–61

hospitals, 14, 25, 49; avoidance of, 26, 45, 52, 54; conditions in, 52–55, 59; effectiveness of, 50, 56–57; expansion of, 48, 51, 55, 125; modernization of, 51; rules and routines of, 59–61; scarcity of resources and, 27, 52–54, 56; services of, 51–52, 54, 59, 61, 127; tubercular, 52–54; urban, 51

Hospital Tornú, 24, 55–56, 58–59, 123, 126

housing: apartments, 219–20, 330; conditions of, 18–19, 326, 343; tenements, 18, 214–17, 219, 334, 338, 340; tuberculosis linked to, 15. *See also* living conditions

hygiene, 15, 134, 136–38; acceptance of, 135, 141–43, 346–47; consensus on, 15, 139, 143; culture of, 140, 143, 346; discourses of, 118–19, 142–43; in educational campaigns, 116, 142, 146–50, 155, 283; exercise and, 289–90, 296, 300; hygienic cure, 71; hygienic excess, 183–86; instruction in health care institutions on, 50, 70–71, 115; limitations of hygienic code, 139, 345–46; morality and, 135, 139, 143, 144, 154, 183, 302, 305, 340; recommendations on, 15, 135, 148, 156–59; sexuality and, 173–75; social, 143–44, 308; in urban plans, 307–11, 314–17, 324–25, 327–30, 334–41; women and, 156

hygiene home visitors, 283

hygiene reformism, 127, 311, 324; ideological organizations and, 119; modernization's impact on, 118–19

hygienic citizenship, 50, 139, 142, 156, 160–61; of patients, 61, 75, 81, 95, 155

hygienic housing, 16, 314, 316, 334–44

hygienic neighborhood, 335, 342

public health initiatives (*continued*) in, 119–20, 123–27; health care services and, 51–52, 54, 59, 61, 117, 123, 126–27, 130–31; hygiene and, 135–39; in schools, 146–50, 289–93, 298

public health system, 125

Pueyo, Jesús, 101–7, 111

Pueyo vaccine, 99, 101–11

quackery, 24, 38–39, 41, 48

race: racial and ethnic mixing, 223–28, 244–45, 248–50; tuberculosis and, 223–24, 232–50

"racial" stereotypes, 16, 226, 250; of Basques, 238–40; of *criollo* women, 247–49; of Galicians, 232–38; of Indians, 244–47, 249; of Jews, 240–44

radio: in antituberculosis campaigns, 132; home medicine and, 28; hygienic culture influenced by, 115, 116

rape, 92

reformism, 301–2, 311; agendas of, 121–22; municipal, 127, 283; tuberculosis and, 122

religion, 61, 91

remedies. *See* therapies

reproduction, 176, 177–79, 282

respiratory exercise, 276, 278–79, 281, 290

rest cure, 14, 25, 55, 58–61, 64, 71–72, 79–83; locations for, 67–69; noncompliance and, 95–96, 111; unsupervised, 70, 77–78

right to health, 91, 97, 105–6, 111–12, 119, 125, 347; in workplace, 114

Sanatorio Santa María, 72–73, 86–95, 127

sanitariums, 25, 49, 55; achievements of, 75–76; administration of, 88, 94; conflicts in, 88–97; criticisms of internment experience in, 96–97; daily life in, 71–72, 75; effectiveness of, 73, 75; hygienic education and, 70–71, 75; political aspects of, 88–89, 94; publicity campaigns of, 69; punishments used in, 73, 91–94, 109

sanitary villages, 78–80

Sarmiento, Domingo Faustino, 67, 142, 276

Sarmiento, Santos, 70, 108

schools: antituberculosis campaigns in, 116; hygienic programs in, 146–50, 155, 289–90; physical education and, 16, 283, 289–98; for pretubercular children, 298–306

self-discipline: in hygienic habits, 155; in treatment, 71, 78

self-exile, of tuberculars, 70, 72, 80–82

self-medication, 24, 25, 84; advertisements' encouragement of, 35; reasons for, 29, 38

sewage systems, 119, 315, 340

sex: risk of contagion and, 175, 194–95; in sanitariums, 96, 111

sexuality: discourses of, 163, 172–73, 191, 193; excesses of, 15, 173, 193–96; tuberculosis linked to, 15, 191–96; women and, 195

soccer, 277–78, 290, 296–98, 331–32

social engineering, 301–2

social hygiene, 143–44, 308

socialists: alcohol and, 200–201; coverage by *La Vanguardia* and, 93, 110; health care and, 47; hygienist programs and, 119, 142; tuberculosis linked to, 121, 187; urban living and, 335, 340; workers' rights and, 20, 123

social mobility, 273–74

social welfare system, 121

socioeconomic status: access to green spaces and, 327–28, 333; access to hospitals and, 56; housing and, 215–17; hygienic recommendations and, 157, 160; rest cure and, 64–65; susceptibility to

disease and, 205, 303; treatment influenced by, 25, 26, 45, 50, 64, 84
sociomedicine, 189
soldiers, 249–50
Sontag, Susan, 8
sports, 277, 280, 289, 296–98, 330
sputum, 15, 150, 153–56, 232–34, 345
state-run agencies, 119, 123–27, 129
stereotypes: of doctors, 39; of healers, 38–39; of tuberculosis, 16. *See also* "racial" stereotypes
sterilization, 176–78
stigma: avoidance of, 49, 65; consequences of, 26, 45, 70, 72; hospital authorities' creation of, 92–93
streptomycin, 347
strikes: efficacy of, 90–91; by hospital employees, 88; by patients, 14, 88, 90; by workers, 20, 114
summer camps, 16, 64, 298–306, 323–24, 331
surgery, 57
syphilis, 194

tango, 261–63, 265–69, 274–75; masculinity in, 272; tuberculosis linked to, 271–72
theater, 252
therapies, 36–37, 85; climotherapies, 68–69; failures of, 45; lack of, 24, 39, 55, 101, 117; self-medication, 24, 25, 29, 35, 38, 84. *See also* home care
tísicas, 16, 260–63
tonics, 35–38
tourism, 83
tubercular psychology, 97, 114, 258–59
tuberculars: demographics of, 48; isolation of, 52, 53, 55, 59, 70, 72, 91; surveillance of, 61; treatment options for, 24, 26, 38, 47, 49, 100–101, 114
tuberculin test, 8, 285
tuberculosis: biomedicine challenged by, 24; excessive behaviors and, 188–97,

201; historiography of, 6–8, 9–13; interpretations of, 1, 2, 8, 23, 163, 173, 186–87, 236, 250–54, 260, 269, 272, 275; pathology of, 8–9, 24; as public health issue, 16, 119, 129; reemergence of, 16, 348–49; social dimensions of, 70, 98, 119–25, 128, 183, 187–90, 192, 202–9, 211, 220, 261; symptoms of, 8–9, 24; in workplace, 114, 121, 124
Tuberculosis Elimination Law, 98
tuberculosis phobia, 15, 183–84; criticisms of, 186–88; print media's contribution to, 185

Unión Cívica Radical, 21, 121; in health care facilities, 88–89
unions, 121–23, 133–34
universal health care, 125
unskilled workers, 206–7, 210–11
urbanization, 16–17, 125, 302, 308–26, 334–41; hygienic culture influenced by, 143, 307; regulation of, 310, 316, 318, 325

vaccines, 97; BCG, 59, 64, 98, 287, 345; crusades for, 106; doctors' views of, 102, 104, 108–10; governmental regulation of, 105–7; patients' reaction to, 101, 105, 107–9, 111; print media's coverage of, 102–11; as public health issue, 98–111; Pueyo, 99, 101–11; Villar serum, 99–101
via crucis, 23
Villar serum, 99–101
vitalism, 47

wet nurses, 283, 286–87
women: admissions of, to tubercular hospitals, 58; in antituberculosis campaigns, 156–60; in *criollos*, 248–49; discourses against contagion and, 161–63; exercise and, 278–81; as health-care workers, 62; as migrants, 249;

Diego Armus is associate professor of Latin American history at Swarthmore College. He is the author of *La ciudad impura: Salud, tuberculosis y cultura en Buenos Aires, 1870–1950* (2007). He is also the editor of *Disease in the History of Modern Latin America: From Malaria to Aids* (Duke, 2003); *Mundo urbano y cultura popular: Estudios de historia Social Argentina* (1990); *Huelgas, habitat y salud en el Rosario del Novecientos* (1995); *Entre médicos y curanderos: Cultura, historia y enfermedad en la América Latina moderna* (2002); and *Avatares de la medicalización en América Latina (1870–1970)* (2005); and the editor, with Gilberto Hochman, of *Cuidar, controlar, curar: Ensaios históricos sobre Saúde e doença na América Latina e Caribe* (2004).

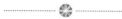

Library of Congress Cataloging-in-Publication Data
Armus, Diego.
The ailing city : health, tuberculosis, and culture in Buenos Aires, 1870–1950 / Diego Armus.
p. cm.
Includes bibliographical references and index.
ISBN 978-0-8223-4999-0 (cloth : alk. paper)
ISBN 978-0-8223-5012-5 (pbk. : alk. paper)
1. Tuberculosis—Argentina—Buenos Aires—History. 2. Public health—Argentina—Buenos Aires—History. I. Title.
RA644.T7A768 2011
614.5′42098211—dc22   2011015529